# Historical Review

P. Lechat

Institut de Pharmacologie, 15 rue de l'Ecole de Médecine,
75006 Paris, France

The aim of this historical review is to recall briefly the main steps of the pharmacological studies carried out on aminopyridines (AP) and related compounds. Initial works describing a given effect or proposing a mechanism of action or a therapeutic application are cited here as important milestones in our story.

Pyridine was isolated from coaltar by Anderson in 1846, and picoline (methylpyridine) appeared to be the first heterocyclic compound obtained by synthesis through the work of Klaus in 1862.

It is interesting to note that the first pharmacological investigation using pyridine concerned its action on neuromuscular transmission. The results were presented in 1883 to the Société de Biologie by Bochefontaine, who worked in Vulpian's laboratory in the Paris School of Medicine, where my own laboratory is now located. At that time Bochefontaine reported the depressive action of pyridine on neuromuscular transmission, just the opposite to what we know to be the effect of aminopyridines today.

The three isomeric aminopyridines were obtained in 1894 by Meyer, who used the Hofmann procedure (treatment of the amides of pyridine monocarboxylic acids by alcaline hypobromites). In 1915 Tchitchibabine obtained 2-AP by heating pyridine with sodamide. The six possible diaminopyridines were synthetised later.

In 1925 Mr. Dohrn from Charlottenburg wrote a short paper entitled "Pharmakologie einiger Pyridinderivate" in the famous German Journal "Naunyn Schmiedeberg's Archiv für experimentelle Pathologie und Pharmakologie". In a few lines, the author described the following effects of amino-2 pyridine:

. convulsions in frogs, mice and rabbits, which were not suppressed by decapitation, disappeared immediately after the spinal cord was destroyed, although fascicular tremors continued to persist. These tremors did not cease after cutting of the innervating nerves, but disappeared after their degeneration.

. stimulation of isolated gastrocnemius, as with guanidine.

. strong rise in blood pressure.

. strong elevation of isolated gut tonus.

The introduction of a second amino group leading to 2,6-diaminopyridine did not modify the activity, but an acetyl group reduced the toxicity.

This was indeed a remarkable achievement to which there is little to add today.

Our present knowledge of the mechanism of AP action is much deeper, but it was Dr. Dohrn who described concisely and with great precision the main pharmacological properties of 2-AP, and that was 56 years ago.

In order to be more clear, I wish to go through the sequence of discoveries by examining one after the other the different actions of AP on the organism.

Aminopyridines and central nervous system.

Clonic convulsions, the major sign of acute intoxication by AP, were mentioned by all workers who administered drugs to animals: Dingemanse and Wibaut (1928) with 3-AP in the frog, then many others in mammals. The first quantitative assays were made by von Haxthausen (1955) who determined $LD_{50}$ of 4-AP in mice and found it somewhat low (5 mg/kg s.c.). Local applications of 4-AP to the spinal cord of cats threw some light on the mechanism of its convulsant effects since spontaneous repetitive discharges were registered on both the dorsal and the ventral roots by Chanelet and Lemeignan (1969). Furthermore an increase in evoked monosynaptic and polysynaptic activity under the influence of 4-AP was observed in the same material again by Lemeignan (1972). The central synapses of Invertebrates were also shown to be sensitive to AP, when Hue and co-workers (1975, 1976) observed in cockroach abdominal ganglions that 4-AP increased the amplitude of both excitatory and inhibitory synaptic potentials, an effect attributed by the authors to a presynaptic action. Only very recently, man too was discovered to be sensitive in this regard when Ball and co-workers (1979) reported epileptic seizures in patients receiving 4-AP. A special mention should be made of Goodhue who discovered that birds ingesting 4-AP became desoriented and emitted distress calls that caused other, non-intoxicated birds, to leave the area (1964). This frightning effect has subsequently been used to reduce damage caused by urban and rural populations of many bird species.

A number of other aminopyridines were tested later, but it must be emphasized that till now 4-AP remains the most toxic of them. Cytotoxicity of aminopyridines has been found to run parallel to their convulsant potency by Lechat and co-workers (1968). Von Haxthausen (1955) was also the first to notice the stimulating respiratory effect of 4-AP. Much more recently See and co-workers (1978) showed that atropine blocked it, indicating an involvement of central muscarinic cholinoceptors. A therapeutic application of this data occurred when Sia and co-workers (1979) used 4-AP to restore normal breathing in fentanyl respiratory depressed patients.

A consequence of the central stimulating action of AP is the reduction of sleeping time following the administration of hypnotic agents, observed in mice by Abernethy and Fastier (1958).

Another manifestation of a central action of 4-AP is the analgesic activity, which von Haxthausen demonstrated in mice in 1955. Many related compounds were found later to share this action the mechanism of which is not yet fully understood. The local anesthetic property of 4-AP described by Dingemanse and Wibaut (1928) is similarly not clearly understood either.

Aminopyridines and cardiovascular system.

The pioneer here was Fastier (1948) who studied a series of amidine derivatives in dogs and rats; with Reid (1948) he noticed the similar effects of methylisothiourea, 2-AP and iminoazole, i.e. hypertension in dogs, vasoconstriction in rats with sensitization to the vasoconstrictor action of adrenaline. The cardiac inotropic effect of AP was subsequently observed by von Haxthausen (1955) and 4-methyl-2-AP (or 2-amino 4-picoline) was marketed in Germany under the trade-name Ascensil[R], as an analgesic drug.

Aminopyridines and neuromuscular junction.

In 1953, at the instigation of Charonnat, I was studying the mechanisms by which injection of thiamine induced shocks in some patients. Hypothesising there was some relationship between the chemical structure of aminopyrimidine moiety of thiamine and of 4-aminopyridine, we injected animals with the latter. As Dohrn had previously found in frog with 2-AP, we observed a strong convulsant effect of 4-AP in mice and rabbits (Charonnat et al., 1953). We were however more interested then in the thiazole moiety of thiamine, which led us to discover the anticonvulsant properties of clomethiazole, but that is another story... 14 years later Mrs. Lemeignan and I (1967) again turned our attention to 4-AP and we observed that it antagonized d-tubocurarine but not suxicurarium.

We were in fact unaware at the time of two earlier works, the first one of Tsobkallo (1942) in which he described the anticurare action of 2-aminopyridine and the second one of Vohra and Pradhan (1964) reporting very briefly that 3,4-diaminopyridine antagonized d-tubocurarine. In our laboratory a pharmacological analysis of this antagonism was performed on the isolated rat phrenic-diaphragm preparation by Sobek and co-workers (1968). On the basis of our experiments on anesthetized cats and rabbits, we proposed that 4-aminopyridine enhances the release of acetylcholine evoked by nerve impulses at the neuromuscular junction. This view was confirmed when it was demonstrated that 4-AP raised EPP amplitude by increasing the EPP mean quantal content (Lundh and co-workers, 1977a; Molgo and co-workers, 1975, 1977). Such a mechanism accords with the lack of anticholinesterase activity of AP at concentrations where they increase neurotransmitter release. This was shown by Shaw and Bentley (1953) and by Lemeignan and Lechat (1967). Therapeutic applications based on this mechanism concern anesthesia (hastening the return of spontaneous movements after the blocking of d-tubocurarine (Paskov and co-workers, 1973), and some neuromuscular diseases: Eaton-Lambert syndrome (Lundh and co-workers, 1977b), myasthenia gravis (Lundh and co-workers, 1979) and botulism (Ball and co-workers, 1979). In addition to their presynaptic actions at the neuromuscular juuction, a direct action of AP on skeletal muscle contractility was first described by Fastier and McDowall (1958) and was confirmed by Bowman and co-workers (1976) and Harvey and Marshall (1977). An increased release of calcium ions from intracellular stores was proposed by Khan and Edman (1979) to account for this enhanced contractility.

Aminopyridines and nervous autonomic system.
The initial observation of Dohrn in 1925 demonstrating that AP increased the tone of isolated ileum preparations was confirmed by Fastier and McDowall (1958). Subsequent studies by Vizi and co-workers (1977) demonstrated that AP enhanced the release of acetylcholine from nerve terminals of ileum Auerbach plexus.

AP have also been shown to enhance nerve impulse evoked release of other neurotransmitters:
. noradrenaline in the cat spleen by Kirpekar and co-workers (1975) and in the rabbit vas deferens by Johns and co-workers (1976).
. and glutamate and GABA at the lobster neuromuscular junction by Schauf and co-workers (1976).

Aminopyridines and excitable membranes.
In many excitable membranes, 4-AP specifically blocks the voltage-dependent potassium channels. The first voltage-clamp studies in this field were made on the cockroach giant axon by Pelhate and co-workers (1974). Two years later Llinas and co-workers (1976) demonstrated the blocking of potassium channels by 4-AP in the presynaptic terminals of the squid giant synapse. A similar action of 4-AP on potassium conductance was described in skeletal muscle membranes by Gillespie and Hutter (1975) and in cardiac muscle membranes by Kenyon and Gibbons (1979).

The ability of 4-AP to block potassium channels seems to contribute substantially to its action in facilitating the influx of calcium ions through the voltage-sensitive calcium channels in the nerve terminals that are opened by the action potential (Molgo and co-workers, 1977; Illes and Thesleff, 1978). However there might well be another mechanism underlying 4-AP's facilitating on transmitter release. Lundh and Thesleff (1977) put forward the possibility that AP may facilitate calcium influx by direct action on voltage-sensitive calcium channels, although this hypothesis needs further investigation.

I have tried in a few minutes to indicate the development of our knowledge of aminopyridines and their related compounds. I have no doubt that the new data presented in this Symposium will advance our understanding of compounds the importance of which has grown and continues to grow so rapidly at this time.

## REFERENCES

Abernethy, J.C. and F.N. Fastier (1958). Aust. J. Exp. Biol., 36, 487-490.
Bowman, W.C., A.L. Harvey and I.G. Marshall (1976). J. Pharm. Pharmacol., 28, suppl. 79P.
Ball, A.P., R.B. Hopkinson, I.D. Farrell, J.P.G. Hutchinson, R. Paul, R.D.S. Watson, A.J.F. Page, R.G.F. Parker, C.W. Edwards, M. Snow, D.K. Scott, A. Leone-Ganado, A. Hastings, A.C. Ghosh and R.J. Gilbert (1979). Quart. J. Med. New Series, 48, 473-491.
Bochefontaine, M. (1883). C. R. Soc. Biol., 35, 5-8.
Chanelet, J. and M. Lemeignan (1969). C. R. Soc. Biol., 163, 365-372.
Charonnat, R., P. Lechat and J. Chareton (1953). Ann. Pharm. Fr., 11, 26-30.
Dingemanse, E. and J.P. Wibaut (1928). Arch. exp. Path. Pharmakol., 132, 365.
Dohrn, M. (1925). Arch. exp. Path. Pharmakol., 105, X-XI.
Fastier, F.N. (1948). Brit. J. Pharmacol., 3, 198-204.
Fastier, F.N. and C.S.W. Reid (1948). Brit. J. Pharmacol., 3, 205-210.
Fastier, F.N. and M.A. McDowall (1958). Austral. J. Exp. Biol. Med. Sci., 36, 365-372.
Gillespie, J.I. and O.P. Hutter (1975). J. Physiol. (London), 252, 70 P.
Goodhue, L.D., A.J. Reinert and R.P. Williams (1964). U. S. Pat., 3, 150.041.
Harvey, A.L. and I.G. Marshall (1977). Comp. Biochem. Physiol., 580, 161-165.
Haxthausen von, E. (1955). Arch. exp. Path. Pharmakol., 226, 163-171.
Hue, B., M. Pelhate, J.J. Callec and J. Chanelet (1975). C. R. Soc. Biol., 169, 876-883.
Hue, B., M. Pelhate, J.J. Callec and J. Chanelet (1976). J. Exp. Biol., 65, 517-527.
Illes, P. and S. Thesleff (1978). Br. J. Pharmac., 64, 623-629.
Johns, A., D.S. Golko, P.A. Lauzon and D.M. Paton (1976). Eur. J. Pharmacol., 38, 71-78.
Kenyon, J.L. and W.R. Gibbons (1979). J. Gen. Physiol., 73, 139-157.
Khan, R.A. and K.A.P. Edman (1979). Acta Physiol. Scand., 105, 443-452.
Kirpekar Madhuri, S.M. Kirpekar and J.C. Prat (1976). Pharmacologist, 18, 208.
Lechat, P., G. Deysson, M. Lemeignan and M. Adolphe (1968). Ann. Pharm. Fr., 26, 345-349.
Lemeignan, M. and P. Lechat (1967). C. R. Acad. Sci. (Paris), Ser. D 264, 169-172.
Lemeignan, M. (1972). Neuropharmacol., 11, 551-558.
Llinas, R., K. Walton and V. Bohr (1976). Biophys. J., 16, 83-86.
Lundh, H., S. Leander and S. Thesleff (1977a). J. Neurol. Sci., 32, 29-43.
Lundh, H., O. Nilsson and I. Rosen (1977b). J. Neurol. Neurosurg. Psychiat., 40, 1109-1112.
Lundh, H. and S. Thesleff (1977). Eur. J. Pharmacol., 42, 411-412.
Lundh, H., O. Nilsson and I. Rosen (1979). J. Neurol. Neurosurg. Psychiat., 42, 171-175.
Molgo, J., M. Lemeignan and P. Lechat (1975). C. R. Acad. Sci. (Paris), Ser. D 281, 1637-1639.
Molgo, J., M. Lemeignan and P. Lechat (1977). J. Pharmacol. exp. Ther., 203, 653-663.
Molgo, J., M. Lemeignan and P. Lechat (1979). Eur. J. Pharmacol., 53, 307-311.
Paskov, D.S., E.A. Stojanov and V.V. Mitzov (1973). Eksp. Khir. Anaesthesiol., 18, 48-52.
Pelhate, M., B. Hue, Y. Pichon and J. Chanelet (1974). C. R. Acad. Sci. (Paris), Ser. D, 278, 2807-2809.
Schauf, C.L., C.A. Colton, J.S. Colton and F.A. Davis (1976). J. Pharmacol. exp. Ther. 197, 414-425.
See, W.R., H. Folgering and M.E. Schläfke (1978). Pflügers Arch., 377, R20.
Shaw, F.H. and G.A. Bentley (1953). Austr. J. Exp. Biol. Med. Sci., 31, 573-576.
Sia, R.L., P.J. Salt, D. Langreh, S. Agoston and W. Erdmann (1979). Acta Anaesth. Belg., 30 suppl., 195-199.

Sobek, V., M. Lemeignan, G. Streichenberger, J.M. Benoist, A. Goguel and P. Lechat
  (1968). Arch. int. Pharmacodyn., 171, 356-367.
Tsobkallo, G.I. (1942). Farmakol. i Toksikol., 5, n°6, 32-39.
Vizi, E.S., J. Van Dijk and F.F. Foldes (1977). J. Neurol. Transm., 41, 265-274.
Vohra, M.M. and S.N. Pradhan (1964). Arch. int. Pharmacodyn., 150, 413-424.

# Aminopyridines and Ionic Currents in Excitable Membranes

*Chairman:* C. Bergman

# General Review on Potassium Currents in Excitable Membranes of Nerve and Muscle

H. Meves

I. Physiologisches Institut der Universität des Saarlandes, D-6650 Homburg/Saar, Federal Republic of Germany

ABSTRACT

The paper describes the physiological and pharmacological properties of the delayed potassium outward current in nerve and muscle.

KEYWORDS

Potassium current; nerve; muscle; single channel conductance; 4-aminopyridine; tetraethylammonium; barium.

TIME COURSE OF POTASSIUM CURRENTS

In nerve and muscle fibres, depolarization produces a delayed K outward current $I_K$ which rises to a maximum and then declines slowly. Fig. 1 shows examples of $I_K$ from frog muscle fibres and from a mouse neuroblastoma cell recorded with the voltage-clamp method. The currents are displayed on fast and slow time scale. The time course of the rising phase is approximately fitted by an activation variable n (which increases exponentially with time) raised to the second or a higher power (Hodgkin and Huxley, 1952; Cole and Moore, 1960; Frankenhaeuser, 1963). A hyperpolarizing prepulse delays the onset of $I_K$ (Cole and Moore, 1960; Goldman and Schauf, 1973; Palti, Ganot and Stämpfli, 1976; Begenisich, 1979; Keynes and Kimura, 1980). To describe the delay mathematically, a larger exponent of n or a time shift $\Delta t$ is required. The secondary decline of $I_K$ in Fig. 1B and D has been attributed to the slow inactivation of the K conductance, a process which occurs also in squid giant axons (Ehrenstein and Gilbert, 1966) and myelinated nerve fibres (Schwarz and Vogel, 1971). With the inactivation variable k and the driving force $(V-V_K)$ the equation for the delayed K current becomes

$$I_K = \bar{g}_K \, n^a k (V-V_K)$$

where $n = n_\infty (1-\exp(-(t-\Delta t)/\tau_n))$ .

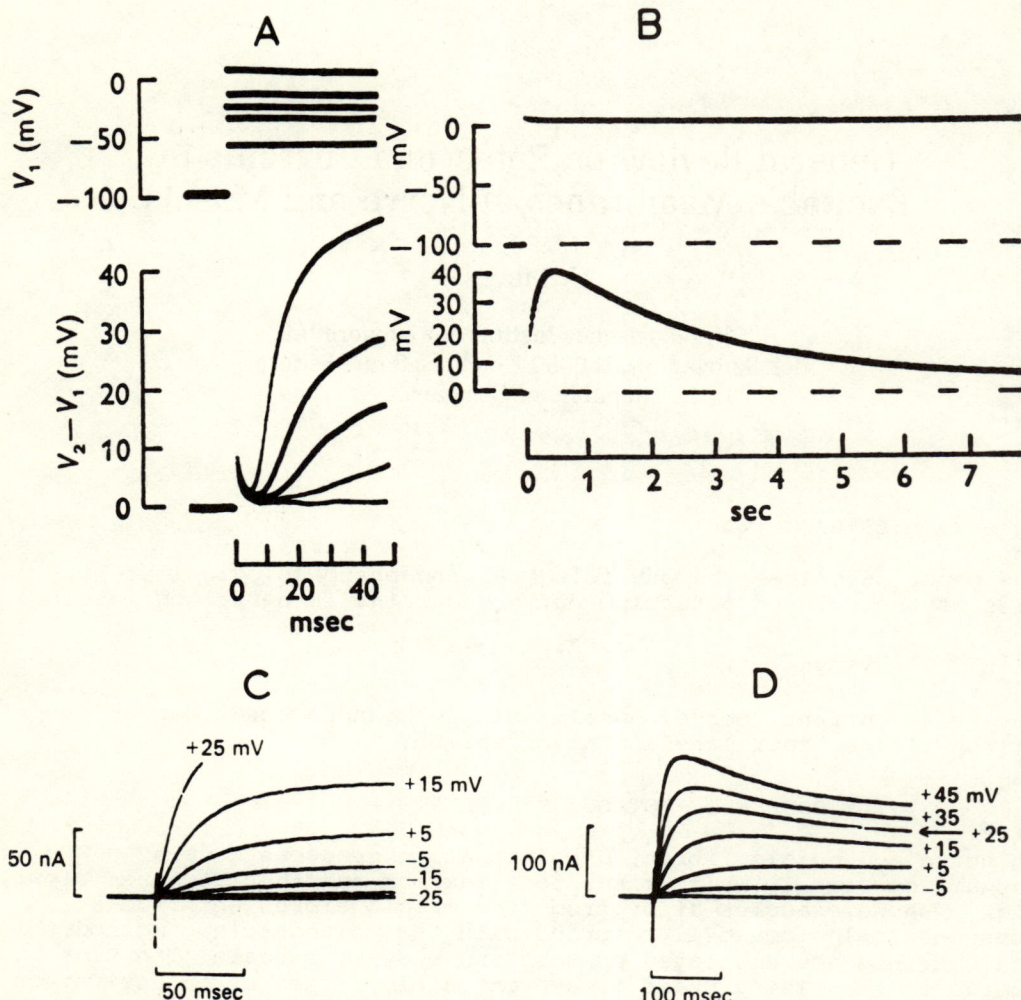

Fig. 1. Potassium outward currents in frog muscle fibres (A,B) and in a mouse neuroblastoma cell (C,D) under voltage clamp. A,B: membrane potentials, above, and currents, below, in two frog muscle fibres at 2 °C in Ringer + 350 mM sucrose and tetrodotoxin, $10^{-6}$ g/ml. Three-microelectrode voltage-clamp with the membrane current given as $(V_2-V_1)$ in mV; 1 mV = 13 and 21 $\mu A/cm^2$ in A and B, respectively. From Adrian, Chandler and Hodgkin (1970). C,D: membrane currents in a cultured mouse neuroblastoma cell at 20 °C. Holding potential -85 mV, pulse potentials indicated next to the current traces. From Moolenaar and Spector (1978).

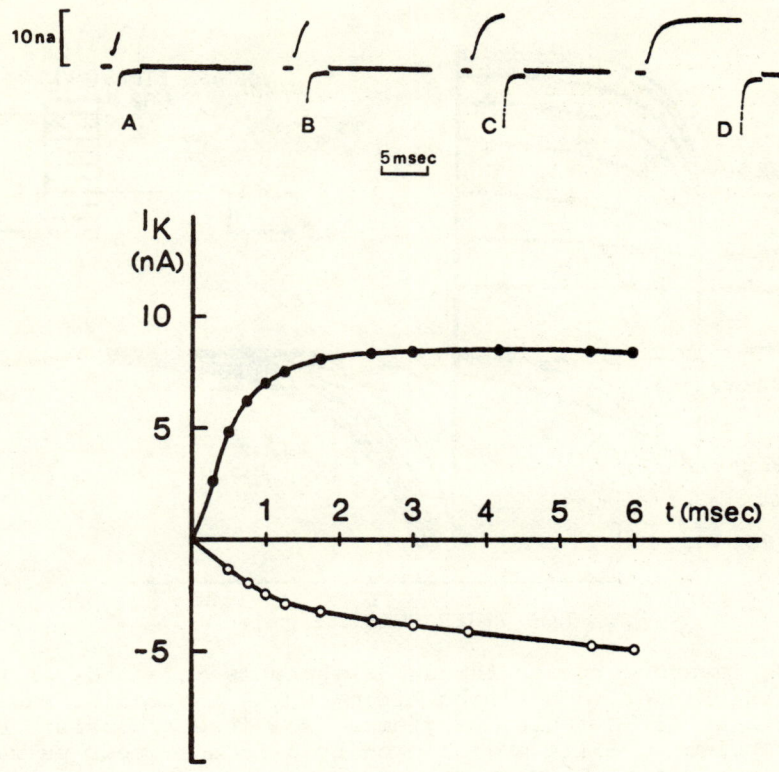

Fig. 2. Potassium outward current and tail inward current in a node of Ranvier superfused with Ringer + tetrodotoxin at room temperature. Above: voltage clamp currents associated with depolarizing pulses of different duration. Holding potential -70 mV, potential during pulse + 70 mV, repolarized to -120 mV. Below: outward current at end of depolarizing pulse (upper curve, filled circles) and initial value of inward tail current (lower curve, open circles) plotted against duration of depolarizing pulse. From Dubois and Bergman (1975).


A decline of $I_K$ during a depolarizing pulse can also result from the accumulation of K ions near the outer surface of the membrane, leading to a positive shift of $V_K$. K accumulation manifests itself in the occurrence of an inward tail current when clamping the potential back to the holding potential. The inward tail current becomes larger with increasing duration of the depolarizing pulse (Fig. 2). K accumulation near the outer surface of the membrane has been demonstrated in squid giant axons (Frankenhaeuser and Hodgkin, 1956; Adelman and Palti, 1972) and in nodes of Ranvier (Dubois and Bergman, 1975; Moran, Palti, Levitan and Stämpfli, 1980).

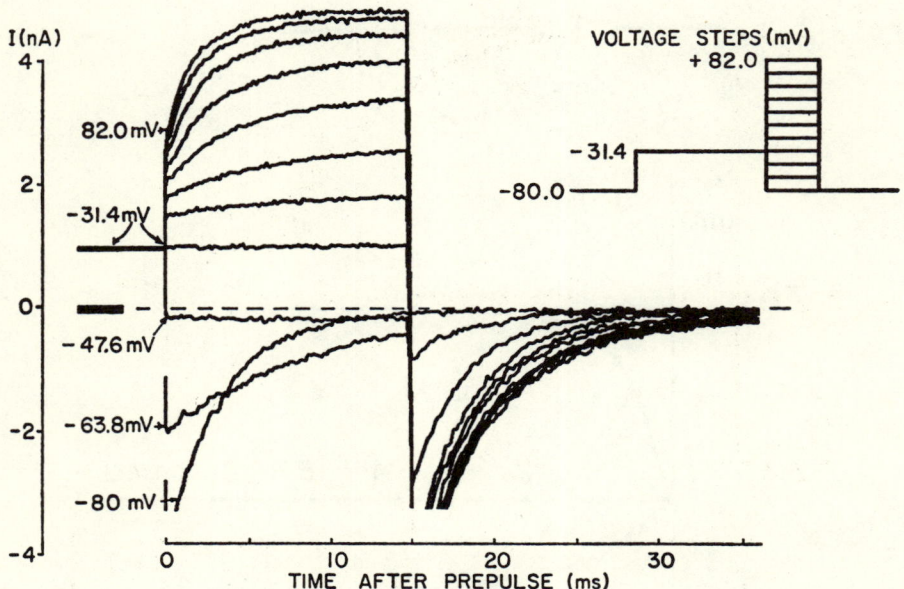

Fig. 3. $NH_4$ inward currents through K channels in a node of Ranvier bathed in $NH_4$ Ringer (containing 115 mM $NH_4Cl$ instead of NaCl) with tetrodotoxin at 15 °C. Pulse programme (see inset) consists of a 40 msec prepulse to -31.4 mV followed by a 15 msec test pulse to different potentials. Current records show current at end of prepulse, during test pulse and after return to the holding potential. From Hille (1973).

## DIAMETER AND CONDUCTANCE OF SINGLE POTASSIUM CHANNELS

Not only K but also Rb, Tl and $NH_4$ ions can pass through K channels (Lüttgau, 1961; Binstock and Lecar, 1969; Hille, 1973). In addition, Ca currents through K channels have been found in internally perfused squid giant axons (Inoue, 1980). As an example, records of $NH_4$ inward currents through K channels in a node of Ranvier bathed in $NH_4$ Ringer are illustrated in Fig. 3. Following a prepulse to -31.4 mV (which produces a small K outward current) the potential is stepped to more positive values (producing larger K outward currents) or to more negative values (producing transient $NH_4$ inward currents); finally, the potential is returned to the holding potential, causing large tails of $NH_4$ inward current. For a quantitative analysis, the zero current potential (at which the outward flux of K and the inward flux of $NH_4$ are equal) is determined. In the experiment of Fig. 3 the test pulse to -47.6 mV is just a few millivolts below the zero current potential. A 3 mV smaller zero current potential is measured when the external solution contains 14 mM KCl instead of 115 mM $NH_4$. From the equation

$$\Delta V = 3 = 58 \log(P_{NH_4} \, 114/P_K \, 14) \quad mV$$

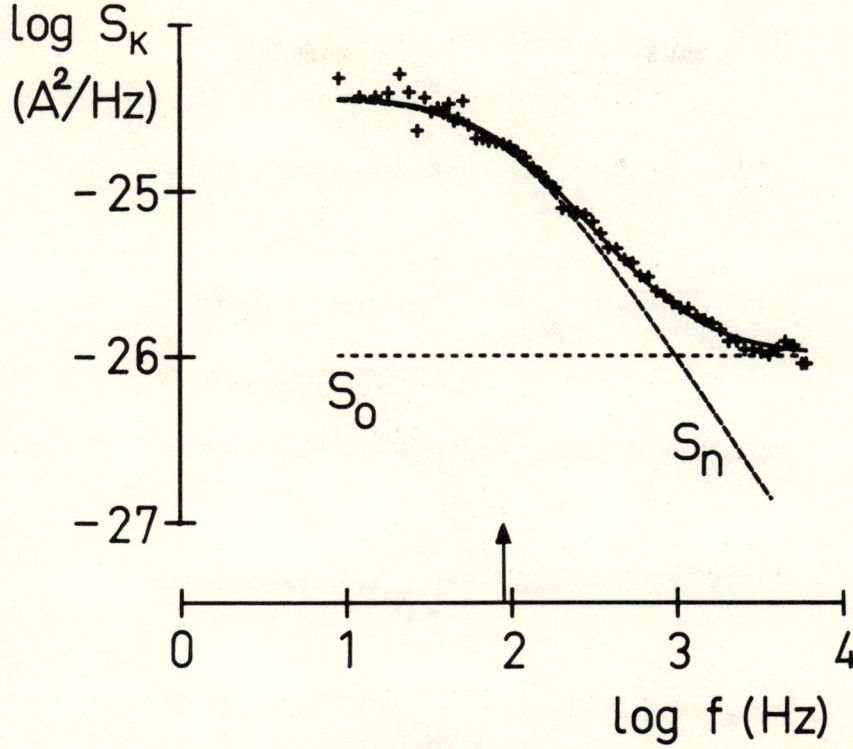

Fig. 4. Spectral density $S_K$ of K current fluctuations in a myelinated nerve fibre of the frog. Points (+) calculated from K current fluctuations during the last 315 msec of a 460 msec depolarization to V = 24 mV. Temperature 18 °C. The solid curve through the points is a fit by the sum of a diffusion spectrum $S_n = S_1/(1+(f/f_c)^{1.5})$ and a frequency-independent plateau $S_o$. The location of the corner frequency $f_c$ of $S_n$ (93 Hz) is indicated by an arrow. From Neumcke (1981).

a permeability ratio $P_{NH_4}/P_K = 0.13$ is obtained, i.e. the permeability of the K channel for $NH_4$ is about 8 times smaller than for K. Similar experiments with Tl and Rb in the external solution showed that the relative permeabilities of the K channel for Tl, K and Rb are in the ratio 2.3:1.00:0.92; organic cations like hydrazine and guanidine do not permeate (Hille, 1973). From the size of the permeating and the non-permeating ions Hille (1973) estimated the diameter of the narrowest part of the K channel as 3 Å.

The conductance of a single K channel is obtained from the current through a single K channel which can be calculated from the variance of K current fluctuations or recorded directly with a patch electrode. Fig. 4 shows the spectral density of K current fluctuations in a node of Ranvier whose Na currents have been blocked by

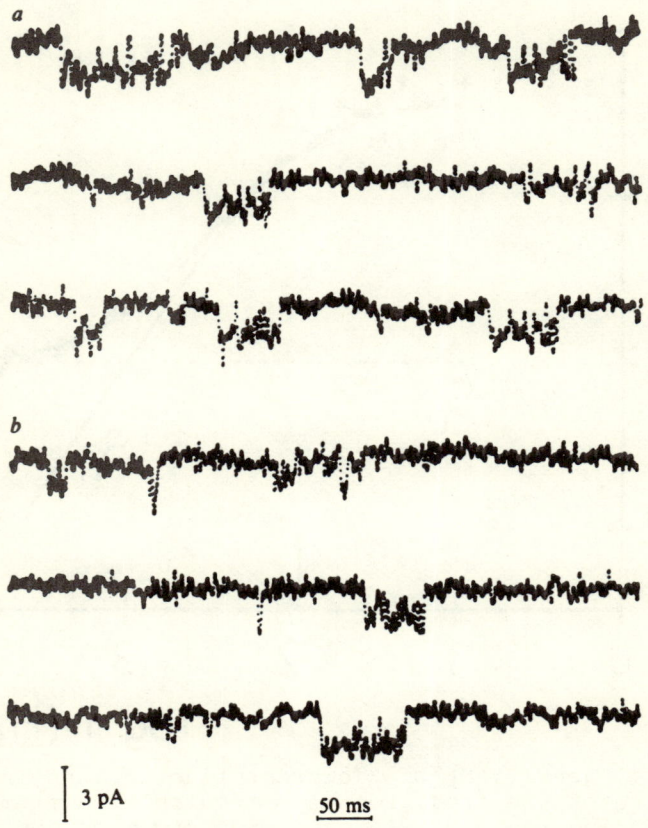

Fig. 5. Single channel recordings of K currents in an intracellularly perfused squid giant axon at two different membrane potentials (a, -25 mV; b, -35 mV). External solution: 460 mM KCl, 50 mM $CaCl_2$, $3 \times 10^{-7}$ M tetrodotoxin, pH 8. Internal solution: 15 mM NaF, 1 mM KCl, pH 7.8-8. Temperature 5.5 °C. From Conti and Neher (1980).

tetrodotoxin (Neumcke, Schwarz and Stämpfli, 1980). The curve $S_K(f)$ exhibits a plateau at low frequencies, decays with increasing frequency and reaches another plateau at high frequencies. It can be fitted by the sum of two components $S_n$ and $S_o$. Only the frequency-dependent component $S_n$ is attributed to the open-close kinetics of K channels. Integration of this component gives the variance of K current fluctuations and the conductance $\gamma$ of a single K channel. Neumcke, Schwarz and Stämpfli (1980) obtained $\gamma = 2.7$ pS for motor fibres and $\gamma = 4.6$ pS for sensory fibres. Measurements on other nerve preparations gave $\gamma$ values between 2 and 12 pS (see review by Neumcke, 1981). The larger $\gamma$ value for sensory fibres is consistent with the observation that sensory fibres produce larger K currents than motor fibres. The different $\gamma$ values suggest that there are different types of K channels.

Currents through single K channels have been recorded directly by Conti and Neher (1980). They introduced an L-shaped pipette for

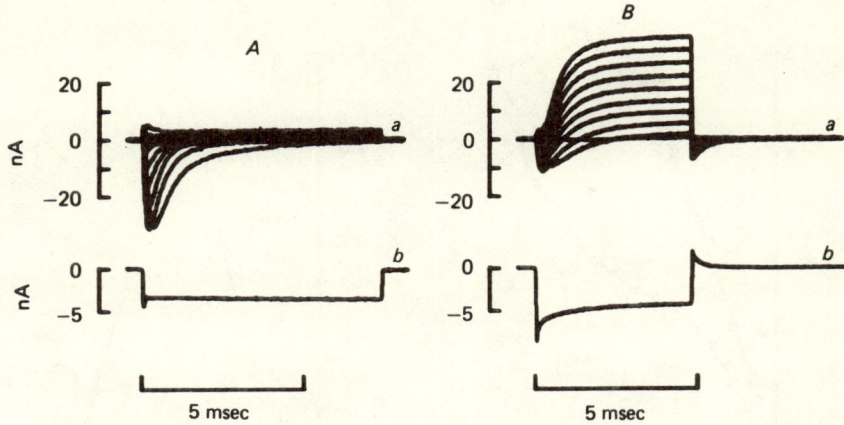

Fig. 6. Voltage clamp currents from a normal myelinated nerve fibre of a rabbit (A) and from a fibre which has been deliberately stretched during dissection (B). a, series of depolarizations from holding potential (-80 mV) to +70 mV in 15 mV increments. b, hyperpolarization from holding potential (-80 mV) to -125 mV. Note delayed outward currents and slow capacity transient in B. Temperature 25 °C. From Chiu and Ritchie (1981).

recording from a small patch of membrane into the interior of an intracellularly perfused squid giant axon. To improve the resolution of their measurements they converted the normal K concentration gradient across the membrane and chose K concentrations of 460 and 1 mM in the external and internal solution, respectively. Under these conditions and in a certain range of membrane potentials they observed bursts of closely spaced current pulses with short interruptions (Fig. 5). The bursts are interpreted as currents through individual K channels. From the amplitude of the currents they determined the single channel conductance $\gamma$ as 17.5 pS. This value is higher than the $\gamma$ values deduced from fluctuation measurements (see above); possible reasons for this discrepancy are discussed by Neumcke (1981).

## PECULIARITIES OF THE K PERMEABILITY IN CERTAIN TISSUES

In certain excitable tissues special properties of the K system have been observed. Four examples are worth mentioning:

(1) Mammalian myelinated nerve fibres have little $I_K$ (Horackova, Nonner and Stämpfli, 1968; Chiu, Ritchie, Rogart and Stagg, 1979; Brismar, 1980) but produce $I_K$ when subjected to mechanical stress or osmotic shock, presumably because K channels present under the myelin in the paranodal region are uncovered (Chiu and Ritchie, 1981) (see records a in Fig. 6A,B). As shown by records b in Fig. 6A, B, the appearance of large delayed outward currents is accompanied by the appearance of a slow capacity transient. The latter is thought to reflect charging of the newly exposed axonal membrane in the paranodal region.

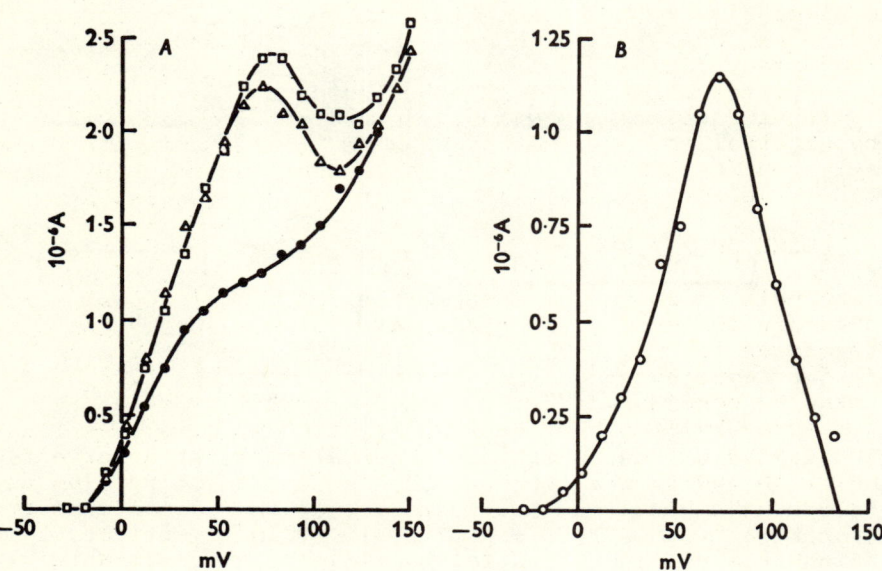

Fig. 7A. Effect of Ca-free saline on the potassium outward current in a <u>Helix</u> <u>aspersa</u> neurone. Abscissa: membrane potential. Ordinate: membrane current measured 80 msec after the beginning of voltage clamp pulse. □ , normal saline with 10 mM $CaCl_2$; ● , after 3 min in Ca-free saline ($CaCl_2$ replaced by $MgCl_2$); △ , 4-5 min after return to normal saline. B: Ca-dependent component of $I_K$, obtained by subtraction of currents recorded in Ca-free saline from those in normal saline. Holding potential -48 mV. Temperature 21.5 °C. From Meech and Standen (1975).

(2) In molluscan and vertebrate neurones, a component of $I_K$ has been observed which is activated by Ca entry (Meech, 1978). Presumably, Ca interacts with a site on the inner membrane surface that controls the permeability of the membrane for K. As shown in Fig. 7, the Ca-mediated $I_K$ disappears in Ca-free solution and at large depolarizations which bring the potential towards the Ca equilibrium potential. The Ca-mediated $I_K$ can be elicited by intracellular injection of Ca or some other divalent cations (Gorman and Hermann, 1979; Hofmeier and Lux, 1981).

(3) Metabolic exhaustion of frog sartorius muscle fibres leads to a large increase of the K conductance, reflecting a permanently open state of the K channels (Fink and Lüttgau, 1976; Fink and Wettwer, 1978). In muscles poisoned with 2 mM cyanide + 1 mM monoiodoacetate and stimulated at 1 Hz until loss of visible contractions the normally delayed K outward currents turn on instantaneously and are larger than in normal fibres. The effect may be due to the increase of intracellular free Ca in exhausted muscle fibres.

(4) Squid axons bathed in K-free sea water and internally perfused with a K-free solution (e.g. NaF) irreversibly loose the K conductance, i.e. K outward currents fail to reappear when internal K is readmitted (Chandler and Meves, 1970; Almers and Armstrong, 1980). The effect (which requires the <u>simultaneous</u> absence of external and internal K) develops slowly with a time constant of about 11 min at 8 °C. K channels can be protected against this effect by external or internal Cs, $NH_4$, Rb. That K channels become permanently non-functional in the total absence of permeant ions may also be true for preparations other than the squid axon.

BLOCK OF K CHANNELS

Like Na channels, K channels can be blocked by local anaesthetics, but much larger concentrations are required. As shown by the dose-response curves for $P_{Na}$ and $P_K$ in Fig. 8, the concentration necessary for reducing $P_K$ to half its normal value is 12.5-95 times larger than the concentration required for a 50 % block of $P_{Na}$. By contrast, tetraethylammonium (TEA) and 4-aminopyridine (4-AP) have a strong blocking effect on K channels with little or no effect on Na channels. In squid giant axons, TEA is only effective from the inside (Armstrong and Binstock, 1965) whereas in myelinated nerve fibres (Hille, 1967; Koppenhöfer, 1967; Koppenhöfer and Vogel, 1969; Armstrong and Hille, 1972) and skeletal muscle fibres (Stanfield, 1970; Fink and Wettwer, 1978) it acts from outside and inside. The effect of externally and internally applied TEA on the nodal membrane is illustrated in Fig. 9. With externally applied TEA, the concentration necessary for reducing $I_K$ to half its normal value is 0.4 mM in myelinated nerve fibres (Hille, 1967) and 8 mM in skeletal muscle fibres (Stanfield, 1970).

Replacing one of the four $C_2H_5$ groups of TEA by the hydrophobic group $C_9H_{19}$ leads to nonyltriethylammonium (abbreviated $C_9$). Whereas the blocking effect of external TEA does not vary with time or with voltage, the effect of internal TEA and especially of internal $C_9$ is strongly dependent on time and voltage. With $C_9$ inside a squid axon, potassium current during a maintained depolarization first increases to an almost normal value, but then spontaneously decreases to a small fraction of its peak value (Fig. 10). The phenomenon is explained by assuming that $C_9$ ions are driven by diffusional and electrical forces from the axoplasm into the K channels once the latter are opened by depolarization (Armstrong, 1971; Armstrong and Hille, 1972).

The same explanation applies to the block of K channels by internal Na or Cs, a phenomenon seen on myelinated nerve fibres (Bergman, 1970) and on squid giant axons (Bezanilla and Armstrong, 1972; French and Wells, 1977). The onset of block by monovalent cations is very fast. As shown in Fig. 11, the voltage-dependent blocking of the K channels produces a region of negative slope in the instantaneous I-V plot, i.e. increasing the pulse height leads to a <u>decrease</u> of $I_K$. However, at V > 160 mV the current increases again, presumably because the K channels become permeable to Na ions.

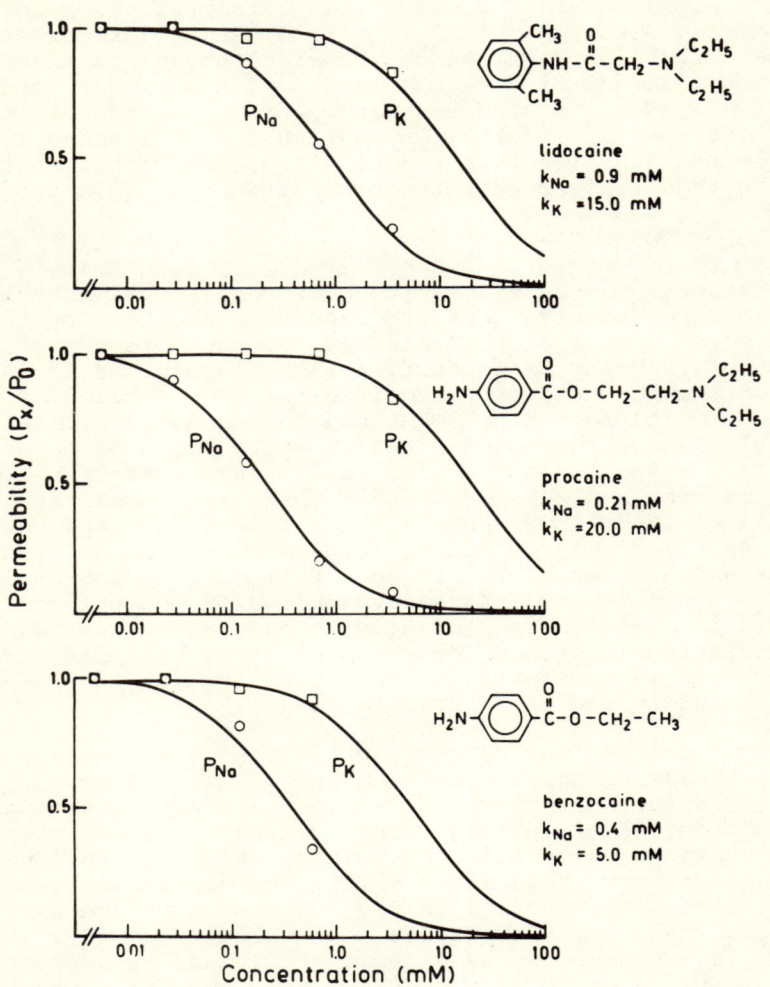

Fig. 8. Effect of three local anaesthetics on Na permeability $P_{Na}$ and K permeability $P_K$ in a myelinated nerve fibre of <u>Xenopus laevis</u>. $P_{Na}$ and $P_K$ were calculated by the constant-field equation from peak $I_{Na}$ and steady-state $I_K$ associated with large depolarizing pulses. The permeabilities $P_{Na}$ and $P_K$ are expressed as fractions of the permeability without local anaesthetic (i.e. $P_x/P_0$). Holding potential -90 to -110 mV. Temperature 15 °C. Smooth curves drawn from the equation
$$P_x/P_0 = k/(k + x)$$
where x is concentration of local anaesthetic; values for k indicated. From Århem and Frankenhaeuser (1974).

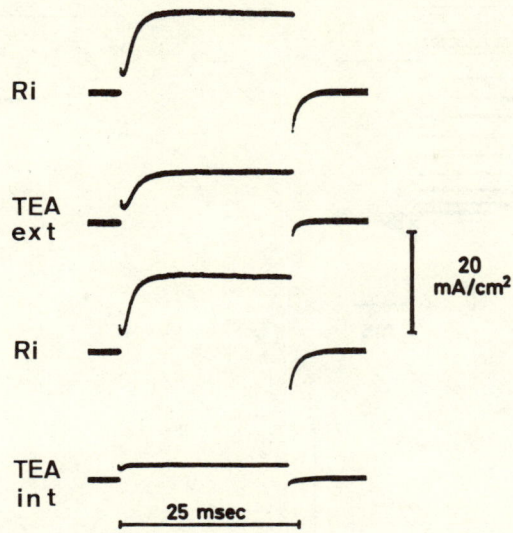

Fig. 9. Effect of TEA on the outer and inner side of the nodal membrane of <u>Xenopus laevis</u>. Traces show current associated with a 130 mV pulse in Ringer's solution (Ri), in Ringer's solution + 0.3 mM TEA (TEA ext), again in Ringer's solution (Ri) and after application of 97 mM KCl + 20 mM TEA to one of the cut ends of the fibre (TEA int). Holding potential -70 mV. Temperature 17.5 °C. From Koppenhöfer and Vogel (1969).

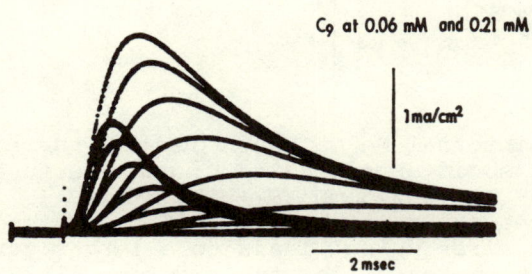

Fig. 10. K outward currents in squid giant axon injected with the TEA derivative $C_9$. Two sets of records: the larger currents are for 0.06 mM and the smaller for 0.21 mM axoplasmic $C_9$. Pulse potential -30 to +90 mV in 20 mV steps. Temperature 9 °C. From Armstrong (1971).

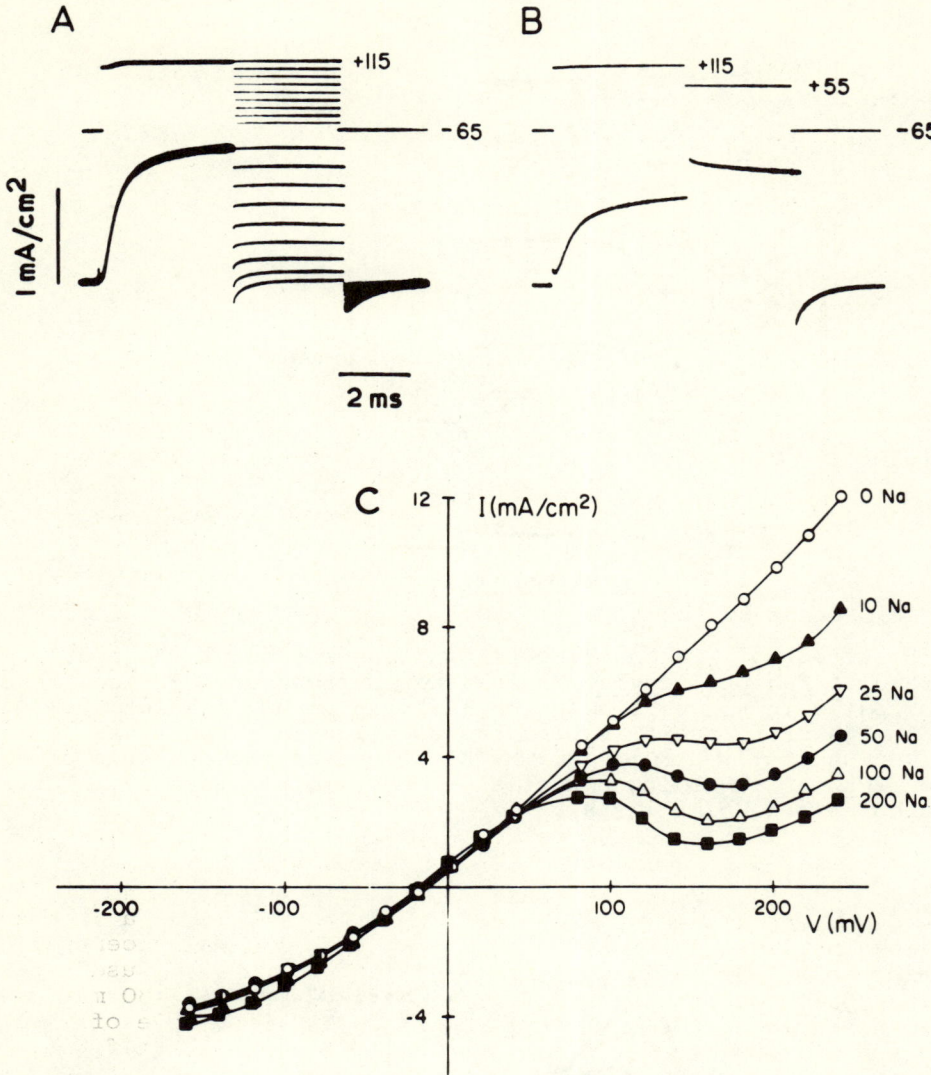

Fig. 11. Effect of internal Na on the K outward current of intracellularly perfused squid axons. A and B: axon perfused with 275 mM KF + 400 mM sucrose (A) or 275 mM KF + 100 mM NaF + 225 mM sucrose (B); pulse programmes shown in insets. In B the second pulse (which is smaller than the first pulse) leads to a larger current; this is not the case in A. From Bezanilla and Armstrong (1972). C: family of instantaneous IV curves for an axon perfused with solutions containing 300 mM K and a series of Na concentrations ranging from 0 to 200 mM as indicated in the figure; pulse programme similar to that in A; current at beginning of second pulse plotted against potential during second pulse. From French and Wells (1977). External solution in A-C: sea water with tetrodotoxin; temperature 8-10 °C.

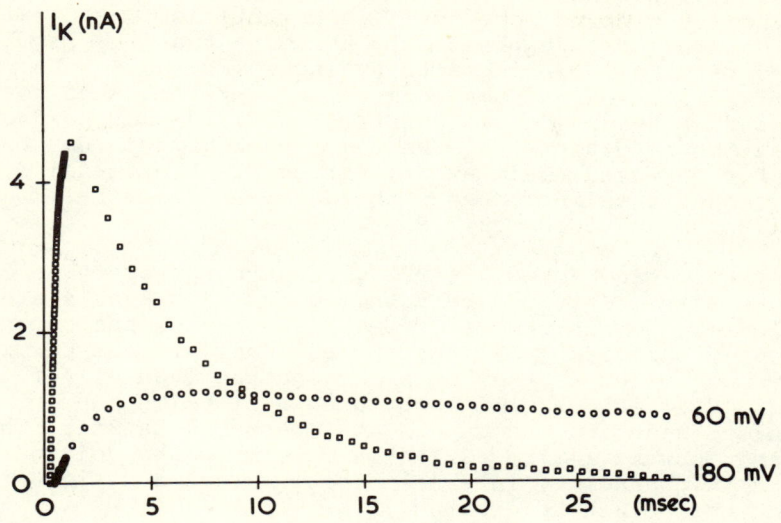

Fig. 12. Effect of internal Ba on the K currents of a node of Ranvier. Depolarizing pulse of 60 or 180 mV amplitude, holding potential -70 mV. Ringer's solution with tetrodotoxin, cut ends of fibre in 120 mM KCl + 0.6 mM $BaCl_2$. Sampling rate 10 μsec at beginning, 570 μsec later. Leakage current subtracted by means of an analogue circuit. Temperature 15 °C. From K. H. Woll (unpublished).


The most potent blocker of the K channel is internal Ba. Its effect has been studied on perfused squid axons (Eaton and Brodwick, 1980; Armstrong and Taylor, 1980) and on myelinated nerve fibres (K. H. Woll, unpublished). Eaton and Brodwick (1980) described a time and voltage dependent block of K channels by internal Ba concentrations as small as 0.1-50 nM while Armstrong and Taylor (1980) used internal Ba concentrations of 3-5 mM. Fig. 12 (record 180 mV) depicts the rapid decay of the potassium current in a node of Ranvier after application of 0.6 mM $BaCl_2$ to the cut ends of the fibre. No decay is seen with small pulses (Fig. 12, record 60 mV). Plotting the final values of $I_K$ against voltage yields an I-V plot similar to those in Fig. 11. The degree of block (estimated from the initial and the final value of $I_K$) and the time constant of decay are strongly dependent on voltage. According to the authors quoted above, the association constant of the reaction between Ba and its receptor increases e-fold per 17, 20 or 27 mV potential change. The time constant of decay is smallest for strong pulses (e.g. 5.5 msec in Fig. 12, record 180 mV). The strong voltage dependence of the Ba block suggests that the blocking site is deep inside the K channel. The similarity in crystal radius (1.33 Å for K, 1.34 Å for Ba) supports the view that Ba penetrates far into the K channel.

The block of $I_K$ by internal mono- or divalent cations is antagonized by external K, i.e. raising external K shifts the region of negative slope in the I-V plot to more positive potentials. The clearing action of external K is explained by assuming that the blocking ions are knocked off their binding site by inward moving K ions. The requirement for at least a small amount of external K to get maximal $I_K$ in nodes of Ranvier (Dubois and Bergman, 1977) may be due to this clearing action of external K. The reverse phenomenon has been described for perfused squid axons: for constant external K, the potassium conductance increases with increasing internal K up to a maximum (Eaton and Brodwick, 1980).

As shown by Hille and Schwarz (1978), the known properties of K channels are best understood by assuming that K channels are "multi--ion single-file pores": two or three sites inside the channel are simultaneously occupied by K ions and the ions are not permitted to pass by each other as they move through the channel (cf. Hodgkin and Keynes, 1955). Block will occur when a blocking ion enters the channel on one side and encounters an impassable barrier. The model of Hille and Schwarz (1978) correctly describes the voltage-dependent block of the K channel by internal blocking ions and the partial reversal of this block by external K.

REFERENCES

Adelman, W.J., and Y. Palti (1972). Some relations between external cations and the inactivation of the initial transient conductance in the squid axon. In Perspectives in Membrane Biophysics, ed. Agin, D.P. pp. 101-128. London: Gordon and Breach.

Adrian, R.H., W.K. Chandler and A.L. Hodgkin (1970). Voltage clamp experiments in striated muscle fibres. J. Physiol. 208, 607-644.

Almers, W., and C. M. Armstrong (1980). Survival of $K^+$-permeability and gating currents in squid axons perfused with $K^+$-free media. J. gen. Physiol. 75, 61-78.

Århem, P., and B. Frankenhaeuser (1974). Local anesthetics: effects on permeability properties of nodal membrane in myelinated nerve fibres from Xenopus. Potential clamp experiments. Acta physiol. scand. 91, 11-21.

Armstrong, C.M. (1971). Interaction of tetraethylammonium ion derivatives with the potassium channels of giant axons. J. gen. Physiol. 58, 413-437.

Armstrong, C.M. and L. Binstock (1965). Anomalous rectification in the squid giant axon injected with tetraethylammonium chloride. J. gen. Physiol. 48, 859-872.

Armstrong, C.M., and B. Hille (1972). The inner quaternary ammonium ion receptor in potassium channels of the node of Ranvier. J. gen. Physiol. 59, 388-400.

Armstrong, C.M., and S.R. Taylor (1980). Interaction of barium ions with potassium channels in squid giant axons. Biophys. J. 30, 473-488.

Begenisich, T. (1979). Conditioning hyperpolarization-induced delays in the potassium channels of myelinated nerve. Biophys. J. 27, 257-266.

Bergman, C. (1970). Increase of sodium concentration near the inner surface of the nodal membrane. Pflügers Arch. 317, 287-302.
Bezanilla, F., and C.M. Armstrong (1972). Negative conductance caused by entry of sodium and cesium ions into the potassium channels of squid axons. J. gen. Physiol. 60, 588-608.
Binstock, L., and H. Lecar (1969). Ammonium ion currents in the squid giant axon. J. gen. Physiol. 53, 342-361.
Brismar, T. (1980). Potential clamp analysis of membrane currents in rat myelinated nerve fibres. J. Physiol. 298, 171-184.
Chandler, W.K., and H. Meves (1970). Sodium and potassium currents in squid axons perfused with fluoride solutions. J. Physiol. 211, 623-652.
Chiu, S.Y., and J.M. Ritchie (1981). Evidence for the presence of potassium channels in the paranodal region of acutely demyelinated mammalian single nerve fibres. J. Physiol. 313, 415-437.
Chiu, S.Y., J.M. Ritchie, R.B. Rogart and D. Stagg (1979). A quantitative description of membrane currents in rabbit myelinated nerve. J. Physiol. 292, 149-166.
Cole, K.S., and J.W. Moore (1960). Potassium ion current in the squid giant axon: dynamic characteristic. Biophys. J. 1, 1-14.
Conti, F., and E. Neher (1980). Single channel recordings of $K^+$ currents in squid axons. Nature 285, 140-143.
Dubois, J.M., and C. Bergman (1975). Potassium accumulation in the perinodal space of frog myelinated axons. Pflügers Arch. 358, 111-124.
Dubois, J.M., and C. Bergman (1977). The steady-state potassium conductance of the Ranvier node at various external K-concentrations. Pflügers Arch. 370, 185-194.
Eaton, D.C., and M.S. Brodwick (1980). Effect of barium on the potassium conductance of squid axon. J. gen. Physiol. 75, 727-750.
Ehrenstein, G., and D.L. Gilbert (1966). Slow changes of potassium permeability in the squid giant axon. Biophys. J. 6, 553-566.
Fink, R., and H.C. Lüttgau (1976). An evaluation of the membrane constants and the potassium conductance in metabolically exhausted muscle fibres. J. Physiol. 263, 215-238.
Fink, R., and E. Wettwer (1978). Modified K-channel gating by exhaustion and the block of internally applied $TEA^+$ and 4-aminopyridine in muscle. Pflügers Arch. 374, 289-292.
Frankenhaeuser, B. (1963). A quantitative description of potassium currents in myelinated nerve fibres of Xenopus laevis. J. Physiol. 169, 424-430.
Frankenhaeuser, B., and A.L. Hodgkin (1956). The after-effects of impulses in the giant nerve fibres of Loligo. J. Physiol. 131, 341-376.
French, R.J., and J.B. Wells (1977). Sodium ions as blocking agents and charge carriers in the potassium channel of the squid giant axon. J. gen. Physiol. 70, 707-724.
Goldman, L., and C.L. Schauf (1973). Quantitative description of sodium and potassium currents and computed action potentials in Myxicola giant axons. J. gen. Physiol. 61, 361-384.
Gorman, A.L.F., and A. Hermann (1979). Internal effects of divalent cations on potassium permeability in molluscan neurones. J. Physiol. 296, 393-410.

Hille, B. (1967). The selective inhibition of delayed potassium currents in nerve by tetraethylammonium ion. J.gen.Physiol. 50, 1287-1302.

Hille, B. (1973). Potassium channels in myelinated nerve: selective permeability to small cations. J.gen.Physiol. 61, 669-686.

Hille, B., and W. Schwarz (1978). Potassium channels as multi-ion single-file pores. J.gen.Physiol. 72, 409-442.

Hodgkin, A.L., and A.F. Huxley (1952). A quantitative description of membrane current and its application to conduction and excitation in nerve. J.Physiol. 117, 500-544.

Hodgkin, A.L., and R. D. Keynes (1955). The potassium permeability of a giant nerve fibre. J.Physiol. 128, 61-88.

Hofmeier, G., and H.D. Lux (1981). The time courses of intracellular free calcium and related electrical effects after injection of $CaCl_2$ into neurons of the snail, Helix Pomatia. Pflügers Arch. in press.

Horackova, M., W. Nonner and R. Stämpfli (1968). Action potentials and voltage clamp currents of single rat Ranvier nodes. Proc. Int. Union Physiol. Sci. 7, 198.

Inoue, I. (1980). Separation of the action potential into a Na-channel spike and a K-channel spike by tetrodotoxin and by tetraethylammonium ion in squid giant axons internally perfused with dilute Na-salt solutions. J.gen.Physiol. 76, 337-354.

Keynes, R.D., and J.E. Kimura (1980). The effect of starting potential on activation of the ionic conductances in the squid giant axon. J.Physiol. 308, 17P.

Koppenhöfer, E. (1967). Die Wirkung von Tetraäthylammoniumchlorid auf die Membranströme Ranvierscher Schnürringe von Xenopus laevis. Pflügers Arch. 293, 34-55.

Koppenhöfer, E., and W. Vogel (1969). Wirkung von Tetrodotoxin und Tetraäthylammoniumchlorid an der Innenseite der Schnürringsmembran von Xenopus laevis. Pflügers Arch. 313, 361-380.

Lüttgau, H.C. (1961). Weitere Untersuchungen über den passiven Ionentransport durch die erregbare Membran des Ranvierknotens. Pflügers Arch. 273, 302-310.

Meech, R.W. (1978). Calcium-dependent potassium activation in nervous tissues. Ann. Rev. Biophys. Bioeng. 7, 1-18.

Meech, R.W., and N.B. Standen (1975). Potassium activation in Helix aspersa neurones under voltage clamp: a component mediated by calcium influx. J.Physiol. 249, 211-239.

Moolenaar, W.H., and I. Spector (1978). Ionic currents in cultured mouse neuroblastoma cells under voltage-clamp conditions. J. Physiol. 278, 265-286.

Moran, N., Y. Palti, E. Levitan and R. Stämpfli (1980). Potassium ion accumulation at the external surface of the nodal membrane in frog myelinated fibers. Biophys. J. 32, 939-954.

Neumcke, B. (1981). Fluctuation of Na and K currents in excitable membranes. Intern.Rev.Neurobiology 23, in press.

Neumcke, B., W. Schwarz and R. Stämpfli (1980). Differences between K channels in motor and sensory nerve fibres of the frog as revealed by fluctuation analysis. Pflügers Arch. 387, 9-16.

Palti, Y., G. Ganot and R. Stämpfli (1976). Effect of conditioning potential on potassium current kinetics in the frog node. Biophys.J. 16, 261-273.

Schwarz, J.R., and W. Vogel (1971). Potassium inactivation in single myelinated nerve fibres of Xenopus laevis. Pflügers Arch. 330, 61-73.

Stanfield, P.R. (1970). The effect of tetraethylammonium ion on the delayed currents of frog skeletal muscle. J. Physiol. 209, 209-229.

# Effects of Aminopyridines on Potassium Currents of the Nodal Membrane

W. Ulbricht, H.-H. Wagner and J. Schmidtmayer

Physiologisches Institut der Universität Kiel, Olshausenstrasse 40-60,
D-2300 Kiel, Federal Republic of Germany

ABSTRACT

Block of potassium channels by 4-aminopyridine (4-AP) and 3,4-diaminopyridine (3,4-DAP) was studied in voltage clamp experiments on myelinated frog nerve fibres. Onset of action was slow ($\tau_{on}$ = ca. 3 min in 30 µM 4-AP, ca. 10 min in 100 µM 3,4-DAP) and after equilibration the block was partially removed during long depolarizing pulses with time constant $\tau_r$ = ca. 0.2 s. A formal description of voltage- and concentration-dependent block is given. Re-establishment of block by 4-AP at the resting potential was very slow with a time constant, $\tau_r'$, of ca. 60 s. $\tau_r'$ was much reduced at weak steady depolarizations suggesting that the channel gates must be open for rebinding of drug to an intra-channel site. Because of $\tau_r' \gg \tau_r$ block removal was cumulative during a series of frequent short pulses until a new stationary level of block was reached. On addition of tetraethylammonium ions (TEA) a steady level was reached faster which may indicate some kind of 4-AP-TEA interaction.

KEYWORDS

Node of Ranvier; frog nerve; 4-aminopyridine; 3,4-diaminopyridine; potassium channel; voltage-dependent block; partial removal of block.

INTRODUCTION

Few chemicals are known that selectively block potassium channels on external application. In nodes of Ranvier of frog nerve fibres two types of such agents have been studied in more detail, tetraethylammonium ions (TEA) and the aminopyridines. Block by TEA is prompt, reversible and little affected by membrane potential although large depolarizations seem to reduce the effect. The aminopyridines, in particular 4-aminopyridine (4-AP) and 3,4-diaminopyridine (3,4-DAP) act slowly and essentially irreversibly on Ranvier nodes; block by these drugs is clearly voltage dependent.

We are interested in these drugs mainly as tools to explore potassium channels. In a previous study we have investigated 4-AP block as a function of membrane potential and drug concentration (Wagner and

Ulbricht, 1975 a; Ulbricht and Wagner, 1976). This paper will be in part review of these earlier findings but also present new results with 3,4-DAP, on restoration of 4-AP block at rest and on possible 4-AP-TEA interaction. Interpretation of the results has become more difficult with the recent recognition of several types of potassium channels that differ in their gating kinetics and susceptibility to drugs (Dubois, 1981 b). Another complication may arise from $K^+$ ion accumulation outside the nodal membrane during the flow of outward $I_K$ (Dubois, 1981 a; Dubois and Bergman, 1975; Moran and others, 1980). Therefore, the observed $I_K$ inhibition is not necessarily a quantitative expression of receptor occupancy and we rather give an operational description in the form of current ratios "r" i.e. $I_K$ in drug solution over $I_K$ before treatment.

METHODS

The experiments were done on single nerve fibres of the frog, Rana esculenta. The voltage clamp arrangement used has been described in detail by Nonner (1969). Leakage and capacity currents were either corrected on-line by an analog device (see Wagner and Ulbricht, 1975b) or with a signal averager (Nicolet 1170). The fast exchanging chamber for current clamp experiments is described in Vierhaus and Ulbricht (1971). If not noted otherwise, membrane potentials are given as deviations, V, from the normal resting potential, depolarizations being positive. In the earlier experiments current densities were calculated according to Frankenhaeuser (1962), in recent experiments currents were usually normalized to the control values. - Mean values are given ± S.E.M.

All solutions were buffered with a mixture (7 mM each) of piperazine dihydrochloride and glycylglycine, the pH being adjusted to 7.2 with NaOH (Smith and Smith, 1948). The total $Na^+$ concentration was brought to 118 mM by adding crystalline NaCl. The Ringer solution also contained (in mM): KCl, 2.5; $CaCl_2$, 2.0. Aminopyridine-containing solutions were freshly prepared from 10 mM stock (4-AP: Fluka, Buchs, Switzerland; 3,4-DAP: EGA-Chemie, Steinheim, Germany). These solutions also contained either 300 nM tetrodotoxin (Calbiochem/Sankyo) or 100 nM saxitoxin (gift of Prof. E. J. Schantz, Madison, Wisconsin).

RESULTS

Onset of Action

In our voltage clamp the node under investigation is continuously superfused and exchange of solutions is prompt. Nevertheless the action of aminopyridines sets in relatively slowly. Figure 1 shows that the onset follows an exponential time course; that on applying 100 µM 3,4-DAP was about 3 times slower ($\tau_{on}$ = 9.70 ± 0.37 min; n = 5) than that following a change to 30 µM 4-AP ($\tau_{on}$ = 3.00 ± 0.20 min; n = 3) although the (estimated) final reduction in $I_K$ was to 0.17 of the control as compared to 0.11 in 3,4-DAP. These equilibrium values are at variance with observations on squid giant axons where 3,4-DAP was about 50 times more potent than 4-AP (Kirsch and Narahashi, 1978).

Our present 4-AP results (mean temperature 16°) compare well with our earlier results with 53 µM 4-AP at 14.5° C where $\tau_{on}$ was 2.65 ± 0.20

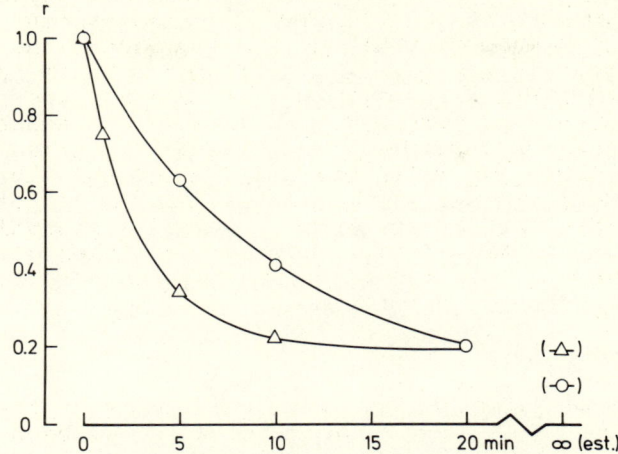

Fig. 1. Onset of action of 100 μM 3,4-DAP (○) and of 30 μM 4-AP (△). Ordinate, normalized value "r" of $I_K$ 25 ms after the start of 0.8-s pulses (V = 120 mV). Abscissa, time after change of solutions in min; equilibrium values ("∞") estimated. Onset time constant was 9.38 min in 3,4-DAP and 2.96 min in 4-AP. Different fibres, both at 16° C.

min (159 ± 12 s; n = 4; Ulbricht and Wagner, 1976). These latter results were obtained with 10-ms depolarizing pulses applied every minute. In the present series no clear difference in onset was observed between measurements of $I_K$ at the end of infrequent short (20 ms) pulses or of $I_K$ measured at t = 20 ms during long (0.8 s) pulses. Obviously, prolonged but infrequent depolarizations did not affect onset. Figure 2 shows the time course of $I_K$, obtained with a signal

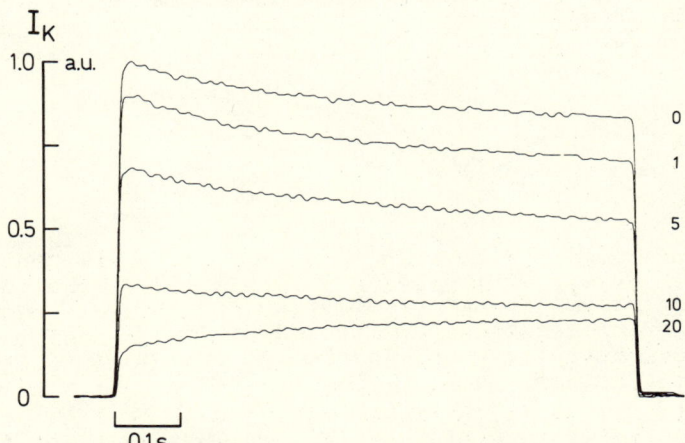

Fig. 2 Time course of $I_K$ (arbitrary units, a.u.) during 0.8-s pulses before ("0") and during the onset of action of 100 μM 3,4-DAP; numbers on right margin are min after solution change. 18.2°C.

averager, during such long pulses (V = 120 mV) before and after changing to 100 μM 3,4-DAP. Not until after ca. 20 min did the typical aminopyridine block become apparent which is partially relieved during sustained depolarization (see next section). With 53 μM 4-AP this state is reached in less than 5 min.

The marked slowness of 3,4-DAP action was also observed with very high drug concentrations in current clamp experiments where the prolongation of action potentials served as a measure. Thus with 1 mM 3,4-DAP half of the final increment in duration (ca. 3 times the control) was not reached until after 2-3 min whereas the half-time in 4-AP was ca. 5 s. In these as well as in the voltage clamp experiments the effect of 4-AP was poorly reversible, that of 3,4-DAP completely irreversible.

Voltage-Dependent Block

Effects of long pulses. Block of potassium channels by 4-AP is partially removed during strong depolarization. Details of this phenomenon are best demonstrated with pairs of long depolarizing impulses (V = 145 mV; 0.8 s duration) with an interval of 0.8 s. Figure 3 shows superimposed original $I_K$ records during such pulses. In Ringer solution (upper pair of traces) $I_K$ during the 2nd pulse differed only little from $I_K$ during the 1st pulse, the slight difference being due to some potassium channel inactivation. After equilibration in 53 μM 4-AP (lower pair of traces) $I_K$ at the beginning of the 1st pulse was very much depressed but recovered with a time constant of 0.20 s to more than half of the control. During the 2nd pulse $I_K$ virtually started at the value observed at the end of the 1st pulse

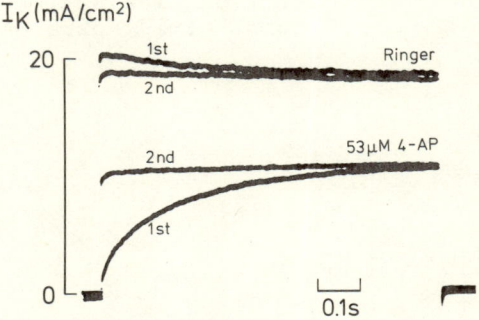

Fig. 3. $I_K$ during pairs of 0.8-s impulses at 0.8 s intervals in Ringer solution and in 53 μM 4-AP. Superimposed original records at 14.6° C. From Ulbricht and Wagner (1976), by permission of copyright holder.

indicating no restoration of block within the 0.8-s interval at the resting potential. Actually it took several minutes at rest for full re-establishment of block. This current pattern, however, was observed only after equilibration in 4-AP; at earlier stages $I_K$ during the paired pulses resembled, at a reduced scale, that in Ringer solution. In 100 μM 3,4-DAP partial relief from block was not seen until after ca. 20 min (see Fig. 2).

Our earlier results were conveniently described by the ratio "r" formed, at any instant, of $I_K$ in 4-AP over $I_K$ in Ringer solution (Ulbricht and Wagner, 1976). In the case of Fig. 3 this yielded, for the 1st pulse, a starting value $r(0) = 0.12$ rising exponentially with a time constant $\tau_r = 0.21$ s to a final value of 0.57. This latter value was close to $r(\infty)$ which, as a rule, was determined from $I_K$ at the end of the 2nd 0.8-s pulse. $r(\infty)$ increased with increasing depolarization; it was e.g. $0.41 \pm 0.04$ (n = 16) for V = 50 mV and $0.66 \pm 0.02$ (n = 15) for V = 120 mV. At V = 0, $r(\infty) = r(0)$ of the test pulse; it was $0.24 \pm 0.02$ (n = 23). To obtain $r(0)$ a pulse was applied after 6 min at rest and $r(t)$ during the pulse was extrapolated to t = 0 on the assumption that 4-AP did not affect the gating parameter "n" of the channels not blocked. This notion was confirmed in nearly all fibres of a recent test employing a signal averager at an expanded time scale. Thus relief from 4-AP block during depolarization is satisfactorily described by a single time constant which, incidentally, was nearly independent of pulse potential (Ulbricht and Wagner, 1976). With extremely long impulses (5 s; V = 120 mV) a second slower phase of relief was observed which increased r another 14% on the average with a time constant of ca. 8 times $\tau_r$. This phase was most likely "caused" by a continuing slow $I_K$ inactivation in Ringer solution (Schwarz and Vogel, 1971) leading to an increase in the ratio $r = (I_K)_{4-AP}/(I_K)_{Ri}$ (Ulbricht and Wagner, 1976). And indeed a recent study revealed several types of potassium channels one of which does not inactivate and is not blocked by 4-AP (Dubois, 1981 b).

The double-pulse experiment of Fig. 2 suggests that block restoration at the resting potential is very slow. To study its time course, block was first relieved by a pair of long (0.8 s) impulses. The subsequent re-establishment was determined with short (10 ms) pulses applied every 30 s that yielded a mean time constant, $\tau_r'$, of $67 \pm 2$ s which is more than 300 times $\tau_r$. The possible significance of this large difference is discussed later.

<u>Trains of short pulses</u>. As a consequence of $\tau_r' \gg \tau_r$ block removal is cumulative during a train of frequent short pulses. This is illustrated in Fig. 4 which gives $I_K$ at the respective ends of 10-ms and 20-ms impulses during 10-Hz trains. Exponential functions were fitted to the points with time constants, $\tau$, of 1.98 s and 1.16 s, respectively. Other runs on this fibre yielded $\tau_r = 0.21$ s and $\tau_r' = 98$ s so that no restoration of block could be expected during $t_R$, the time at rest between pulses. Hence the process of block removal continued during each consecutive pulse from where it was left at the end of the preceding pulse. For pulses of duration $t_D$ and time constant $\tau_r$ of block removal we can approximate $\tau = \tau_r(t_D + t_R)/t_D$. The expected values of $\tau$ are 10 $\tau_r = 2.10$ s for $t_D = 10$ ms = 0.01 s (vs. $\tau = 1.98$ s observed) and $\tau = 5\ \tau_r$ for $t_D = 0.02$ s (vs. $\tau = 1.16$ s observed). For lower pulse frequencies (e.g. 0.5 Hz) and hence much larger values of $t_R$, $\tau_r'$ has to be considered in calculating $\tau$; the exact calculations are given in the original paper which also contains a list of observed and computed values of $\tau$ for several fibres (Ulbricht and Wagner, 1976)

<u>Concentration dependence</u>. Block by 4-AP increases with increasing concentration as illustrated in Fig. 5 which shows $r(\infty)$ in 3 solutions and in each at 3 different membrane potentials, here given in absolute values E (resting potential E = -70 mV). The points are mean values, the vertical bars denote ± S.E.M. of 4 preparations. Because of the irreversible effect each fibre was treated successively with

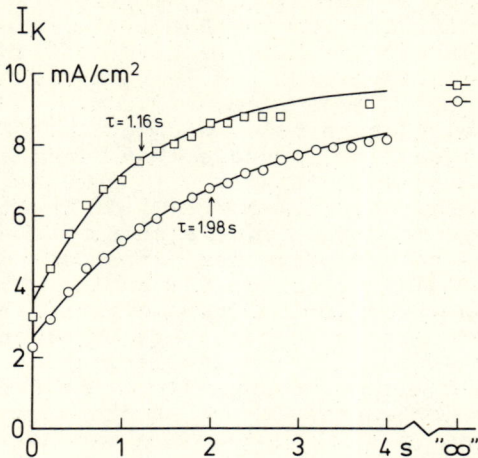

Fig. 4. Cumulative block removal during 10-Hz trains of impulses of 10 ms (○) and 20 ms (□) duration (V = 144 mV) Points give $I_K$ (in mA/cm²) at the end of each pulse. Abscissa, time after start of train, "∞" when steady state is reached. 14.6° C. From Ulbricht and Wagner (1976), by permission of copyright holder.

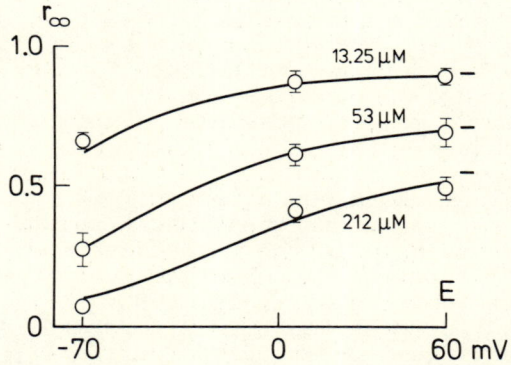

Fig. 5. 4-AP effect as a function of absolute membrane potential E and [4-AP]. $r_\infty = r(\infty)$ of text. Curves and bars at right margin were calculated as explained in text. From Ulbricht and Wagner (1976), by permission of copyright holder.

increasing concentrations between 13.3 and 848 μM (not shown). The curves were calculated with the empirical equation $1/r_\infty = 1/r(\infty) = 1 + c_t + c_v \exp(-\delta EF/RT)$ with $\delta = 0.77$ and the dimensionless constants $c_t$ and $c_v$ which depend on concentration and represent the "tonic" (i. e. voltage-independent) and voltage-dependent component, respectively. At rest or on hyperpolarization, $c_v$ dominates; it was linearly related to [4-AP] being 0.06, 0.25, and 1.0 in 13.3, 53, and 212 μM but, less satisfactorily, only 2.0 in 848 μM. Nevertheless, at E = -70 mV (V = 0), a Hill plot of log $[(1 - r_\infty)/r_\infty]$ vs. log [4-AP] has a slope close to unity (0.92; 16 pairs of observations, correlation coeff. = 0.94) At very large depolarizations $r_\infty$ is determined by $c_t$ which is not linearly related to [4-AP]; it was 0.11, 0.40, 0.82, and 1.3 for 13.3, 53, 212, and 848 µM, respectively. Hence a Hill plot for $r(\infty)$ at E = 60 mV has a slope of much less than unity (0.64). In Fig. 5, block at infinite depolarization i.e. $r(\infty) = 1/(1 + c_t)$ is indicated by the bars at the right margin. Tested with pulses of V = 130 mV (E = 60 mV) $\tau_r$ decreased from 0.25 s in 13.3 µM to 0.10 s in 848 µM (at 17° C on the average).

3,4-DAP effects were not systematically investigated but the mean $r(\infty)$ values obtained after a 20-min treatment with 100 µM were 0.18 at E = -70 mV and 0.29 at E = 50 mV (measured after 0.8 s); $\tau_r$ was 0.23 s at 16-18° C. For E = -70 mV the value lies between that in 53 and 212 µM 4-AP (0.27 and 0.07) whereas for E = 50 mV the mean $r(\infty)$ is near that in 848 µM 4-AP (0.34).

<u>Further evidence in favour of voltage dependence</u>. Finally a few more points concerning removal of block by 4-AP should be added. 1. Block and its removal were also observed in 118 mM K⁺ at potentials where $I_K$ flows inward. This excludes the possibility that, at normal K⁺ concentration, outward $I_K$ "flushes out" the channels that are occupied by 4-AP. 2. Block removal depends on previous potential history rather than on the size of $I_K$. This is demonstrated in Fig. 6. which again shows superimposed current traces during two runs with pairs of 0.7-s pulses, 10 s apart. In the first run both pulses were applied in 53 µM 4-AP. In the subsequent run the 1st pulse was applied in a

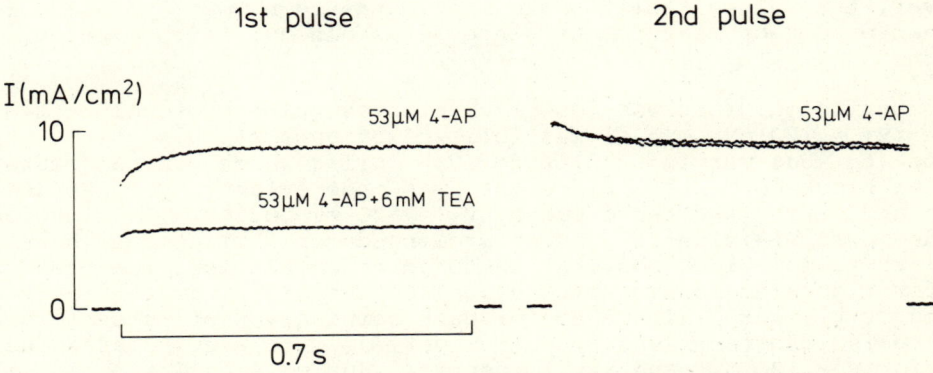

Fig. 6. Current during 2nd pulse is independent of current during 1st pulse (either pulse, V = 93 mV; 10 s interval). Currents not corrected for leakage. First run in 4-AP exclusively; in the second run the 1st pulse was applied in 4-AP + TEA while TEA was washed out completely in the pulse interval. 22° C. From Ulbricht and Wagner (1976), by permission of copyright holder.

4-AP + TEA mixture which reduced the current almost to the leakage component (not subtracted in this figure). 4-AP nevertheless must have come off its blocking site since the 2nd pulse, applied 10 s later after complete exchange for pure 4-AP solution, gave the same current pattern as in the first run. 3. If, for a given drug concentration, block solely depends on membrane potential, $r(\infty)$ should be independent of the value with which r starts at the beginning of a pulse. This was indeed found but attaining equilibrium took considerably longer than expected from $\tau_r$, due to the appearance of slower phases of equilibration. The pertinent experiments required rather complicated pulse protocols and the reader is referred to the original paper for details (Ulbricht and Wagner, 1976).

## The Possible Reason for $\tau_r' \gg \tau_r$

The preceding section presented evidence that equilibrium block by 4-AP depends on membrane potential. How this comes about is still unknown but it appears reasonable to assume that block is the consequence of a drug-site reaction and that relief from block on depolarization (time constant $\tau_r$) is due to a decreasing site affinity for 4-AP. Conversely, re-establishment of block at the resting potential (time constant $\tau_r'$) should reflect an increased affinity and we would expect $\tau_r' < \tau_r$. However, the reverse is true and the deviation is extreme with $\tau_r'$ being about 300 $\tau_r$ as reported in the previous section.

A possible explanation of this puzzling fact is to assume that rebinding of 4-AP is prevented or much impeded if the channel gates are closed at the resting potential. Hence restoration of block should be enhanced even at weak depolarizations at which the probability, N, of gates to be open is much larger than at rest. For Xenopus fibres, N = $n_\infty^2$ (Frankenhaeuser and Huxley, 1964); at 20° C N increases from 0.0006 at V = 0 to 0.0067 at V = 10 mV and to 0.0522 at V = 20 mV. The values given for Rana nodes (N = $n_\infty^4$; Hille, 1967) change less: N = 0.0107, 0.0279, and 0.0745 for V = 0, 10, and 20 mV. For either preparation, however, the values seem to have been obtained by extrapolation rather than by direct measurement since $I_K$ is minimal in this potential region.

The experimental test was done with a three-pulse protocol; a test pulse ($V_1$ = 120 mV; 0.5 s) was followed by another pulse of 0.8 s duration ($t_2$) but varying amplitude ($V_2$) during which partial restoration of block could take place that was made evident by $I_K$ at the start and during the third pulse ($V_3$ = 120 mV; 0.5 s). This protocol avoided possible side-effects of prolonged depolarizations (however weak) to follow block restoration to go to completion. The protocol was first applied in Ringer solution and then in 50 μM 4-AP; current ratios, r(t), were calculated for each combination of pulses. The three-pulse programme was repeated every 10 s to keep r large (near r(∞) for V = 120 mV) and $r(t_1)$ identical during each 1st pulse. $I_K$ at the start of the 3rd pulse characteristically depended on $V_2$; it was lowest following $V_2$ = 20 mV, lower than after $V_2$ = 0 or $V_2 \geq$ 40 mV. For an interpretation we term $r_2(0.8)$ = r at the end of the 2nd pulse of 0.8 s duration. Because of the assumed continuity of r, $r_2(0.8)$ = $r_3(0)$ = r at the start of the 3rd pulse where $I_K$ is large enough to be measured with accuracy. We then introduce $r_2(\infty)$ = equilibrium value at $V_2$ and have, for an exponential time course of block restoration, $r_2(0.8) = r_2(\infty) - [r_1(0.5) - r_2(\infty)] \exp(-t_2/\tau_r')$. A decrease in $r_3(0)$ following $V_2$ = 20 mV must then be due to a decrease in $\tau_r'$ because $r_2(\infty)$ increases with increasing $V_2$ (see previous section). Increase in $r_2(\infty)$, incidentally, is the reason why $r_3(0)$ increases again for $V_2$ = 40 or 80 mV although $\tau_r'$ continues to decrease.

Actually, to obtain a good estimate of $\tau_r'(V_2)$ it is sufficient to measure the respective currents in 4-AP thus saving the tedious

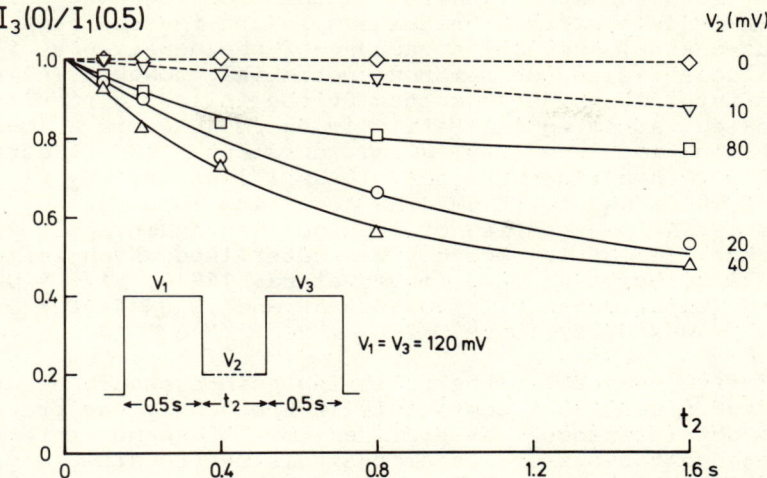

Fig. 7. Time course of re-establishment of block by 50 μM 4-AP as a function of membrane potential ($V_2$). Pulse protocol shown by inset. Ordinate, $I_K$ at $V_3$ extrapolated to t = 0, $I_3(0)$, normalized to $I_K$ at the end of 1st pulse, $I_1(0.5)$. Abscissa, duration, $t_2$, of 2nd pulse.. For $V_2$ = 0 (◇) there was nearly no, for $V_2$ = 10 mV (▽) only a slight re-establishment of block. Only lower limits of $\tau_r'$ = 30 and 8 s, respectively, can be estimated; points connected by interrupted lines. Other points connected by exponentials with $\tau_r'$ = 1.02, 0.60, and 0.46 s for $V_2$ = 20, 40, and 80 mV. The respective values of $r_2(\infty)$ are 0.36, 0.40, and 0.73. 16.4° C.

calculation of r(t). Currents were also measured in a modified experiment illustrated in Fig. 7 where $t_2$ was varied for different $V_2$ and $I_3(0)/I_1(0.5)$, corresponding to $r_3(0)/r_1(0.5)$, was plotted as a function of $t_2$. The graph shows a clear difference already between $V_2$ = 0 and $V_2$ = 10 mV; the values of $\tau_r'$, decreasing with increasing $V_2$, are given in the legend. Obviously, re-establishment of block is greatly enhanced at relatively weak depolarizations where equilibrium block differs little from that at the resting potential (V = 0) but where the probability of open gates is markedly increased.

## Comparison of the Effects of 4-AP and TEA

In the previous study (Ulbricht and Wagner, 1976) the effects of 4-AP, TEA and a 4-AP-TEA mixture were measured at the end of 0.8-s pulses (V = 110 mV; 19° C). In 53 μM 4-AP $r(\infty)$ was 0.67 ± 0.05; in 3 mM TEA $I_K$ was reduced to $p_{TEA}$ = 0.14 ± 0.01, in 53 μM 4-AP + 3 mM TEA to p'= 0.12 ± 0.01 (n = 5). In the case of two independent blocking sites per channel for 4-AP and TEA one would expect (see Wagner and Ulbricht, 1976) $p_{TEA} \times r(\infty)$ = p'; however one calculates 0.14 × 0.67 = 0.09 i.e. less, but not significantly so, than the mean observed p'. Does this mean that the actions of 4-AP and TEA are not completely independent? The question is difficult to answer since proof of drug interaction or even competition for the same receptor (in contrast to the two-site hypothesis) requires specification of the blocking reaction. In the case of 4-AP this clearly is not a simple one-to-one reaction of a homogeneous channel population because of the dependence of the apparent Hill coefficient on membrane potential. However, there appears to be some interaction as suggested by the following results. Nodes were subjected, after equilibration in 53 μM 4-AP, to a 10-Hz series of depolarizing impulses (V = 120 mV, duration = 15 ms) during which $I_K$ recovered with a time constant, $\tau$, as illustrated by Fig. 4. Then 0.75 mM TEA was added to 53 μM 4-AP resulting in a further marked reduction of $I_K$. A 10-Hz series of impulses was again applied and the time constant, $\tau'$, of $I_K$ recovery was determined which was consistently smaller. We found in 4 fibres at ca. 16° C, $\tau'/\tau = 0.62 \pm 0.03$. In another 2 experiments with 30 μM 4-AP and 30 μM 4-AP + 0.5 mM TEA, the mean $\tau'/\tau$ was 0.78 (18.5° C).

For a tentative evaluation the following points should be considered. 1. If the two drugs block completely independently the presence of TEA should not influence $\tau$ as e.g. saxitoxin does not interfere with the use-dependent block of sodium channels by procaine (Wagner and Ulbricht, 1976). 2. If two drugs, A and B, directly compete for the same site in a one-to-one reaction, changing the concentration of A to $c_A$ leads to an exponential change in receptor occupation with a time constant $\tau_A = [k_{2A}(c_A + 1)]^{-1}$ where $c_A = [A]/K_A$, $K_A$ = equilibrium dissociation constant and $k_{2A}$ = dissociation rate constant. In the presence of drug B which we assume to react "instantaneously", the same change in $c_A$ now leads to a change in receptor occupation with a time constant $\tau_{A+B} = [k_{2A}(c_A + c_B + 1)]^{-1}$ where $c_B$ is defined in analogy to $c_A$ (Rang and Ritter, 1970); hence we obtain $\tau_{A+B}/\tau_A = (c_A + 1)/(c_A + c_B + 1)$. TEA acts so fast on external application to the node (Vierhaus and Ulbricht, 1971) that it satisfies the requirements for drug B. Because of the uncertainties about the 4-AP-receptor reaction we cannot simply assign 4-AP to the role of drug A whose effective concentration, $c_A$, is reduced on depolarozation; therefore we cannot simply equate $\tau_r$ with $\tau_A$. Nevertheless, the measured ratio $\tau'/\tau < 1$ could reflect $\tau_{A+B}/\tau_A < 1$ since $\tau \approx \tau_r(t_D + t_R)/t_D$ as discussed in connexion with Fig. 4.

Another test for drug interaction proved inconclusive: after equilibrating a fibre in 4-AP we changed the perfusate to a 4-AP-TEA mixture and back and watched for transients in block during a 1-Hz series of test pulses (see Wagner and Ulbricht, 1975 b, for the rationale of the experiment). Transients were observed but not consistently so. Similar experiments in our fast exchanging current clamp chamber, too, yielded variable results. We measured the duration of action potentials of a 1-Hz series on changing from 1 mM 4-AP + 1 mM TEA to 1 mM 4-AP. In some (but not all) preparations a transient shortening was observed which could indicate some drug interaction. Incidentally, 1 mM TEA was more effective in increasing the duration than 1 mM 4-AP but less effective than the mixture.

## DISCUSSION

The prominent feature of block by 4-AP in myelinated frog nerve fibres is its dependence on membrane potential so that a fraction of potassium channels becomes unblocked during a long depolarizing impulse. This relief from block proceeds with a time constant of about 200 ms which is much larger than the time constant with which channel gates open on depolarization. While there is no indication that 4-AP affects gating of channels which are not blocked, the rate of block restoration on repolarization seems to be highly dependent on the probability that the gates are open. This could mean that closed gates either impede access to the receptor or drastically reduce receptor affinity. We favour the first possibility which could be realized by a site located inside the channel and a gate at its axoplasmic mouth, with the adjacent axoplasm forming the pool of drug molecules. The pool must be filled during onset and this slow process appears to be rate limiting since occasional long depolarizing pulses during onset of action did not noticeably enhance it. Since 4-AP molecules are too large to pass the selectivity filter of the potassium channel (see discussion in Ulbricht and Wagner, 1976) we must assume that they penetrate the lipid matrix of the membrane. Reversing this already slow process on washing the small nodal area may be extremely slow after equilibration of the interior of sizeable parts of the adjacent internodes. This may explain the poor reversibility of 4-AP effects on nodes in contrast to those on intracellularly perfused squid axons which can be washed both externally and internally (Meves and Pichon, 1977). In squid axons, incidentally, 4-AP acts from either side (Meves and Pichon, 1977; Yeh and others, 1976 a, 1976 b); so does 3,4-DAP which, however, is clearly more effective on internal application (Kirsch and Narahashi, 1978). It is not clear whether this finding is related to the extremely slow onset of 3,4-DAP action in nodes of Ranvier. In either preparation the reversibility of 3,4-DAP effects is poor (squid) to nonexistent (frog).

4-AP action in other nerve preparations such as the axons of Myxicola (Schauf and others, 1976) and the cockroach, Periplaneta americana, (Pelhate and Pichon, 1974; Pelhate and others, 1974, 1975) is comparable to that in frog fibres. In squid axons an extensive study of rates of block removal and restoration has led to a simple model where aminopyridine binds to closed channels and is released from open channels in a voltage-dependent fashion; no change in the gating parameter "n" had to be assumed (Yeh and others, 1976 b). Our results, too, speak against a change in n(t) but they also suggest that closing the channel gates prevents rather than favours binding. A quantitative formulation of gate interference with block appears premature as long as the basic blocking reaction is uncertain. The recent realization that some potassium channels are not blocked by 4-AP and do not inactivate (Dubois, 1981 b) only partially improves the description. We have "corrected" our earlier results by substracting from $r(\infty)$ at various concentrations the value of $r(\infty)$ in 848 µM 4-AP on the assumption that it in fact constitutes the fraction of slow drug-resistant channels. The Hill coefficient for $V = 130$ mV ($E = 60$ mV) nevertheless remained far below 1.0 which makes it unlikely that there exists a true one-to-one 4-AP-receptor reaction that is masked by the presence of slow channels. Obviously, further experiments are required to elucidate this reaction and the possible influence of TEA on it.

### ACKNOWLEDGEMENTS

We thank Miss E. Dieter for technical help, Dr. J. M. Dubois (Paris) for making avaliable to us manuscripts before publication and the Deutsche Forschungsgemeinschaft for financial support.

## REFERENCES

Dubois, J. M. (1981a). Simultaneous changes in the equilibrium potential and potassium conductance in voltage clamped Ranvier nodes. J. Physiol. (Lond.), (in press)

Dubois, J. M. (1981b). Evidence for the existence of three types of potassium channels in the Ranvier node membrane. J. Physiol. (Lond.), (in press)

Dubois, J. M. and C. Bergman (1975). Potassium accumulation in the perinodal space of frog myelinated axons. Pflügers Arch., 358, 111-124.

Frankenhaeuser, B. (1962). Delayed currents in myelinated nerve fibres of Xenopus laevis investigated with voltage clamp technique. J. Physiol. (Lond.), 160, 40-45.

Frankenhaeuser, B. and A. F. Huxley (1964). The action potential in myelinated nerve fibres of Xenopus laevis as computed on the basis of voltage clamp data. J. Physiol. (Lond.), 171, 302-315.

Hille, B. (1967). A pharmacological analysis of the ionic channels of nerve. Thesis. The Rockefeller University. University Microfilms, Inc., Ann Arbor (No. 68-9584).

Kirsch, G. E. and T. Narahashi (1978). 3,4-Diaminopyridine. A potent new potassium channels blocker. Biophys. J., 22, 507-512.

Meves, H. and Y. Pichon (1977). The effect of internal and external 4-aminopyridine on the potassium currents in intracellularly perfused squid giant axons. J. Physiol. (Lond.), 268, 511-532.

Nonner, W. (1969). A new voltage clamp method for Ranvier nodes. Pflügers Arch., 309, 176-192.

Pelhate, M., B. Hue, Y. Pichon and J. Chanelet (1974). Action de la 4-aminopyridine sur la membrane de l'axone isolé d'Insecte. C. R. Acad. Sci. Paris, Série D, 278, 2807-2809.

Pelhate, M., L. Mony, B. Hue and J. Chanelet (1975). Modifications des courants potassium par la 4-aminopyridine. Cas de l'axone géant isolé de la Blatte (Periplaneta americana). C. R. Soc. Biol., 169, 1436-1441.

Pelhate, M. and Y. Pichon (1974). Selective inhibition of potassium current in the giant axon of the cockroach. J. Physiol. (Lond.), 242, 90-91 P.

Rang, H. P. and J. M. Ritter (1970). On the mechanism of desensitization at cholinergic receptors. Mol. Pharmacol., 6, 357-382.

Schauf, C. L., C. A. Colton, J. S. Colton and F. A. Davis (1976). Aminopyridines and sparteine as inhibitors of membrane potassium conductance. Effects on Myxicola giant axons and the lobster neuromuscular junction. J. Pharmacol. Exp. Ther., 197, 414-425.

Schwarz, J. R. and W. Vogel (1971). Potassium inactivation in single myelinated nerve fibres of Xenopus laevis. Pflügers Arch., 330, 61-73.

Smith, M. E. and L. E. Smith (1948). Piperazine dihydrochloride and glycylglycine as non-toxic buffers in distilled and in sea water. Biol. Bull., 96, 233-237.

Ulbricht, W. and H.-H. Wagner (1976). Block of potassium channels of the nodal membrane by 4-aminopyridine and its partial removal on depolarization. Pflügers Arch., 367, 77.87.

Vierhaus, J. and W. Ulbricht (1971). Rate of action of tetraethylammonium ions on the duration of action potentials in single Ranvier nodes. Pflügers Arch., 326, 88-100.

Wagner, H.-H. and W. Ulbricht (1975a). 4-Aminopyridine block of K channels and its partial relief on depolarization. Abstr. 5th Int. Biophys. Congr. 1975, p. 138.

Wagner, H.-H. and W. Ulbricht (1975b). The rates of saxitoxin action and of saxitoxin-tetrodotoxin interaction at the node of Ranvier. Pflügers Arch., 359, 297-315.

Wagner, H.-H. and W. Ulbricht (1976). Saxitoxin and procaine act independently on separate sites of the sodium channel. Pflügers Arch., 364, 65-70.

Yeh, J. Z., G. S. Oxford, C. H. Wu and T. Narahashi (1976a). Interactions of aminopyridines with potassium channels of squid axon membranes. Biophys. J., 16, 77-81.

Yeh, J. Z., G. S. Oxford, C. H. Wu and T. Narahashi (1976b). Dynamics of aminopyridine block of potassium channels in squid axon membrane. J. Gen. Physiol., 68, 519-539.

# Properties and Physiological Roles of K+ Currents in Frog Myelinated Nerve Fibres as Revealed by 4-Amino Pyridine

J. M. Dubois

Laboratoire de Neurobiologie, Ecole Normale Supérieure,
46, rue d'Ulm, 75230 Paris Cedex 05, France

ABSTRACT

On repolarization, the $K^+$ conductance in frog Ranvier node turns off in two phases: a large and fast phase followed by a smaller and very slow phase. 4-amino pyridine (4-AP) blocks the fast phase but does not affect the slow phase. In the presence of 4-AP (1 mM), there remains a slow $K^+$ current, distinct from the fast familiar $K^+$ current. It is shown that the slow $K^+$ current plays an important role in the resting potential and spike frequency limitation. The differences between spike frequency adaptation in motor and sensory fibres are discussed in relation to differences in $K^+$ conductance-voltage relationships of both types of fibres.

KEYWORDS

Frog Ranvier node ; 4-amino pyridine ; $K^+$ conductance ; $K^+$ channels ; spike frequency adaptation.

INTRODUCTION

4-amino pyridine (4-AP) is known to block the $K^+$ current in cockroach axons (Pelhate & Pichon, 1974), squid axons (Yeh, Oxford, Wu & Narahashi, 1976 ; Meves & Pichon, 1977), frog myelinated nerve fibres (Ulbrich & Wagner, 1976) and mammalian non-myelinated or demyelinated nerve fibres (Bostock, Sears & Sherratt, 1981). It is shown here that 4-AP can be used on frog myelinated nerve fibres as an efficient tool to separate different K+ current components and to study their physiological roles.

METHODS

All methods were as described elsewhere (Dubois, 1981a). In normal KCl Ringer, the resting potential was assumed to be - 70 mV. In isotonic KCl Ringer, the absolute zero potential was determined as the reversal potential for the $K^+$ current. The sodium current was blocked by tetrodotoxin $(10^{-6}$ M). Symmetrical leakage and capacity currents were compensated for automatically.

## RESULTS

### Evidence for the Existence of Different $K^+$ Currents

During depolarizations in normal Ringer, the outward $K^+$ current gives rise to a marked accumulation of $K^+$ ions in the perinodal space (Dubois & Bergman, 1975 ; Attwell, Dubois & Ojeda, 1980 ; Dubois, 1981a). As a consequence of this accumulation, the time course of the $K^+$ current not only reflects the change in $K^+$ conductance but also the change in driving force on $K^+$. In K-rich media, the effects of accumulation are minimized (Dubois, 1981a). In these conditions, after activation of the $K^+$ conductance by depolarization, the $K^+$ current that flows upon repolarization (tail current) decreases in two phases : a large and fast phase followed by a smaller and very slow phase (Ilyin, Katina, Lonskii, Makovsky & Polishchuk, 1980 ; Dubois, 1981a,b). This observation suggests that the $K^+$ conductance is composed of two components whose kinetics are very different. This hypothesis is confirmed by the observation that 4-AP blocks the fast phase of the tail current with an apparent dissociation constant of $10^{-5}$ M but does not affect the slow phase (Dubois, 1981b).

Figure 1 presents $K^+$ current traces recorded in isotonic $K^+$ solutions without and with 4-AP (1 mM). Whereas the fast phase of the tail current recorded upon repolarization to - 90 mV after a depolarization to - 40 mV (a) or + 40 mV (b) is blocked by 4-AP, the slow phase remains unaffected. In the presence of 1 mM 4-AP, the block of the fast $K^+$ current is not removed by depolarizations or repetitive pulsing. In such conditions, the slow $K^+$ current can be studied separately.

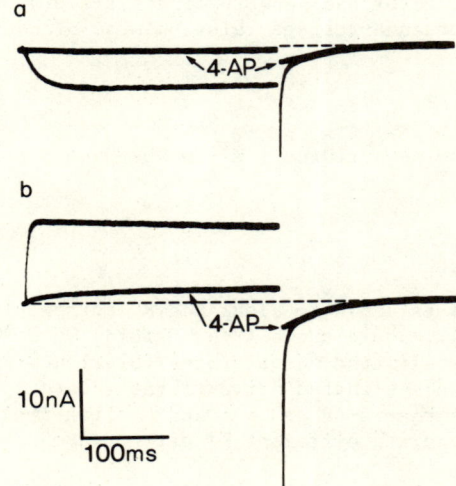

Figure 1. Superimposed $K^+$ current traces recorded during and after depolarizations to - 40 mV (a) and + 40 mV (b) in isotonic $K^+$ Ringer and isotonic $K^+$ Ringer + 1 mM 4-AP (arrows). In the presence of 4-AP, the remaining slow current is activated during depolarizations and de-activated upon repolarization. The tail current recorded in 4-AP corresponds to the slow phase of the tail current recorded without 4-AP. Holding potential : - 90 mV. Temperature : 13.5 °C. Fibre : 7-11-80.

In the experiment presented Fig. 2, the tail current was recorded in isotonic $K^+$ Ringer at - 90 mV after activation of the conductance by 300 ms depolarizations of various amplitudes. In the presence of 4-AP (1 mM), the fast phase is fully blocked whereas the slow phase remains unchanged whatever the amplitude of the conditioning depolarization. Taking into account the observation that the instantaneous fast and slow current-voltage relationships are linear (Dubois, 1981a,c) the amplitude of the instantaneous currents recorded upon repolarization without or with 4-AP are directly proportional to respectively the total and slow $K^+$ conductances at the end of depolarizations. Consequently, the envelopes of peak currents in Fig. 2 represent the variation of the slow (with 4-AP) and total (without 4-AP) $K^+$ conductances as a function of voltage. The fast conductance can be calculated as the difference between the total and the slow conductance, this latter being calculated from the instantaneous slow current recorded in the presence of 4-AP or extrapolated to the time of repolarization in the presence of 4-AP.

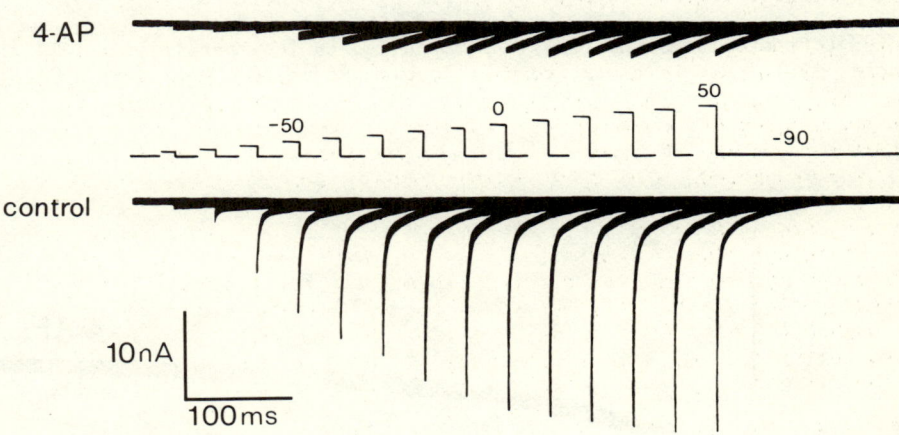

Figure 2. Tails of $K^+$ current recorded in isotonic $K^+$ Ringer without or with 4-AP (1 mM) at - 90 mV after 300 msec conditioning depolarization of various amplitudes. The amplitude of depolarizations (middle traces and numbers) was increased by 10 mV steps and the origin of the current traces was shifted to the right by an amount proportional to the amplitude of depolarizations. The envelopes of the peak currents respectively represent the slow (with 4-AP) and total (without 4-AP) $K^+$ conductances-voltage curves. Temperature : 13.5 °C. Fibre : 7-11-80.

During depolarizations in the presence of 4-AP (1 mM), the slow $K^+$ current is activated alone (Fig. 1). It has been shown previously that the time and voltage dependence of this current differs from those of the fast $K^+$ current (Dubois, 1981a,b). Whereas the kinetics of the fast current activation are sigmoid, the activation kinetics of the slow current are described by a single exponential ; b) a hyperpolarizing prepulse delays the fast current but has no effect on the activation kinetics of the slow current ; c) whereas the fast current can be completely inactivated during large and long lasting depolarizations, the slow current does not inactivate.

An analysis of the voltage and time dependent properties of the fast current revealed that the fast conductance can be decomposed further into two components ($g_{Kf1}$ and $g_{Kf2}$) which both activate over different voltage ranges (- 80 to - 30 mV for $g_{Kf1}$ and - 40 to + 30 mV for $g_{Kf2}$) and inactivate with different time constants (45 sec for $g_{Kf1}$ and 2 sec for $g_{Kf2}$ at E = 0 mV and t = 12 °C) (Dubois, 1981b ; see also Fig. 6).

From these observations, it is concluded that the $K^+$ conductance of the frog nodal membrane is composed of three components which correspond to three classes of distinct voltage dependent $K^+$ channels.

## Physiological Roles of the Different $K^+$ Currents

Following the demonstration of the existence of several $K^+$ currents, it was of interest to investigate their respective physiological roles. For this purpose, the electrical activity of the fibres was studied in current clamp conditions after successive blockade of the different $K^+$ currents. Since, at the present time, no pharmacological agent has been found to specifically block the slow $K^+$ current ($I_{Ks}$), its role was studied by comparing the electrical activity of the fibres after blockade of only $I_{Kf}$ by 4-AP and after blockade of both $I_{Kf}$ and $I_{Ks}$ by 4-AP and tetraethylammonium (TEA). Although $I_{Ks}$ is less sensitive to TEA than $I_{Kf}$ (Dubois, 1981b), it is almost completely blocked by 20 mM TEA (Fig. 3).

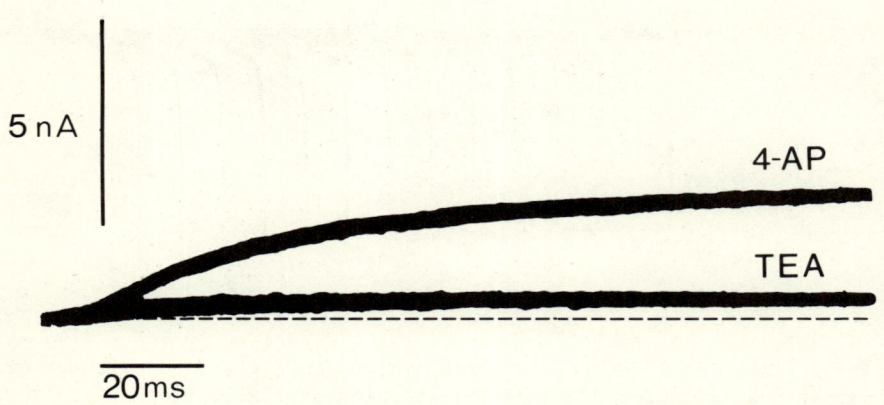

Figure 3. Blockade of the slow $K^+$ current by TEA. Superimposed traces of slow $K^+$ current recorded during depolarizations to + 68 mV in Ringer + 4-AP (1 mM) and Ringer + 4-AP + TEA (20 mM). Holding potential : - 70 mV. Temperature : 13 °C. Fibre : 6-4-81c.

The change in resting potential, the spike amplitude and the spike duration were measured in Ringer, Ringer + 1 mM 4-AP and Ringer + 1 mM 4-AP + 20 mM TEA (Fig. 4 and Table 1).

In each solution, the resting $Na^+$ inactivation was maintained constant by repolarization of the fibres to their resting potential in Ringer. This was done in order to minimize secondary effects of $K^+$ current blockade on $Na^+$ permeability.

However, during the action potentials, the rate and extent of Na⁺ inactivation will be modified by 4-AP and TEA because of the increase in spike duration due to the blockade of K⁺ currents. It is impossible to prevent such voltage dependent effects on Na⁺ current which will necessarily contribute to changes in the spike duration. It must be noted that, in the absence of any control of the resting potential, the depolarization induced by the blockade of fast or slow K⁺ currents should greatly affect the excitability of the fibres by increasing Na⁺ inactivation.

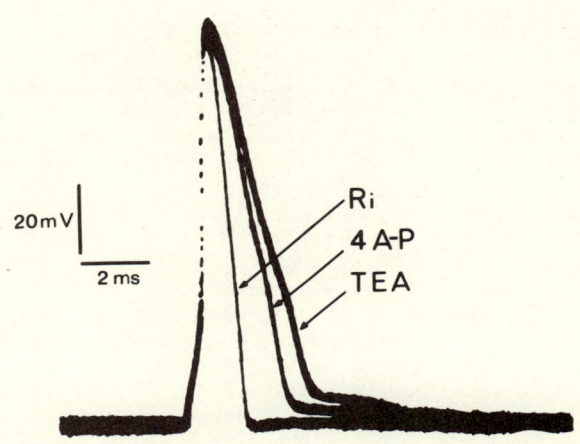

Figure 4. Superimposed action potentials recorded in Ringer, Ringer + 1 mM 4-AP and Ringer + 1 mM 4-AP + 20 mM TEA. In 4-AP and TEA solutions, the fibre was repolarized to its resting potential in Ringer. Temperature : 13 °C. Fibre : 6-4-81c.

TABLE 1. Effect of 4-AP (1 mM) and TEA (20 mM) on the Resting and Action Potentials. Temperature : 12-14 °C

| Fibre | Change in resting potential (mV) | | Spike amplitude (mV) | | | Spike duration (at 0 mV) (msec) | | |
|---|---|---|---|---|---|---|---|---|
| | 4-AP | TEA | Control | 4-AP | TEA | Control | 4-AP | TEA |
| 24-3-81 | + 4.0 | + 6.0 | 105 | 106 | 111 | 1.9 | 3.5 | 3.9 |
| 25-3-81a | 0 | + 2.0 | 116 | 116 | | 0.9 | 1.4 | |
| 25-3-81b | + 4.0 | + 6.0 | 115 | 118 | 118 | 0.9 | 1.7 | 1.9 |
| 25-3-81c | + 4.0 | + 5.0 | 119 | 119 | 119 | 1.0 | 1.6 | 1.8 |
| 6-4-81a | + 2.0 | + 4.0 | 111 | 114 | 114 | 0.9 | 1.2 | |
| 6-4-81c | + 2.5 | + 3.0 | 117 | 119 | 120 | 0.8 | 1.4 | 1.6 |
| mean | + 2.8 | + 4.3 | 114 | 115 | 116 | 1.1 | 1.8 | 2.3 |
| ± S.E. | ± 0.7 | ± 0.7 | ± 2 | ± 2 | ± 2 | ± 0.2 | ± 0.4 | ± 0.6 |

While the threshold, the amplitude and the rate of rise of action potential were not significantly affected, the resting potential and the spike duration were modified by 4-AP or TEA. The results suggest that the slow $K^+$ current plays an important role in the resting potential and the fast $K^+$ current plays an important role in the repolarizing phase of the action potential.

The physiological activity of nerve fibres consists of trains of spikes. One can ask whether the slow current plays a role during high frequency or sustained stimulations. This point was tested and is illustrated in a typical experiment presented Fig. 5. In Figs. 5a and b, the fibre was stimulated at a frequency of 100 Hz by twenty 500 μs supra threshold shocks applied successively after blockade of the fast $K^+$ current by 1 mM 4-AP (a) and the slow $K^+$ current by 20 mM TEA (b). In both solutions, the fibre was polarized to the level of its resting potential in normal Ringer. In the presence of 4-AP, the fibre fires an action potential in response to each of the first six stimuli and then starts to show intermittent failures. These failures were preceded by a progressive decrease in spike amplitude. After blockade of the slow $K^+$ current by TEA, the fibre, stimulated by the same stimuli (in duration, amplitude and frequency), fires an action potential in response to each shock. This experiment suggests that the slow $K^+$ current is slowly activated during high frequency stimulations and limits the spike frequency response by increasing the firing threshold. This view is confirmed in the experiment presented in Fig. 5c and d. The fibre (sensory) was stimulated successively in the presence of 4-AP (c) and TEA (d) by the same long lasting shock. After blockade of the slow $K^+$ current by TEA, the fibre responded to the stimulation by 7-8 spikes while it responded only by 2-3 spikes when the slow $K^+$ current was activated. In some respects, these results support the hypothesis of Krylov & Makovsky (1978) that the spike frequency adaptation (decrease in firing frequency during a sustained stimulus) is due to the slow $K^+$ current. While this hypothesis may account for the spike frequency adaptation of sensory fibres (cf. Figure 5c and d), it cannot explain the difference in spike frequency adaptation of motor and sensory fibres (see next section).

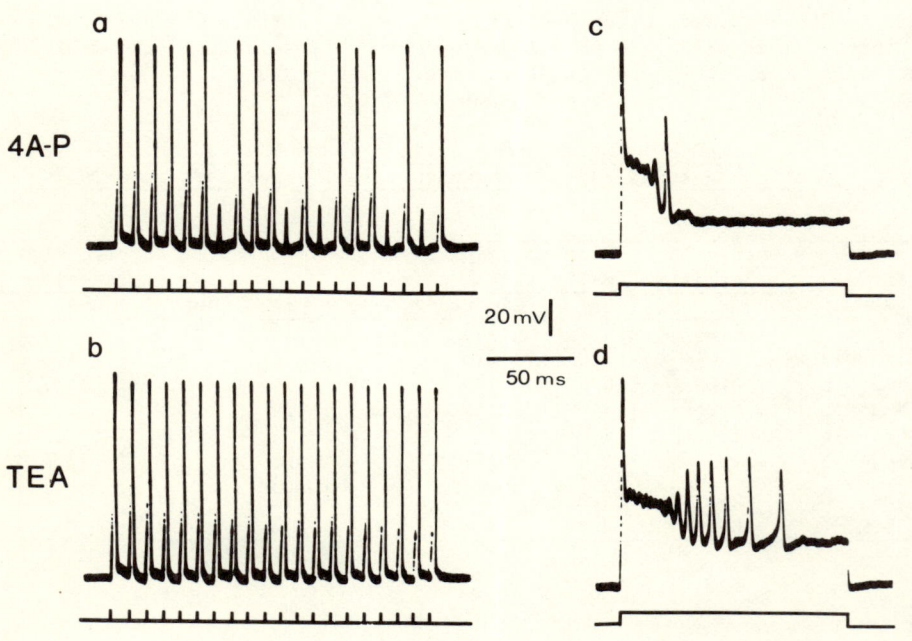

Figure 5. Role of the slow $K^+$ current in spike frequency adaptation. The fibre was stimulated by a train of 20 shocks (f = 100 Hz (a and b) or by a maintained shock (c and d) in Ringer + 1 mM 4-AP (a and c) and Ringer + 1 mM 4-AP + 20 mM TEA (b and d). After blockade of the slow $K^+$ current by TEA, the fibre responded by a spike to each short stimulus (b) or by a prolonged discharge to the maintained stimulation (d). The traces below each membrane potential records denote the stimulation current. Temperature : 13 °C. Sensory fibre : 6-4-81c.

Motor and Sensory Fibres

It is well known that, during a sustained stimulus, motor fibres respond by only one spike and sensory fibres gives a train of spikes. Differences between $K^+$ conductances of the two types of fibres were reported earlier (Bergman & Stämpfli, 1966 ; Bretag & Stämpfli, 1975). Based on the analysis of three different $K^+$ currents, it has been shown (Dubois, 1981b) that the major difference lies in the proportion of fast-1 and fast-2 $K^+$ conductances. While the amplitude of the total, fast and slow, $K^+$ conductances are similar in both types of fibres ($g_{Ks}$ represents about 20 % of the total conductance after 100-200 msec of depolarization for both types of fibres), The proportion of $g_{Kf1}$ versus the total fast conductance is about 55 % in motor fibres but only about 35 % in sensory fibres (i.e. : the proportion of $g_{Kf1}$ versus the total conductance is about 44 % in motor fibres and about 28 % in sensory fibres) (see Fig. 6).

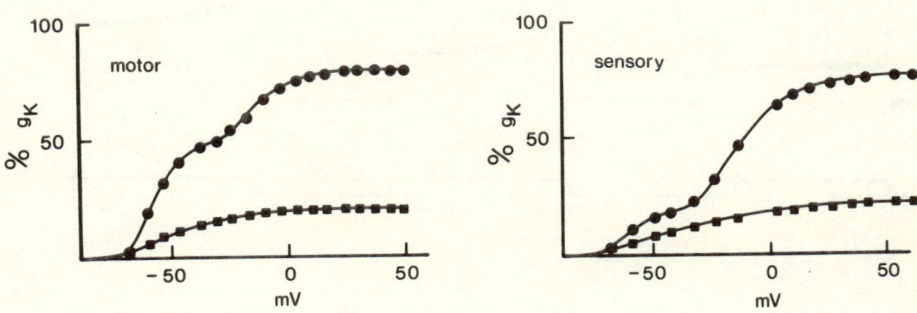

Figure 6. $K^+$ conductance-voltage relationships in a motor and sensory fibre. The relative fast (circles) and slow (squares) $K^+$ conductances were calculated from fast and slow $K^+$ currents recorded in isotonic $K^+$ Ringer at - 90 mV after 150 msec depolarizing pulses of various amplitudes. Both fast conductance-voltage curves present a bend near - 30 mV corresponding to a voltage at which $g_{Kf1}$ (activated between - 80 and - 30 mV) is almost completely activated while $g_{Kf2}$ (activated between - 30 and + 30 mV) is still not activated (for the demonstration of this interpretation, see Dubois, 1981b). Note that $g_{Kf1}$ is smaller in sensory than in motor fibres. Temperature : 12 °C. Motor fibre : 24-5-79. Sensory fibre = 1-6-79.

This observation suggests that the difference in spike frequency adaptation of motor and sensory fibres are somehow related to the different proportions of $g_{Kf1}$ and $g_{Kf2}$ since near the threshold of the action potential (- 50 mV), the activated $K^+$ conductance is larger in motor than in sensory fibres. However, if $g_{Kf1}$, which is smaller in sensory than in motor fibres, is certainly related to some differences in excitability of the two types of fibres, it does not seem to be the sole phenomenon responsable for the repetitive firing of sensory fibres during a sustained stimulation. This conclusion is based on the following demonstration. If one assumes that, during a sustained stimulation, motor fibres cannot fire repetitively because of the activation of the fast $K^+$ conductance, they should respond by several spikes after blockade of this conductance. This hypothesis was tested in the experiment presented Fig. 7. In normal Ringer, the fibre (motor) responded to a maintained stimulus by only one action potential. After blockade of the fast $K^+$ conductance by 4-AP, the depolarization induced by the same stimulation was increased but the fibre still responded by only one spike. After blockade of the slow $K^+$ conductance by TEA, the fibre was largely depolarized during the stimulus but no repetitive firing was observed. It must be noted that these observations are certainly not sufficient to conclude that the $K^+$ conductance is not responsable for the absence of repetitive firing in motor fibres since, with 4-AP, as both $g_{Kf1}$ and $g_{Kf2}$ are blocked. However, in the same conditions, it has been observed (Fig. 5c and d) that sensory fibres continue to respond by several spikes when $g_{Kf}$ or both $g_{Kf}$ and $g_{Ks}$ are blocked. These observations suggest that the difference in spike frequency adaptation of motor and sensory fibres is not due solely to the $K^+$ permeability but also involves the $Na^+$ permeability.

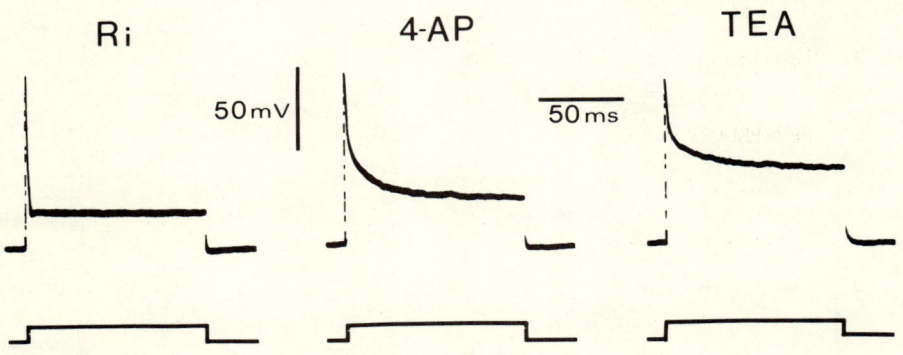

Figure 7. Action potential of a motor fibre recorded in Ringer, Ringer + 1 mM 4-AP and Ringer + 1 mM 4-AP + 20 mM TEA during a sustained stimulation. The blockade of fast $K^+$ current (4-AP) or fast and slow $K^+$ currents (TEA) induced an increase of the after action potential depolarization but did not induce repetitive activity. Temperature : 13 °C. Fibre : 7-5-81.

CONCLUSION

The existence of different types of $K^+$ channels has already been demonstrated in muscles and neurones (see Thompson & Aldrich, 1980). In myelinated nerve fibres, the existence of several types of $K^+$ channels has been proposed by several authors (Schwarz & Vogel, 1971 ; Palti, Ganot & Stämpfli, 1976 ; Ilyin, Katina, Lonskii, Makovsky & Polishchuk, 1977, 1980 ; Krylov & Makovsky, 1978). Although the conclusion of the existence of two types of $K^+$ channels is supported by the observation that the fast and slow components of the tail current are not coupled (Ilyin et al., 1980), the demonstration is not entirely convincing until one of the components is blocked specifically. From this point of view, 4-aminopyridine is an efficient tool since it blocks the fast $K^+$ component without affecting the slow one. Furthermore, 4-AP allows to study the properties of the slow current (Dubois, 1981c) which, during depolarizations, is normally masked by the fast one. The separation of the $K^+$ current into a slow and a fast component furthermore allows the decomposition of the fast $K^+$ current into two components whose relative amplitudes are different in motor and sensory fibres. Finally, the consecutive use of 4-AP (which blocks the fast $K^+$ current) and TEA (which blocks the total $K^+$ current) allows the study of the physiological roles of both fast and slow $K^+$ currents.

ACKNOWLEDGEMENT

I thank S. Siegelbaum for critical reading of the manuscript.

REFERENCES

Attwell, D., Dubois, J.M. and C. Ojeda (1980). Pflügers Arch., 384, 49-56.
Bergman, C. and R. Stämpfli (1966). Helv. Physiol. Pharmacol. acta, 24, 247-258.
Bostock, H., Sears, T.A. and R.M. Sherratt (1981). J. Physiol. (Lond.), 313, 301-305.
Bretag, A.H. and R. Stämpfli (1975). Pflügers Arch., 354, 257-271.
Dubois, J.M. (1981a). J. Physiol. (Lond.), 318, 279-295.
Dubois, J.M. (1981b). J. Physiol. (Lond.), 318, 297-316.
Dubois, J.M. (1981c). J. Physiol. (Paris) (in the press).
Dubois, J.M. and C. Bergman (1975). Pflügers Arch., 358, 111-124.
Ilyin, V.I., Katina, I.E., Lonskii, A.V., Makovski, V.S. and E.V. Polishchuk (1977). Dokl. Akad. Nauk. S.S.S.R., 234, 1467-1470.
Ilyin, V.I., Katina, I.E., Lonskii, A.V., Makovski, V.S. and E.V. Polishchuk (1980). J. Membr. Biol., 57, 179-193.
Krylov, B.V. and V.S. Makovsky (1978). Nature (Lond.), 275, 549-551.
Meves, H. and Y. Pichon (1977). J. Physiol. (Lond.), 268, 511-532.
Palti, Y., Ganot, G. and R. Stämpfli (1976). Biophys. J., 16, 262-273.
Pelhate, M. and Y. Pichon (1974). J. Physiol. (Lond.), 242, 90 P.
Schwarz, J.R. and W. Vogel (1971). Pflügers Arch., 330, 61-73.
Thompson, S.H. and R.W. Aldrich (1980). The cell surface and neuronal function. O.W. Cotman G. Poste & G.L. Nicolson (eds). Elsevier North Holland Biomedical Press, pp. 49-85.
Ulbricht, W. and H.H. Wagner (1976). Pflügers Arch., 367, 77-87.
Yeh, J.Z., Oxford, G.S., Wu, C.H. and T. Narahashi (1976). J. gen. Physiol., 68, 519-535.

# Effects of Aminopyridines on Ionic Currents and Ionic Channel Noise in Unmyelinated Axons

Y. Pichon*, H. Meves** and M. Pelhate***

*Laboratoire de Neurobiologie Cellulaire du C.N.R.S.,
Gif sur Yvette, France
**I-Physiologisches Institut der Universität des Saaralandes,
Homburg/Saar, Federal Republic of Germany
***Laboratory of Physiology, Faculty of Medicine, Angers, France

ABSTRACT

4-amino-pyridine and most of its derivatives block the potassium conductance in the micromolar range of concentration. This blockage is strongly voltage dependent. The time and voltage dependency of the binding of 4-AP has been studied in internally perfused giant axons of the squid. The results suggest that 4-AP molecules can be displaced from their binding site under the effect of the electric field and a simple model which accounts for most data has been proposed. Interaction of 4-AP with the opening and closing of individual potassium channels has been tentatively analysed using spectrum analysis of membrane current fluctuations (noise) of small patches of the axonal membrane of the cockroach. The results suggest that 4-AP molecules block open or closed channels in an all-or-none manner.

KEYWORDS

Unmyelinated axons; potassium channels; aminopyridines; membrane currents; noise analysis; molecular model.

INTRODUCTION

4-aminopyridine (4-AP) is known to increase excitability in isolated vertebrate nerves (Le Meignan, Chanelet and Saade, 1969) and invertebrate connectives (Pelhate Hue and Chanelet, 1972). These effects were analysed on single giant axons of the cockroach by Pelhate, Hue and Chanelet (1974) who found that 10.6 uM of 4-AP decreased delayed rectification and increased spike duration suggesting a decrease in the potassium conductance. This suggestion was soon confirmed by Pelhate, Hue, Pichon and Chanelet (1974) and Pelhate and Pichon (1974) using the voltage-clamp technique This finding was extended one year later to squid axons (Meves and Pichon, 1975) and Myxicola axons (Pichon and Rudy, unpublished). Since then, numerous studies have been devoted to the effects of 4-AP and its derivatives on squid axon (Yeh, Oxford, Wu and Narahashi, 1976a and b; Meves and Pichon, 1977a and b), Myxicola axons (Schauf, Colton, Colton and Davis, 1976) and frog nodes of Ranvier (Ulbricht and Wagner, 1976). Various models have been proposed to explain the effects of aminopyridine on potassium conductance and very recently noise analysis has been used to tentatively analyse the effects of 4-AP on single potassium channels (Lees Pichon, and Poussart, 1981 unpublished).

In this paper, we shall illustrate the most salient features of the effects of aminopyridines on unmyelinated axons. After a short description of the "physiological" effects (i.e. the effects on resting potential, action potential and excitability, we shall report the effects of 4-AP on the membrane currents and membrane current noise. The last paragraph will be devoted to the comparative efficiency of 4-AP and various related molecules on the cockroach axon preparation. In the first part of the discussion, we shall deal with the molecular aspects of potassium channel block whereas the second part of the discussion will be concerned with some aspects of 4-AP induced modifications of axonal membrane excitability and related phenomena.

## METHODS

The experiments described in this paper were done on giant axons of the cockroach, Periplaneta americana L. and on giant axons of the squid, Loligo forbesi L.

Giant axons of Periplaneta americana were isolated from the abdominal connectives and placed in a double oil-gap three electrode systems (Pichon and Boistel, 1966, Pichon, 1970). A small patch of membrane (around $10^4 \mu m^2$) was electrically isolated from the rest of the preparation and studied under current-clamp and voltage-clamp conditions. For the experiments on noise, the output of a specially designed low noise voltage-clamp amplifiers was connected via 1 Hz-3kHz window to a low noise differential amplifier with a gain of 1000. The amplified noise was then fed into the input of a spectrum analyser and spectra between 10 and 2500 Hz were averaged and stored on cartridge tape for subsequent treatment. The saline used for these experiments contained 210.2 mM NaCl, 3.1 mM KCl and 10 mM $CaCl_2$ and was buffered at pH 7.2 using a phosphate carbonate buffer.

Giant axons of Loligo forbesi L. were isolated from fresh or refrigerated mantles. For perfused axon experiments, the axoplasm was removed using the roller technique of Baker, Hodgkin and Shaw (1962). In early experiments, the voltage-clamp technique was the same as that described by Chandler and Meves (1965). In more recent experiments, the technique was similar to that used by Kimura and Meves (1979). The external solution contained 470 mM NaCl, 11 mM $CaCl_2$, 55 mM $MgCl_2$ and was buffered at pH 7.7 using Tris-HCl. The internal solution contained 300 mM KF sucrose and was buffered at pH 7.2 using Tris-HCl.

In early experiments voltage and/or current traces were recorded on film and digitized off-line. In more recent ones, the traces were digitized at the output of the voltage clamp amplifier and stored onto digital tape. Computations were done using Hewlett-Packard 9830 or 9825 dektop computers.

## RESULTS

### Effects of 4-AP on resting potential, action potential and membrane excitability.

Concentrations of 4-AP of the order of 10 μM have little effect on the resting potential of cockroach (or squid) axons. A significant lengthening of the spike is however observed associated with a decrease in delayed rectification (Pelhate, Hue and Chanelet, 1974). Larger concentrations (up to 10 mM) depolarize the membrane, lowers the threshold and increases the spike duration as illustrated in Fig.1. Under normal physiological conditions, 4-AP induces repetitive firing in otherwise silent squid giant axons. For large concentrations (1-10 mM), this firing activity is only transient and disappears when the membrane potential drops below -50 mV. Smaller concentrations (1-100 μM) induce bursts of activity, the frequency and the duration of which increase with time. A short burst is illustrated in Fig. 2. In all cases, the burst itself is preceded and followed by oscillations of the

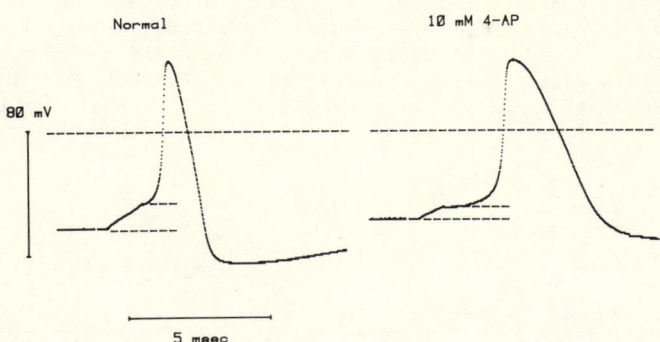

Fig. 1. Effects of 4-AP on resting potential and action potential in a space-clamped squid giant axon. Temperature : 8°C. Note that the threshold is lower in 4-AP than in drug free solution.

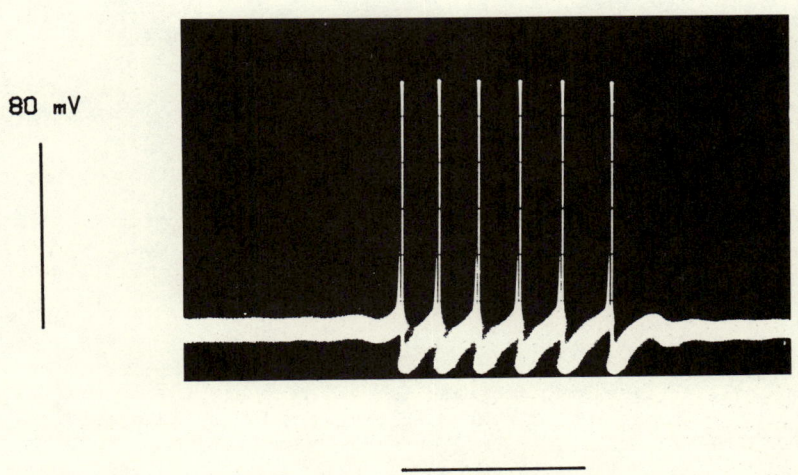

Fig. 2. Burst of activity recorded in a space-clamped giant axon of Loligo 5 min after application of 10 mM 4-AP to the external solution. Intact axon. Temperature : 8°C. From Pichon (1981b).

membrane potential. Even after a long period in large concentrations of 4-AP, the axons failed to depolarize below 35-40 mV.

Effect of 4-AP on membrane currents.

Under voltage-clamp conditions, 4-AP was found to block the potassium current. This is illustrated in Fig.3 where a progressive inhibition of the membrane current elicited by a 110 mV depolarization follows external application of 53 µM 4-AP (Fig. 3A). This effect is only partly reversible (Fig. 3B). This inhibition was observed at all potential values although the efficacy of the drug decreased

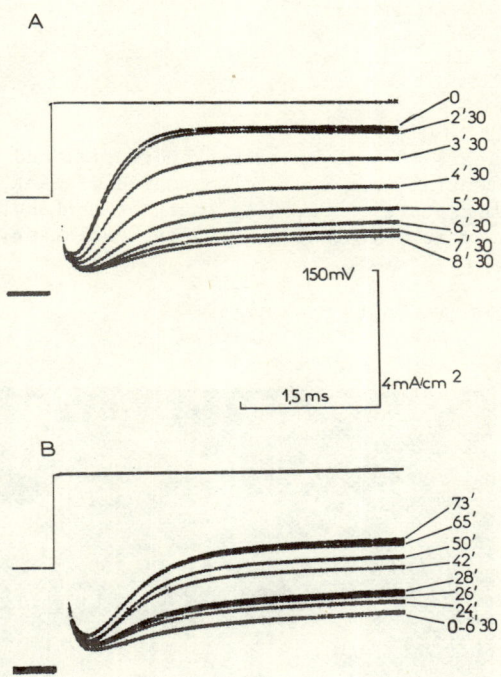

Fig. 3. Progressive decrease (A) and recovery (B) of the potassium current elicited by a 110 mV depolarization of a cockroach axon under voltage-clamp conditions. 4-AP concentration : 53 µM. Upper traces: voltage, lower traces : currents. Figures given at the right of each trace indicate time (in min) following application (A) or removal (B) of 4-AP. Leak not substracted.

with membrane depolarization. The effects of 1 mM 4-AP applied in the bath on the family of membrane currents of a voltage clamped squid giant axon are illustrated in Fig.4. 4-AP was found to have little effect if any, on the sodium current as illustrated in Fig.5 for 21.2 µM. It is now routinely used in several laboratories to isolate pharmacologically the sodium current from the (4-AP sensitive) potassium current.

The effects of 4-AP resemble in some respects those of similar concentrations of tetraethylammonium ions (TEA$^+$) and related compounds (Armstrong, 1966). They differ however from those of TEA$^+$ in three respects : (1) 4-AP act equally well from

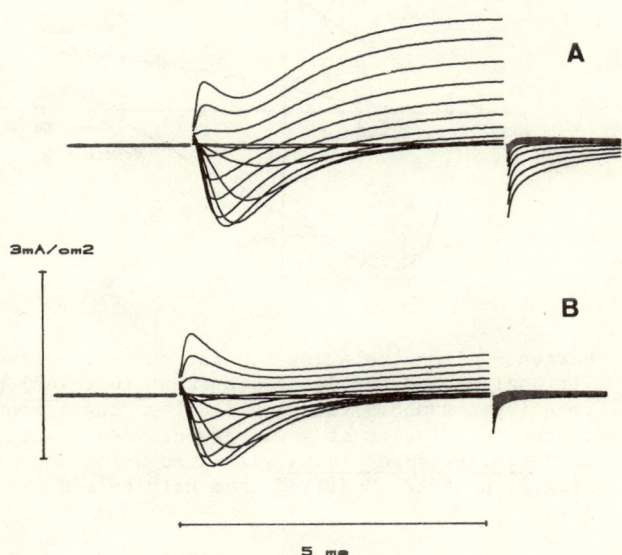

Fig. 4. Family of membrane currents corresponding to 13 step depolarizations of the membrane of a voltage clamped giant axon of <u>Loligo</u> from a holding potential of -60 to respectively -50, -40, -30, -20, -10, 0, 10, 20, 30, 40, 50, 60 and 70 mV before (A) and during bath application of 4-AP (B). Note that the peak current is little affected and that the delayed (potassium) current as well as the tail current (also carried by potassium) are very much reduced by 4-AP.

inside or from outside the nerve fibre; (2) it reduces both the potassium outward current and the potassium inward current (measured with 200 mM KCl) in the external KCl solution; (3) internal or external application of 4-AP markedly delay the turning-on of the potassium current resulting in a slow exponential rise of the potassium current. These effects are illustrated in Fig.6 and Fig.7.

High external potassium as well as long depolarizing prepulses were found to decrease the inhibitory effect of 4-AP.

The slow rise of the potassium current observed in the presence of small concentrations of 4-AP can be accelerated by repetitive pulsing as illustrated in Fig.8. This effect which has been also observed with most 4-AP derivatives has been studied quantitatively by Meves and Pichon (1977a). Several factors are involved : pulse duration, pulse size, pulse frequency and 4-AP concentrations : maximal

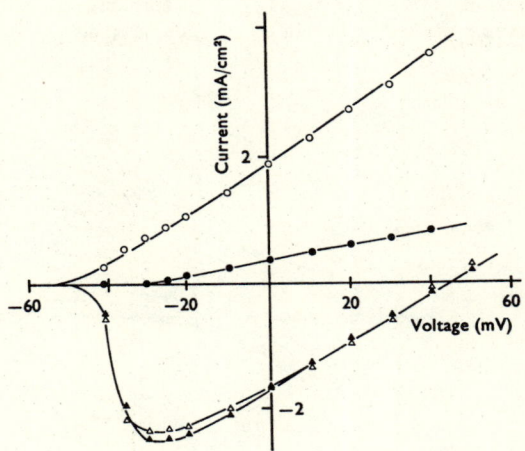

Fig. 5. Current-voltage relationship for the peak current (triangles) and the delayed current (circles) before (open symbols) and 10 min after the beginning of the superfusion of a voltage-clamped giant axon of <u>Periplaneta americana</u> with a solution containing 21 µM 4-AP. Modified from Pelhate and Pichon, 1974.

effects were seen for small concentrations of 4-AP (10-100 µM), large (185 mV depolarizations from a holding of -95.5 mV) and long (up to 100 ms) pulses and high frequencies (10/s). The effects of varying pulse length are illustrated in Fig.9, those of pulses frequency in Fig.10. More quantitative data were obtained using double pulse procedures. In a first set of experiments, a conditioning pulse of variable amplitude and duration was applied 5 s before a test pulse of constant height and length. The amplitude of the potassium current 3.25 ms after the beginning of the test pulse was measured and compared to that obtained in the absence of the conditioning pulse. This difference was found to increase exponentially with membrane depolarization and to vary with prepulse duration with the same time course as the current produced by the conditioning pulse alone (see Fig.8 of Meves and Pichon, 1977a). In a second set of experiments, the effects of repetitive pulsing with various frequencies was analysed quantitatively using a similar double pulse procedure : the difference between the current produced 5 ms after the beginning of the test pulse and that produced 5 msec after the beginning of the conditioning pulse was measured for various pulse intervals and in different 4-AP concentrations. These experiments illustrated in Fig. 11 show that the unblocking effect of the first pulse decays exponentially and that the time constant of the exponential is shorter in higher 4-AP concentrations.

The effect of repetitive pulsing does not seem to depend on the size of the potassium current and the experiments suggest that removal of 4-AP block could result from a voltage and time dependent displacement of the 4-AP molecules from their blocking site. A model based on this assumption is illustrated in the next subchapter.

<u>Descriptive model of the effects of 4-AP on the axonal membrane.</u> If one assumes

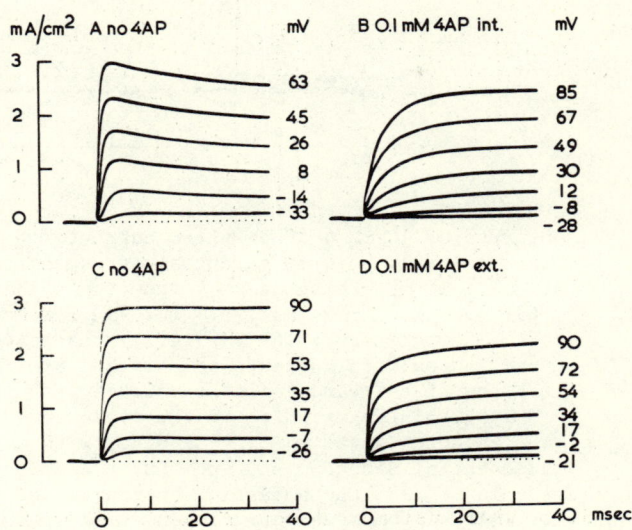

Fig. 6. Effects of internal (B) or external (D) application of 100 μM 4-AP on the potassium currents in a perfused giant axon of Loligo. The axon was depolarized from its holding potential (=resting potential) to the various potential levels indicated at the right of each current trace. Outside solution : Na free, K free seawater with 2 μM tetrodotoxin. Temperature : 16°C. Note that internal and external application are roughly equipotent and that the turning-on of the potassium current is slowed in 4-AP.

that one molecule of 4-AP binds to one receptor R (probably in the enlarged inner portion of the potassium channel) to form a complex 4-AP-R which blocks the channel, the binding reaction can be written :

$$4\text{-AP} + R \underset{k_{-1}}{\overset{k_1}{\rightleftarrows}} 4\text{-AP-R} \qquad (1)$$

(d)       (1-b)         (b)

where d represents the 4-AP concentration, b the proportion of bound receptors (i.e. blocked channels) and $k_1$ and $k_{-1}$ the rate constants of the reaction. The experiments suggest that the affinity of the receptor for 4-AP decreases during membrane depolarization. This results into an increase of the dissociation constant of the reaction ($K_s = k_{-1}/k_1$) and a decrease in b. This decrease in b with membrane potential follows an exponential time course :

$$b(t) = b_\infty - (b_\infty - b_0) \exp(-t/\tau_b) \qquad (2)$$

where $b_0$ and $b_\infty$ are respectively the initial and final values of b and $\tau_b$ the time constant of the reaction which is function of $k_1$, $k_{-1}$ and d. The potassium current in the presence of 4-AP is proportional to the fraction of unoccupied

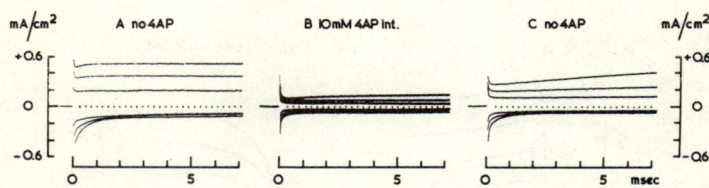

Fig. 7.  Effects of 10 mM 4-AP on the K currents in 200 mM external KCl. Holding potential (=resting potential) : -10 mV. Pulse height (from top to bottom) +69, +50, +30, -33, -52, -74 mV. 2µM TTX in the bath. Temperature : 16°C. Note (1) that both inward and outward currents are blocked by 4-AP. (2) that the inward tails associated with the -74 mV hyperpolarizing pulse in the presence (B) and the absence (A and C) of 4-AP decay with a similar exponential time course, indicating that the turning off of the potassium current is not modified by 4-AP. (From Meves and Pichon, 1977a).

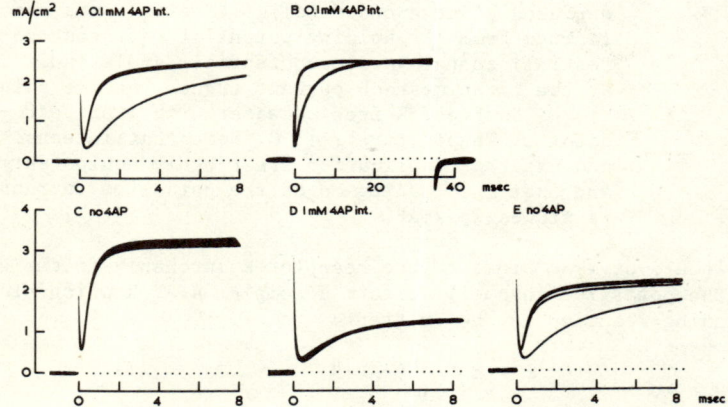

Fig. 8.  Effects of repetitive clamp pulse on the potassium current in perfused squid axons. Frequency of stimulation : 2/sec, pulse duration : 35 ms. Na and K free Tris seawater with 2 µM tetrodotoxin. Voltage pulse to 85 mV in A and B; 89.5 mV in C, 92 mV in D and E. Temperature : 16°C. Note that in A,B, and E, the lower current traces correspond to the first stimulation and the upper current traces to the second and (A and E) third stimulations. From Meves and Pichon, 1975.

receptors (1-b) and is given by the equation

$$lk = \overline{g}_k n4 \ (V-V_k) \ (1-b) \qquad (3)$$

where $\overline{g}_k$ is the maximum potassium conductance, n the K activation variable and $V_K$ the potassium equilibrium potential. Values of $k_1$ and $k_{-1}$ have been calculated from the experiments reported in the previous subchapter and incorporated into a set of equations (the b equations) which are used in conjunction with the classical m, n and h (Hodgkin and Huxley, 1952) equations to reproduce ionic currents in different experimental conditions (Fig.12) and also to reconstruct membrane potential behaviour (Fig. 13 and 14).

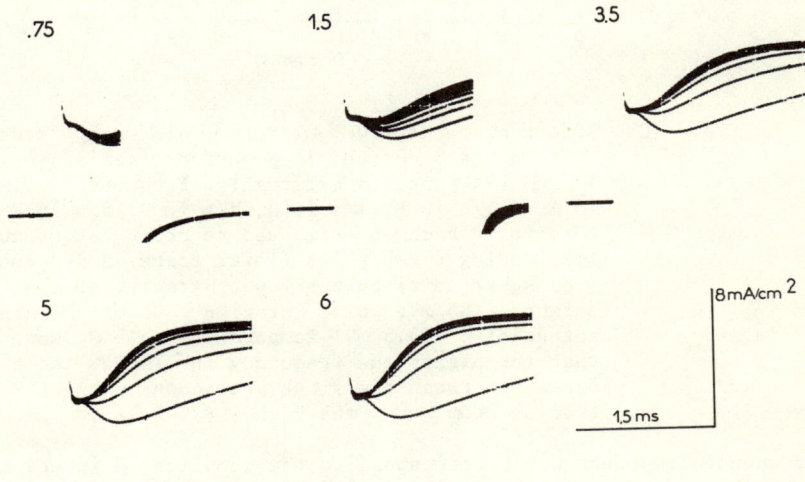

Fig. 9. Effects of repetitive pulsing with pulses of different durations (as indicated on each set of recordings). Pulse amplitude : 100 mV. Pulse frequency: 1/s. 4-AP concentration : 53 µM. Giant axon of Periplaneta. Temperature 20°C. Leak not substracted. Note that the maximum intensity of the current increases with pulse duration.

Effects of 4-AP on membrane current noise.
----

Membrane current noise was recorded from small patches of nerve membrane of Periplaneta. This noise which exceeds the background noise and increases with membrane depolarization was found to be insensitive to TTX and to consist into a 1/f component and Lorentzian component with corner frequencies in good agreement with those calculated from the relaxation time constant of the potassium current (Lees, Pichon and Poussart, 1981). The effects fo 1 mM 4-AP are illustrated in Fig.15. As expected, 4-AP decreases the noise. No high frequency component could be detected in 4-AP, suggesting that unlike $TEA^+$, 4-AP does not bind to open potassium channels. A low frequency component analogous to that described by Fishman, Moore and Poussart (1977) for squid axons might be responsible for the fact that inhibition is larger at high frequencies that at low frequencies. Such a

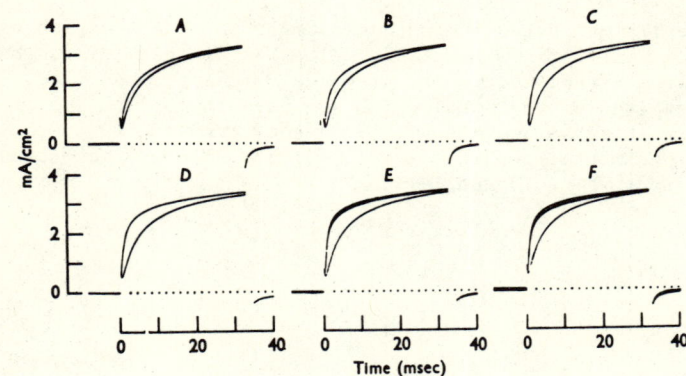

Fig. 10. Effect of repetitive pulsing at different frequencies on the K current in a perfused squid axon. 100 μM 4-AP applied externally. Frequency : 0.2/s in A, 0.4/s in B, 1/s in C, 2/s in D, 5/s in E and 10/s in F. Each superimposed recording shows current during first pulse (lower trace) and second (and subsequent) pulses (upper traces). Pulse height : 185 mV, pulse duration : 35 ms; holding potential : -95.5 mV. Temperature : 15°C. Note that the higher the frequency the larger the difference between the first and second current traces. From Meves and Pichon (1977a).

low frequency component would correspond to the complicated interactions between 4-AP and its receptor site. Indications on the mode of action of 4-AP on a single K channels can be obtained from such experiments as illustrated Table 1. The admittance values were obtained from the transfer function of the nerve membrane in TTX and TTX + 4 AP. The variance values were calculated from the area under the power spectra and the values of p, the probability of opening of a single channel, were calculated from Pichon (1974). It can be seen that although admittance is reduced about three times and noise four times by 4-AP, single channel conductance ($\gamma$) is not significantly modified. This finding can be taken as an indication that 4-AP blocks $K^+$ channels in all-or-none manner.

<u>Compared effects of 4-AP and related molecules on the potassium conductance.</u>

Amongst the 4-AP derivatives, differences in efficiency have been reported by several investigators. The experiments summarized in this subchapter have been performed to compare on a given preparation, the giant axon of the cockroach, the efficacy of 4-AP and its isomers (2-AP and 3-AP) and derivatives (3.4 diaminopyridine, 4-aminoquinoline and 9-aminoacridine). Dose-response curves for 4-AP, 3,4-diaminopyridine (3,4-DAP) and pyridine are illustrated in Fig. 16 A whereas those for 4-aminoquinoline (4-AQ) and 9- aminoacridine (9-AA) are illustrated in Fig. 16 B.

The results can be summarized as follows : (1) Whereas the pyridine nucleus alone has very little effect, even at high concentrations (about 10 % inhibition for 10 mM), 4-AP and its isomers and derivatives all depress the potassium conductance at

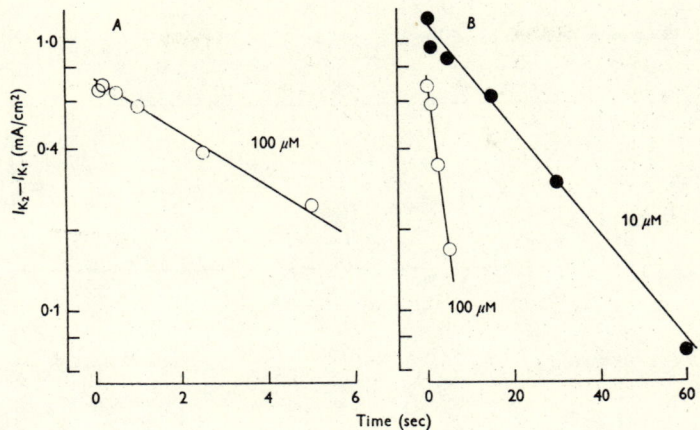

Fig. 11. Analysis of the effects of repetitive pulsing in a perfused squid axon. The difference between the currents produced by two successive identical pulses ($I_{K_2}-I_{K_1}$) decreases exponentially with the interval between the two pulses. The time constant of this decay is shorter in 100 μM (3.3 s in A, 4.35 s in B) than in 10 μM (22.3 s). Pulse duration 32 (1), 35 (B) ms; Pulse size : 185 mV. Temperature : 15°C. 4-AP applied externally in A, internally in B. From Meves and Pichon (1977a).

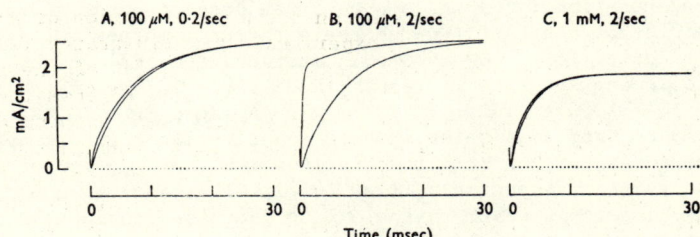

Fig. 12. Computed effects of repetitive pulsing on the K current in 100 μM (A and B) and 1 mM 4AP (C). Pulse frequency 0.2/s in A, 2/s in B and C. Each superimposed recording shows current during first (lower trace) and second pulse (upper trace). Pulse amplitude : 185 mV from a holding potential of -100 mV. Compare with Fig. 8 and 10. Temperature : 15.5°C. From Meves and Pichon (1977a).

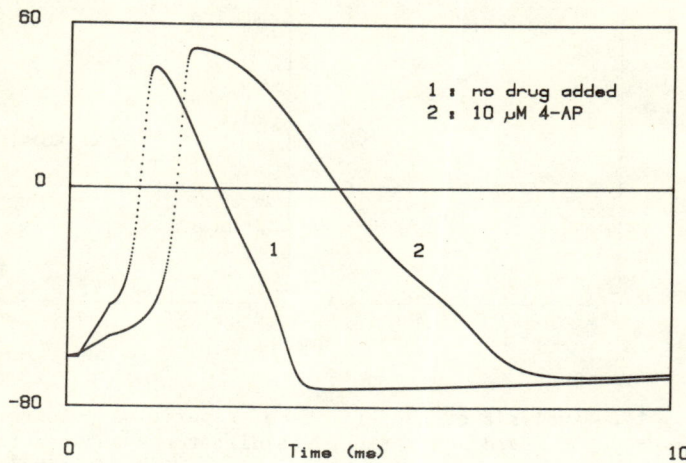

Fig. 13. Computer reconstruction of space-clamped action potential before (1) and in 10 μM 4-AP (2). Original Hodgkin and Huxley (1952) equations. Temperature : 6°C. The effects of 4-AP on the resting potential, threshold and spike duration are well predicted by the model (cf. Fig.1).

micromolar concentrations; (2) the slope of the dose-response curve as well as the apparent dissociation constant (Kd) change with the membrane voltage and the nature of the molecule. For a 100 mV depolarization, the efficacy decreased according to the following sequence : 3,4-DAP (Kd : 1.8   $10^{-5}M$) > 4-AP (Kd : 3   $10^{-5}M$) > 3-AP (Kd : 5   $10^{-5}M$) > 2-AP (Kd : 2   $10^{-4}M$) > 9-AA (Kd : 2.7   $10^{-4}M$) > 4-AQ (Kd 3.7 $10^{-4}M$); (3) Apart from 9-AA which induces inactivation after an apparently normal opening of the potassium channels in very much the same way as internally applied tetraethylammonium (Armstrong and Hille, 1972), all the other compounds can block the potassium channels at rest. This blocking decreases during the course of the depolarization (voltage-dependent "clearing" of Meves and Pichon (1977a);   (4) 4-AQ and 9-AA modify both sodium and potassium conductances whereas the other molecules only affect the latter.

These data indicate that at least three molecular factors are involved in channel blockage : lipid solubility, presence of a quaternary ammonium and size.

DISCUSSION

Our results suggest that opening of the potassium channel "gate" is not prerequisite for 4-AP to bind to its receptor and that the bound molecule sits across the channel with its pyridine nucleus in the walls of the enlarged (inner) portion of the potassium channel and its polar head in the lumen of the channel. Following membrane depolarization, the (positively charged) molecule would tend to leave the channel according to the transmembrane field. Such a movement would be possible

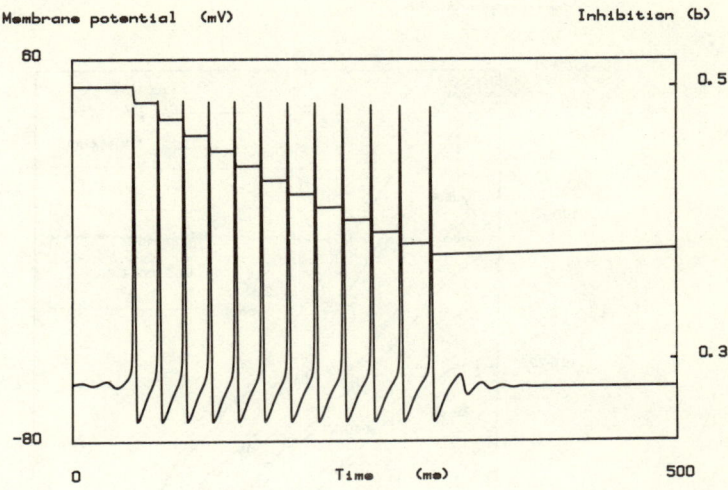

Fig. 14. Computer reconstructed burst of activity induced by 4-AP. Note that the proportion of bound receptors (b) decreases during the burst in a stepwise manner and that oscillations occur before and after the burst as in Fig.2. Temperature : 8°C. (From Pichon, 1981b). 1 μM 4-AP.

because (1) the dehydrated polar head of the molecule ($-NH_3^+$) can cross the narrow part of the channel (2.96 Å) and (2) the walls of the channel are probably partly hydrophobic and let the highly lipid soluble pyridine nucleus still attached to its polar head move through. The fact that channels are blocked in an all-or-none manner by 4-AP are in agreement with the estimated small size of the enlarged portion of the potassium channel. The channels could be blocked while still closed (1) because 4-AP is soluble in lipids,(2) because its polar head is small 4-AP would differ in that respect from blocking agents with larger polar heads such as $TEA^+$ and derivatives (Armstrong, 1969) which must be injected inside the axon and are apparently unable to block $K^+$ channels before they open. Externally applied 9-AA which induces potassium inactivation when applied externally onto the axonal membrane of the cockroach (Pelhate and coworkers, 1976) would be similar to $TEA^+$ in that respect.

The fact that small concentrations of 4-AP can block resting channels has important implications as far as membrane excitability is concerned. Micromolar concentrations of 4-AP are able to transiently unstabilize the nerve membrane and induce repetitive activity. Such an activity might produce unexpected transmitter release if occuring in the presynaptic membrane. In this same preparation, a small concentration of 4-AP can induce a marked increase in the duration of the spike and in turn increase calcium entry manyfolds (as it probably increases sodium entry). Some of the side effects of 4-AP on membrane potential such as repetitive firing can be eliminated using use dependent sodium blocking agents (Pichon, 1981b) and it might be worthwhile to take this aspect into consideration in future experiments.

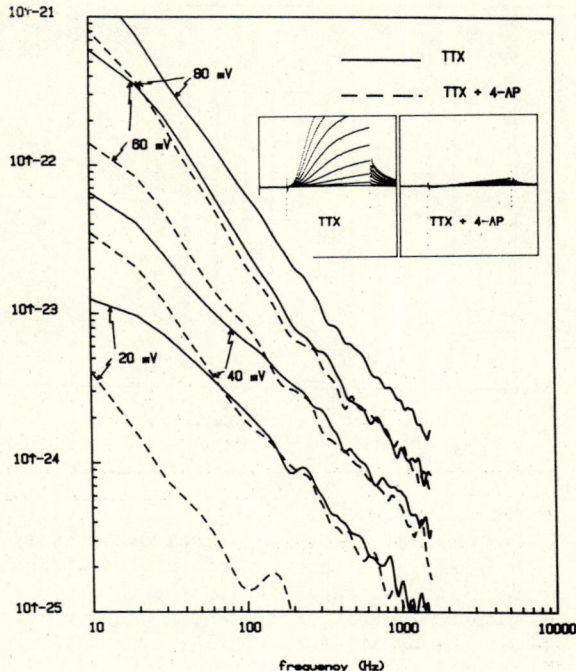

Fig. 15. Effects of 1 mM 4-AP on membrane current noise of a patch of nerve membrane of the giant axon of <u>Periplaneta americana.</u> Inset : effects of 1 mM-4-AP on macroscopic currents. The power density spectrum in 4-AP (interrupted lines) is shifted downwards, the overall noise being reduced by a factor of about 4. Note that no hump is seen at high frequencies but that the inhibition is proportionally larger at high frequencies that at low frequencies. Temperature : 9°C.

ACKNOWLEDGMENTS

The Authors wish to acknowledge the MBA, Plymouth (U.K.) for providing facilities and squid supply. Part of this work has been supported by grants of the D.G.R.S.T. (France). Thanks are due to the Physiological Society for giving permission to reproduce several Fig. from the J. of Physiol.

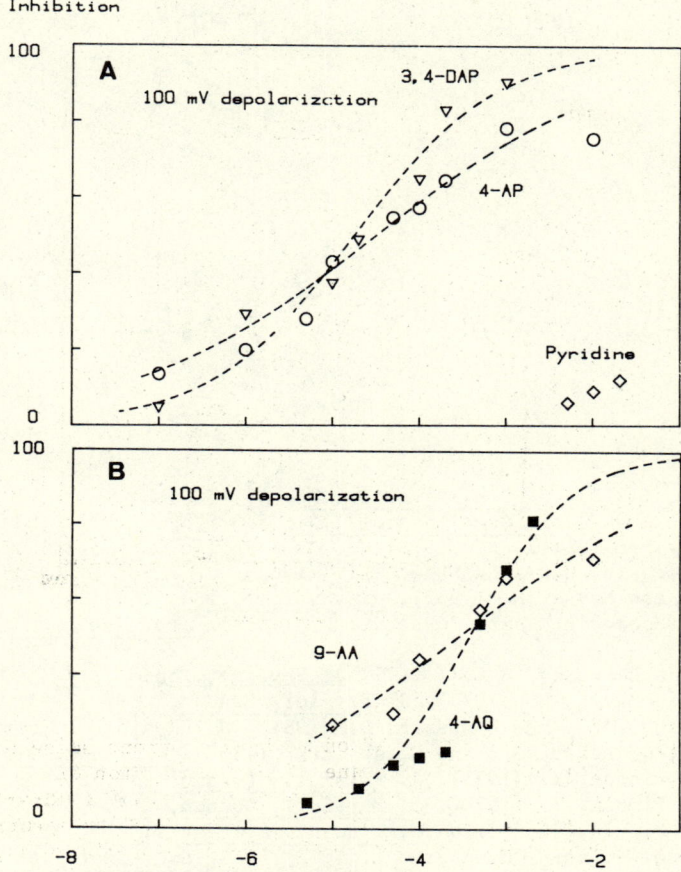

Fig. 16. Dose-response curves for 4-AP and derivatives on the potassium current corresponding to a 100 mV depolarization in the voltage-clamped axon of _Periplaneta americana._

TABLE 1  Effects of 1 mM 4-AP on Admittance and Noise in Cockroach Axons

| Vm (mV) | Admittance ($10^{-6}\,\Omega^{-1}$) | p | $\overline{I^2}$ ($10^{-21}A^2$) | $\gamma$ ($10^{-12}\Omega^{-1}$) |
|---|---|---|---|---|
| TTX | | | | |
| 20 | 3.4 | 0.17 | 1.05 | 0.19 |
| 40 | 5.0 | 0.44 | 3.94 | 0.33 |
| 80 | 9.0 | 0.8 | 50.7 | 2.55 |
| TTX + 4 AP | | | | |
| 20 | 1.05 | 0.17 | 0.142 | 0.08 |
| 40 | 1.5 | 0.44 | 1.41 | 0.39 |
| 80 | 3.4 | 0.8 | 21.3 | 2.8 |
| Ratio | 3 ± 0.5 | | 4.2 ± 2.7 | 1.36 ± 0.83 |

REFERENCES

Armstrong, C.M. (1966). J. Gen. Physiol., 50, 491-503.
Armstrong, C.M. (1969). J. Gen. Physiol., 54, 553-575.
Armstrong, C.M., and Hille, B. (1972). J. Gen. Physiol., 59, 388-400.
Baker, P.F., Hodgkin, H.L., and Shaw, T.I. (1962). J. Physiol. London, 164, 330-354.
Chandler, W.K., and Meves, H. (1965). J. Physiol., 180, 788-820.
Fishman, H.M., Moore, L.E., and Poussart, D. (1977). Ann. New York Acad. Sci., 303 399-423.
Hodgkin, A.L., and Huxley, A.F. (1952). J. Physiol. London, 117, 500-544.
Kimura, J.E., and Meves, H. (1979). J. Physiol. London, 289, 479-500.
Lees, G.V., Pichon, Y., and Poussart, D. (1981). J. Physiol. London (in the press)
Le Meignan, M., Chanelet, J., and Saade, N.E. (1969). C.R. Soc. Biol. 163, 359-365.
Meves, H., and Pichon, Y. (1975). J. Physiol., London, 251, 60-62P.
Meves, H., and Pichon, Y. (1977a). J. Physiol., London, 268, 511-532.
Meves, H., and Pichon, Y. (1977b). C.R. Acad. Sci. Paris, 284, 1325-1328.
Pelhate, M., Hue, B., and Chanelet, J. (1972). C.R. Soc. Biol., 166, 1598.
Pelhate, M., Pichon, Y., Hue B., and Chanelet, J. (1974). C.R. Acad. Sci. Paris, 278, 2807-2809.
Pelhate, M., Mony, L., Hue, B., and Chanelet, J. (1976). C.R. Soc. Biol., 170, 1182-1186.
Pelhate, M., and Pichon, Y. (1974). J. Physiol., London, 242, 50-51 P.
Pichon, Y. (1974). In : "Insect Neurobiology", North Holland:Amsterdam, pp. 73-117.
Pichon, Y. (1981a). J. Physiol., Paris (accepted for publication).
Pichon, Y. (1981b). In "Physiology and Pharmacology of Epileptogenic phenomena", M.R. Klee, H.D. Lux and E.J. Speckmann (Eds). Raven Press : New York (in the press).
Schauf, C.L., Colton, C.A., Colton, J.S., and Davis, F.A. (1976). J. Pharmacol. Exp. Ther., 197, 414-425.
Ulbricht, W., and Wagner, H.H. (1976). Pflügers Arch. 367, 77-87.
Yeh, J.Z., Oxford, G.S., Wu, C.H., and Narahashi, T. (1976a). Biophys. J., 16, 77-81.
Yeh, J.Z., Oxford, G.S., Wu, C.H., and Narahashi, T. (1976b). J. Gen. Physiol., 68, 519-535.

# 3- and 4-Aminopyridine in Synaptic Transmission at the Squid Giant Synapse

R. Llinás, K. Walton, M. Sugimori and S. Simon

Department of Physiology and Biophysics, New York University
Medical Center, 550 First Avenue, New York 10016, USA

ABSTRACT

We have studied the effects of 3- and 4-aminopyridine (3-, 4-AmP) on the process of synaptic transmission using the squid giant synapse. In this in vitro preparation both the pre- and postsynaptic elements are directly accessible for electrophysiological study at the actual site of transmitter release. Following pharmacological blockage of both Na and K conductances with tetrodotoxin (TTX) and tetraethylammonium (TEA) respectively, the amplitude of the presynaptic Ca current may be directly determined (Llinas et al., 1981a) as well as the relationship to amount of transmitter release (Llinas et al., 1981b). Because in these preparations blockage of voltage-dependent K conductance with TEA is incomplete, we supplemented the K blockage produced by intracellular injection of TEA by adding 3- or 4-AmP to the extracellular bathing solution. Following voltage clamp of the presynaptic terminal, it was shown that the Ca current obtained under K blockage by TEA alone and the one obtained following K blockage by combining TEA and 3- or 4-AmP were similar, indicating that aminopyridine did not alter synaptic transmission in a manner different from that by TEA itself. These initial experiments, while important in demonstrating that 3- or 4-AmP did not alter Ca conductance beyond the possible alterations produced by TEA, did not directly demonstrate that 3- or 4-AmP or TEA do not modify the Ca current or the release process directly. In recent experiments, the presynaptic fiber was voltage-clamped with a command pulse exactly resembling the action potential of the fiber prior to blockage of the action potential. It was determined that under these conditions the reconstructed action potential generated in the presence of TEA and 3-AmP could reproduce exactly the latency and amplitude of the postsynaptic response observed prior to blockage of voltage-dependent Na and K conductances. The results fell within the values predicted by the model obtained for transmission in this synapse using square pulses under TEA and 3- or 4-AmP blockage (Llinas et al., 1981b). In conclusion, 3- and 4-AmP seem to have their main action at the voltage-dependent K gate. They do not seem to modify the voltage-dependent Ca conductance or the synaptic release triggered by such inward Ca current.

KEYWORDS

Synaptic transmission; aminopyridines; calcium current; squid synapse.

## INTRODUCTION

3- and 4-AmP have been extensively used in the study of synaptic transmission Among the basic questions concerning the use of these drugs in research dealing with the depolarization-release coupling at chemical junctions has been that of determining whether this drug has a direct effect on the release sequence. Indeed, in addition to blocking voltage-dependent K conductance, AmP could have, of itself, a direct action on either the Ca conductance which triggers synaptic transmitter release or on the release process itself.

## TECHNIQUES

Experimental paradigms were similar to those described in previous publications (Llinas et al., 1976a, 1981 a,b). The stellate ganglion of the squid Loligo pealei, together with its afferent and major efferent axons, was removed from the mantle and placed in a chamber. The preparation was continuously perfused with oxygenated artificial seawater, and the most distal and largest "giant" synapse was exposed with fine dissection. Under direct observation, microelectrodes were then placed in the pre- and postsynaptic elements of this synapse. Routinely 2 or 3 microelectrodes were placed in the presynaptic terminal and 1 electrode penetrated the postsynaptic element. Following the recording of normal pre- and postsynaptic action potentials elicited by extracellular stimulation of the presynaptic nerve bundle, Na and K conductances were blocked by adding TTX and 3- or 4-AmP to the superfusion solution. In some experiments the K conductance in the presynaptic element was further blocked by intracellular injection of TEA. Following these procedures, the presynaptic terminal could be depolarized directly by injecting current through one of the impaling electrodes (henceforth, the current electrode). The potential could then be recorded from the presynaptic terminal by 1 or 2 electrodes depending on whether the penetration was double or triple. The postsynaptic potential evoked by presynaptic depolarization was recorded directly.

The effects of 3- and 4-AmP were studied using three approaches: First, by studying the modifications produced in the presynaptic action potential and the resultant postsynaptic response prior to blockage of the Na conductance. This included a comparison between the K blockage produced by 3- or 4-AmP and TEA. Secondly, in current clamp experiments, the effect of 3- and 4-AmP was studied following the blocking of the Na conductance. Next, voltage clamp results were obtained in which a square voltage step was utilized as a feedback to the current injection system allowing then the study of synaptic transmission under presynaptic voltage control. Since these last experiments have been reported in extenso (Llinas et al., 1981 a,b), we will not cover them in detail. Finally, another technique utilized to study the effect of AmP on synaptic transmission involved recording the presynaptic action potential onto a digital buffer and, following blockage of Na and K conductances, this voltage envelope was reinjected into the terminal and used as a feedback to the current injection system. In this way, a waveform which mimicks the original presynaptic action potential was used as the command voltage for the clamp. This particular technique was utilized to determine whether TEA or 3- or 4-AmP modifies the depolarization-release coupling process.

## RESULTS

Results reported here were obtained using both 3- and 4-AmP. Results obtained with 4-AmP were similar in every way to those obtained using 3-AmP. Also, we found that following an initial partial blockage of K conductance using 3-AmP, the

addition of more 3-AmP could not be distinguished from the addition of an equal
amount of 4-AmP. Therefore, in this paper the term AmP will be used to refer to
3- or 4-AmP. In most of our experiments, 5 mM AmP was utilized.

Effect of AmP on synaptic transmission in the presence of a Na conductance

Upon application of AmP to reach final concentrations of 1-50 mM the most obvious
finding was that AmP tended to depolarize the presynaptic terminal and in some
cases produced spontaneous repetitive activity in both pre- and postsynaptic
fibers. In synapses where this did not occur, it was possible to study the time
course of the effect of AmP treatment on the amplitude and width of the pre- and
postsynaptic spikes. This is illustrated in Fig. 1 A-D. Here action potentials

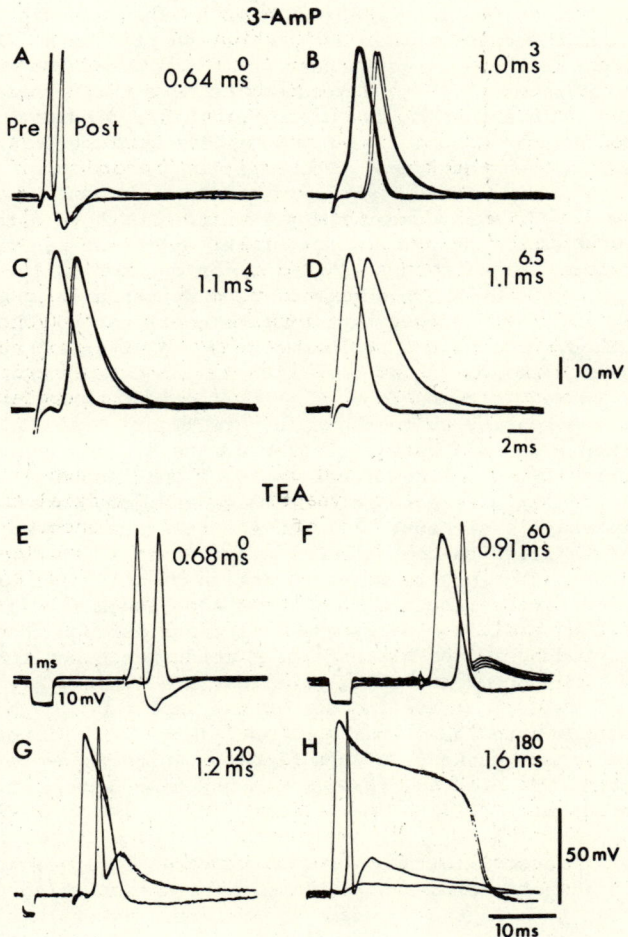

Fig. 1.  Time course of effect of 3-AmP (30 mM) (A-D) and
intraterminal injection of TEA (F-I) on synaptic
transmission. Times after drug application are
given in minutes and synaptic delay in msec at the
upper right corner.

were recorded at 3, 4 and 6 minutes after the addition of AmP (30 mM). Note that under these conditions both the duration and amplitude of the pre- and postsynaptic action potentials increase. This is to be expected as the resting resistance of the membrane is slightly higher as the K conductance is reduced. As shown in the figure, the large change in the duration and amplitude of both spikes occurs within 3 minutes of AmP addition. While the duration of the postsynaptic spike increases after 4 and 6 minutes, the change in the spike in the pre-fiber is not as marked.

A second finding of interest is that synaptic transmission becomes slightly slower in the presence of AmP in the sense that the synaptic delay is prolonged. This occurs soon after addition of the drug, the increased latency being obvious after 3 minutes (Fig. 1 A,B) and not changing significantly thereafter (Llinás, Walton and Bohr, 1976). The increase is related to the fact that the Ca current generated by the presynaptic action potential becomes patent at the falling phase of the spike and thus, given the increased duration of the presynaptic spike and its slower rate of rise, there is an increase in the synaptic delay (Llinás et al., 1976a, 1981b). Note that the largest increase in the pre-spike duration occurs during the same time interval, 0 to 3 minutes, as does the increase in synaptic delay (Fig. 1 A-D). The actual delays are given in the figure. They were measured by extrapolating to the baseline the fast rate of rise of the presynaptic spike, to the onset of the postsynaptic potential.

In order to make a comparison between these results and those obtained with intraterminal injection of TEA, the time course of the effect of TEA is illustrated in Fig. 1 E-H. Here, in another synapse, TEA was iontophoretically injected for a total of 3 hours. Note that the blockage of K conductance is more complete than obtained with AmP and that the presynaptic spike continues to increase in duration for the entire period, producing a prolonged Ca spike after 180 minutes (Fig. 1H). The postsynaptic response, as in the case with AmP, became larger and the synaptic delay increased. Indeed, a comparison of the effects of these two blockages on synaptic transmission becomes quite clear in this figure. As far as the squid synapse is concerned, TEA is a better blocker of the K conductance but, if injected iontophoretically, may take 2 or 3 hours of continuous pulsing (see Katz and Miledi, 1967) to obtain a reasonable blockage and, of course, the effect is limited to the presynaptic element. AmP, on the other hand, produces an incomplete blockage but may be applied to the bath and acts within a few minutes, affecting both terminals. The difference between the action of these two drugs has been studied in detail in squid giant axons by Meves and Pichon (1977) and Yeh et al. (1976). Their results explain clearly the difference between these two compounds. Both 3- and 4-AmP produce a good blockage of K conductance but the blockage is both voltage- and time-dependent; thus, as illustrated in Fig. 1, presynaptic spikes show a rapid return to baseline due to the amplitude of the action potential, which drives the drug out of the K channel (Meves and Pichon, 1977; Yeh et al., 1976) and the time dependence of the blockage which tends to have a similar effect. In contrast, TEA blockage is voltage- and time-dependent but in a different manner (see below).

In short then, AmP produces, in an otherwise untreated synapse, an increase in the amplitude and duration of the presynaptic action potential which produces a clear increase in the amplitude of the postsynaptic response as well as an increase in the latency for the onset of this potential.

## Action of AmP following blockage of Na conductance

As shown in the control traces of Fig. 2, when Na conductance is blocked by addition of TTX to the bath, a square injection of current into the presynaptic terminal produces a depolarization characterized by a delayed rectification which brings the membrane potential down to a plateau level lower than that initially obtained. Under these circumstances, presynaptic depolarization would produce

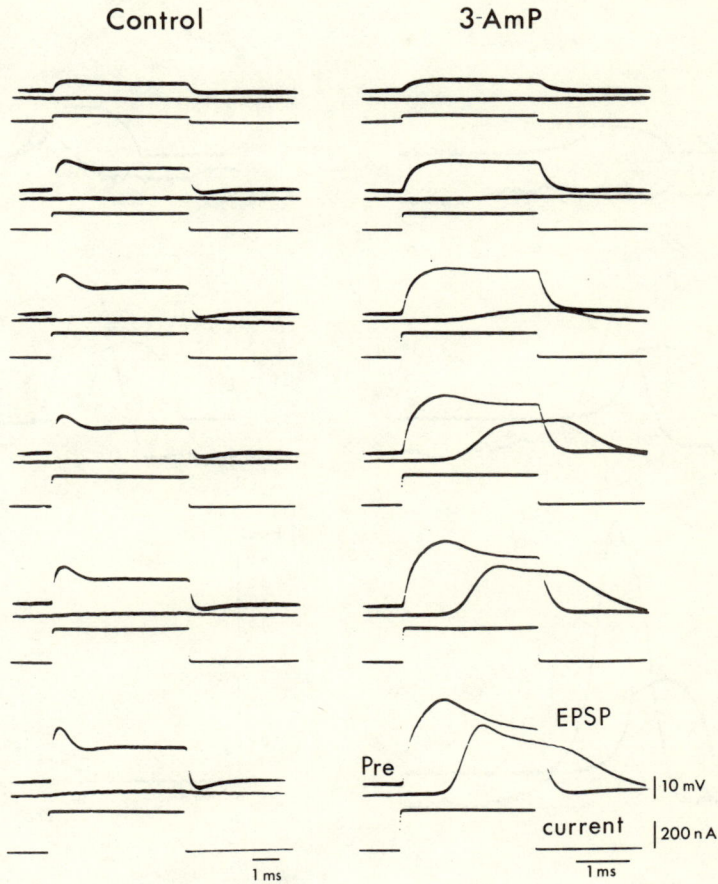

Fig. 2. Effect of 3-AmP (12.5 mM) on presynaptic voltage and postsynaptic potential in a synapse where sodium conductance is blocked with TTX.

synaptic transmission mainly during the onset of the depolarization since during the period of delayed rectification both the potential and the distribution of potential in space are reduced given that the resting conductance of the presynaptic axon is markedly increased. Following the addition of AmP to the bath, delayed rectification is reduced and thus the same amount of current injection produces a larger presynaptic depolarization and an enormous increase in the amount of transmitter release (Fig. 2, 3-AmP). In fact, under these conditions a careful analysis of transmitter release and presynaptic depolarization becomes possible since, due to bath application of the drugs, both the pre- and post-terminals demonstrate blockage of Na and K conductances. This facilitates the study of small postsynaptic potentials following release of low levels of transmitter. A study of the relationship between small presynaptic depolarization and postsynaptic response is shown in Fig. 3 after TTX and AmP treatment. These values illustrate the fact that even small pre-terminal depolarizations may release transmitter, indicating that this transmission process is a continuous function of voltage.

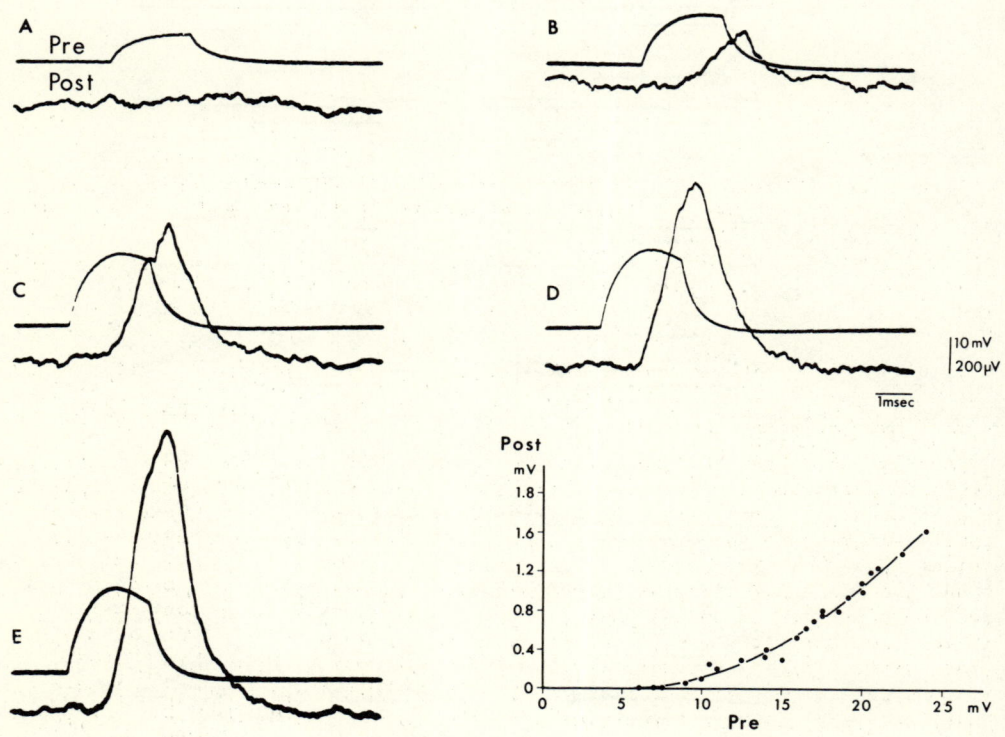

Fig. 3. Transmitter release using low levels of presynaptic depolarization in synapse treated with 3-AmP (5 mM) and TTX. (Modified from Llinas, 1979)

Often in the presence of TTX and AmP, Ca action potentials could be generated by the presynaptic terminal (Llinás et al., 1976). These spikes are shorter and smaller in amplitude than those originally reported by Katz and Miledi (1969) using TEA. However, it is important in analyzing the results obtained with AmP that the possibility of a presynaptic Ca spike be considered, especially with reduced Na conductance. An example of a Ca-dependent spike recorded in high external Ca (40 mM as opposed to the usual 10 mM) following Na conductance blockage and the administration of 5 mM 3-AmP is illustrated in Fig. 4. Note that the Ca spike is followed by a very large and prolonged postsynaptic response which is not present when the stimulus is subthreshold for regenerative Ca activation.

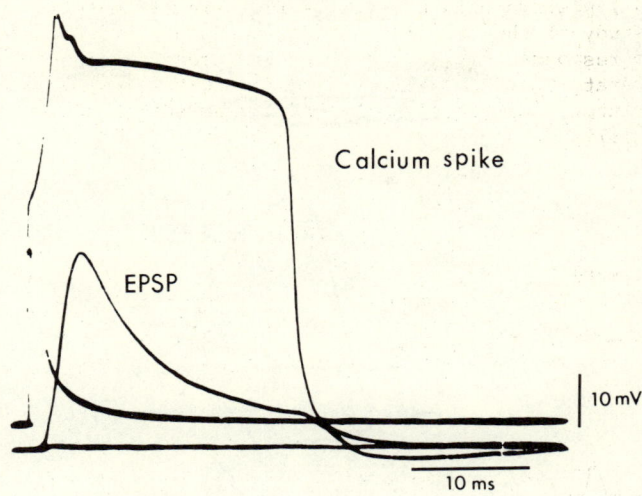

Fig. 4. Transmitter release in presence and absence of Ca spike in 3-AmP (5 mM) treated synapse using 40 mM $[Ca]_o$.

Advantages of using both AmP and TEA in the study of synaptic transmission

In studying the relationship between presynaptic depolarization and Ca entry and between Ca and transmitter release, the squid giant synapse provides a valuable preparation since here it is possible to voltage clamp the presynaptic terminal directly and measure the presynaptic $I_{Ca}$ and the postsynaptic response. This study requires that Na and K conductances be blocked as completely as possible. Regarding the blockage of K conductance, TEA - while being an excellent blocker at potentials above 50 mV from rest (-20 mV absolute) - did not block K conductance as well when lower amplitude pulses were applied. Indeed, a K current could always be seen with smaller depolarizing steps. On the other hand, AmP is especially efficient in blocking K conductance at the lower potential levels (Meves and Pichon, 1977; Yeh et al., 1976; Llinás et al., 1976b). Thus, the blockage of K conductance by these drugs is complementary; used together, K conductance is effectively blocked over the range of voltages from rest (-70 mV) to the "suppression potential" (Katz and Miledi, 1967) (Fig. 5, 130 mV). In conjunction then, using these two pharmacological agents, a complete blockage of the K conductance is achieved.

Voltage clamp studies

Basically our presynaptic voltage clamp studies indicated that, following blockage of Na and K currents, a rapid presynaptic voltage step would produce, after a certain delay, a Ca current having an S-shaped onset. This Ca conductance does not show inactivation for the periods tested in our experiments (up to 100 msec) and at the end of the pulse a rapid Ca tail current is observed (Fig. 5) which is accompanied by the so-called "off" response (Katz and Miledi, 1967). At the suppression potential (130 mV, Fig. 5) only this tail current and the "off" response is present. The largest Ca currents and postsynaptic response ("on" response) were seen with depolarizing steps of 60 mV (Fig. 5). These results allowed us to generate a model for synaptic transmission which related presynaptic depolarization to Ca entry and intracellular Ca to synaptic release (as measured by the postsynaptic response) (Llinás et al., 1981 a,b).

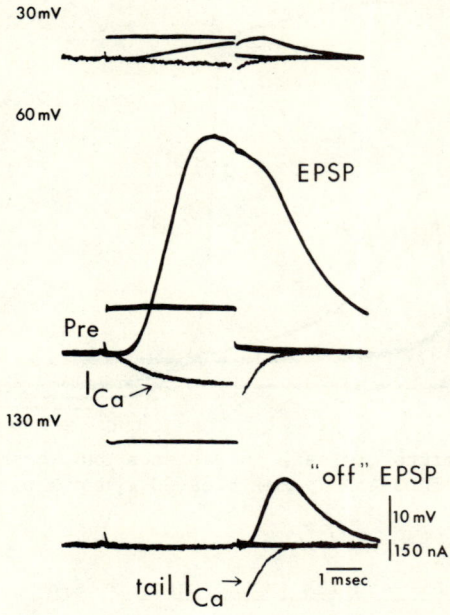

Fig. 5. Calcium currents in presynaptic terminal and postsynaptic potentials recorded using step voltage clamp pulses in AmP (5 mM), TEA and TTX-treated synapse. (Modified from Llinas et al., 1981b)

Transmission with artificial spikes

Two points remain to be tested in this model: (1) the validity of the model itself in explaining the sets of events triggered by the normal presynaptic action potential and (2) the possibility that AmP and/or TEA could have a deleterious effect on the depolarization-release coupling system. With these questions in mind, we developed a new experimental paradigm in which we study synaptic transmission following a presynaptic action potential both before and after the blockage of Na and K conductances (Llinas, Sugimori, and Simon, 1979, and in press). These results, as shown in Fig. 6, indicate that synaptic transmission is unaltered by the use of AmP and/or TEA. A presynaptic action potential evoked either by the normal Na and K conductances (Fig. 6A) or that produced by the artificial injection of current by the command amplifier of a voltage clamp circuit (Fig. 6B) produces essentially the same postsynaptic response. This is illustrated in Fig. 6C where the presynaptic potential and postsynaptic response recorded prior to Na and K conductance blockage and the results obtained with a voltage step which simulates the action potential are superimposed. Because the results indicate that the latency and rate of rise of the post-response is the same as in the original transmission in A, we must conclude that AmP and TEA, while blocking K conductance, do not modify the depolarization-release coupling system in any discernible way. The results demonstrated that, as expected from our model (Llinás et al., 1976a, 1981a), $I_{Ca}$ occurs at the fall of the presynaptic action potential (Fig. 6B).

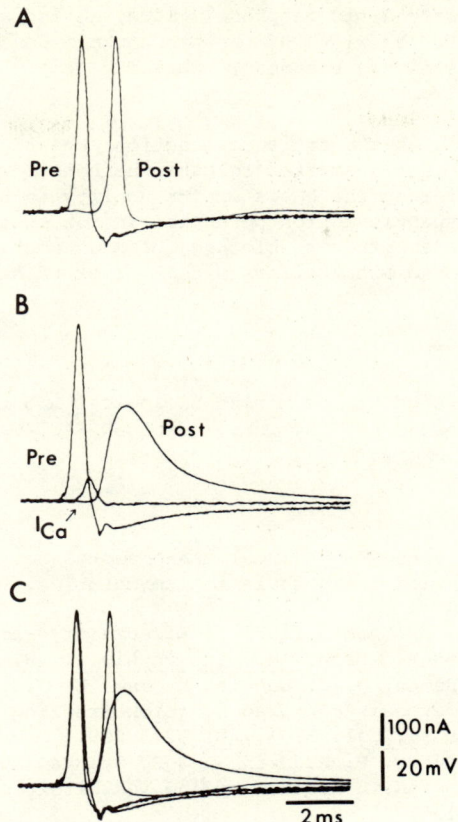

Fig. 6. Synaptic transmission by artificial presynaptic action potentials. (A) Pre- and postsynaptic action potentials. (B) Calcium current and postsynaptic response obtained using presynaptic spike in A as the command signal for the voltage clamp circuit after AmP (5 mM), TEA and TTX. (C) Superposition of A and B.

CONCLUSIONS

The present experiments in squid giant synapse indicate that AmP is a tool of great power in studying synaptic transmission since it seems to be capable of blocking K conductances when applied externally yet does not interfere with depolarization-release coupling. Because this drug has been utilized in both physiological (Jankowska et al., 1977; Lundh, 1978; Klee, 1979; Kawai and Niwa, 1980; Kocsis et al., 1980; Hermann and Gorman, 1981) and anatomical (Heuser et al., 1979; Takunaga et al., 1979 a,b) studies and is becoming an important tool in defining the steps which lead to transmitter release, it is of consequence to determine whether it has a deleterious effect on synaptic transmission per se. We conclude that the action of these compounds, even at the high concentrations utilized in some of these studies, has no obvious effect on depolarization-release coupling. In addition, these results indicate that in preparations where only the postsynaptic element is accessible (such as the neuromuscular junction) some aspects of the modification of the presynaptic spike by these drugs may be inferred from the postsynaptic response. Thus, an increase in synaptic delay reflects an increase in the width of the pre-spike. Concomitant with an increased **amplitude** of the postsynaptic response, there may be prolonged release suggesting presynaptic Ca spikes.

In short, the results with the artificial action potentials indicate that the rather large increase in transmitter release which follows AmP treatment can be completely accounted for on the basis of its ability to block K conductance. Indeed, when the presynaptic action potential is forced to have exactly the same amplitude and duration as prior to blockage of K conductance, the properties of the postsynaptic response are similar to that prior to AmP administration.

ACKNOWLEDGEMENT

Experiments were conducted at the Marine Biological Laboratory in Woods Hole, MA, and research was supported by U.S.P.H.S. grants NS14014 and 13742.

REFERENCES

Armstrong, C. M. and L. Binstock (1965). Anomalous rectification in the squid giant axon injected with tetraethylammonium chloride. J. Gen. Physiol., 48, 859-872.
Hermann, A., and A. L. F. Gorman (1981). Effects of 4-aminopyridine on potassium currents in a molluscan neuron. J. Gen. Physiol., 78, 63-86.
Heuser, J. E., T. S. Reese, M. J. Dennis, Y. Jan, L. Jan, and L. Enams (1979). Synaptic vesicle exocytosis captured by quick freezing correlated with quantal transmitter release. J. Cell Biol., 81, 275-300.
Jankowska, E., A. Lundberg, P. Rudomin, and E. Sykova (1977). Effects of 4-aminopyridine on transmission in excitatory and inhibitory synapses in the spinal cord. Brain Res., 136, 387-392.
Katz, B. and R. Miledi (1967). A study of synaptic transmission in the absence of nerve impulses. J. Physiol. (Lond.), 192, 407-436.
Katz, B. and R. Miledi (1969). Tetrodotoxin-resistant electric activity in presynaptic terminals. J. Physiol. (Lond.), 203, 459-487.
Kawai, N. and A. Niwa (1980). Neuromuscular transmission without sodium activation of the presynaptic nerve terminal in the lobster. J. Physiol. (Lond.), 305, 73-85.
Klee, M. R. (1979). TEA and 4-AP affect separate potassium and calcium channels differently in aplysia S and F cells. Brain Res. Bull., 4, 162-166.
Kocsis, J. D., R. C. Malenka, and S. G. Waxman (1980). Effects of 4-aminopyridine on the frequency following properties of the parallel fibers of the cerebellar cortex. Brain Res., 195, 510-516.
Llinás, R. (1979). The role of calcium in neuronal function. In F. O. Schmitt and F. G. Worden (Eds.), The Neurosciences: Fourth Study Program. M.I.T. Press, Cambridge, MA. pp. 555-571.
Llinás, R., I. Z. Steinberg, and K. Walton (1976a). Presynaptic calcium currents and their relation to synaptic transmission: Voltage clamp study in squid giant synapse and theoretical model for the calcium gate. Proc. Natl. Acad. Sci. (USA), 73, 2918-2922.
Llinás, R., I. Z. Steinberg, and K. Walton (1981a). Presynaptic calcium currents in squid giant synapse. Biophys. J., 33, 289-322.
Llinás, R., I. Z. Steinberg, and K. Walton (1981b). Relationship between presynaptic calcium current and postsynaptic potential in squid giant synapse. Biophys. J., 33, 323-352.

Llinás, R., M. Sugimori, and S. Simon (1979). Presynaptic calcium current and postsynaptic response generated by a presynaptic action potential; a voltage clamp study in the squid giant synapse. Biol. Bull., 157, 380.

Llinás, R., M. Sugimori, and S. Simon (in press). Transmission by presynaptic spike-like depolarization in the squid giant synapse.

Llinás, R., K. Walton, and V. Bohr (1976b). Synaptic transmission in squid giant synapse after potassium conductance blockage with external 3- and 4-aminopyridine. Biophys. J., 16, 83-86.

Lundh, H. (1978). Effects of 4-aminopyridine on neuromuscular transmission. Brain Res., 153, 307-318.

Meves, H. and Y. Pichon (1977). The effect of internal and external 4-aminopyridine on the potassium currents in intracellularly perfused squid giant axons. J. Physiol. (Lond.), 268, 511-532.

Pelhate, M. and Y. Pichon (1974). Selective inhibition of potassium current in the giant axon of the cockroach. J. Physiol. (Lond.) 242, 90-91P.

Takunaga, A., C. Sandri, and K. Akert (1979a). Ultrastructural effects of 4-aminopyridine on the presynaptic membrane in the rat spinal cord. Brain Res., 163, 1-8.

Takanuga, A., C. Sandri, and K. Akert (1979b). Increase of large intramembranous particles in the presynaptic active zone after administration of 4-aminopyridine. Brain Res., 174, 207-219.

Yeh, J. Z., G. S. Oxford, C. H. Wu, and T. Narahashi (1976). Dynamics of aminopyridine block of potassium channels in squid axon membrane. J. Gen. Physiol., 68, 519-535.

# DISCUSSION OF THE FIRST SESSION

Dr. Llinás: Is it, Dr. Meves, the case that under certain conditions when $Ca^{2+}$ moves through gK it will not allow $Ba^{2+}$ to move through gK? If so, what can this tell us about gK?

Dr. Meves: Inoue (J. gen. Physiol., 76, 337, 1980) who studied $Ca^{2+}$ currents through $K^+$ channels in internally perfused squid giant axons did not investigate the question whether the $Ca^{2+}$ currents are blocked by internal $Ba^{2+}$; he merely showed that they are blocked by internal tetraethylammonium. It is also not known whether external $Ba^{2+}$ (like external $Ca^{2+}$) can move through $K^+$ channels.

Dr. Thesleff: Is anything known about interactions between $K^+$ and $Ca^{2+}$ channels in the respect that activation or inactivation of the $K^+$ channel might influence the kinetics of $Ca^{2+}$ channels?

Dr. Meves: Sofar there are only few electrophysiological studies of $Ca^{2+}$ channels (e.g. Adams and Gage, J. Physiol., 289, 115, 1979 and Kostyuk and co-workers, J. Physiol., 310, 403, 1981 on molluscan neuron) and, to my knowledge, they have not revealed any influence of gK on $Ca^{2+}$ channels.

Dr. Bergmann: Regarding the fact that paranodal or internodal channels in the frog nerve are covered by myeline, are they accessible to drugs like aminopyridines?

Dr. Meves: Chiu and Ritchie (J. Physiol., 313, 415, 1981) have speculated that the $K^+$ channels in the paranodal region of mammalian myelinated nerve fibres may have the function to prevent spurious re-excitation of the node after an action potential. $K^+$ ions may accumulate underneath the myeline sheath and the covered K channels may be responsible for the long-lasting excitability changes that follow a single impulse or multiple impulses (see Raymond, J. Physiol., 290, 273, 1979).

Dr. Foldes: You have demonstrated that procaine and lidocaine have similar effects on $Na^+$ and $K^+$ channels. We have observed that the neuromuscular block produced by these compounds in the phrenic nerve-hemidiaphragm preparation of the rat was influenced differently by 4-aminopyridine. While the procaine induced block was antagonized, the lidocaine block was unaffected by 4-aminopyridine. Could you explain this observation?

Dr. Meves: To answer this question properly one would require experimental information about the effect of the two local anesthetics on (a) the presynaptic action potential and (b) the endplate current, both in the absence and in the presence of 4-aminopyridine. The effect of procaine and lidocaine on end-plate currents has been studied by Kordaš (J. Physiol., 209, 689, 1970) and Beam (J. Physiol., 258, 279, 1976). No investigations of the combined effects of local anesthetics and 4-aminopyridine are known to me.

Dr. Khodorov: Have you, Dr. Ulbricht, studied the effect of internal TEA on 4-aminopyridine block? What about the effects of external $Ba^{2+}$ on 4-aminopyridine blocked channels?

Dr. Ulbricht: We have neither tried internal TEA nor $Ba^{2+}$.

Dr. Meves: Does the effect of $V_2$ on the time constant of block restoration saturate when $V_2$ is large and $n_\infty$ approaches unity?

Dr. Ulbricht: Considering the fact that $\tau$ decreased to 1.0, 0.6 and 0.46 s as $V_2$ increased to 20, 40 and 80 mV there is a clear tendency to saturate. This, however, is not easily proved since at larger depolarization, i.e. as $V_2$ approaches $V_1$ there is little increment in equilibrium block.

Dr. Pichon: Why are you not explaining the slow recovery by drug-receptor reaction kinetics?

## Discussion

<u>Dr. Ulbricht:</u> Since the rate of restoration increased at least 4-5 times for a change from $V_2 = 0$ to 10 mV at almost no change in equilibrium block one would have to postulate a large modulation of the dissociation rate constant, which seems rather unusual. A modulation of gate "openness", on the other hand, is well within what one measures in untreated nodes.

<u>Dr. Shahid:</u> What chemical form of 4-aminopyridine was employed in your experiments i.e. was it the neutralised hydrochloride or the base.

<u>Dr. Dubois:</u> I used the base form of 4-aminopyridine. The pH was adjusted to 7.4 with HCl. However, changing the pH from 7.4 to 9 did not seem to modify the blockade of fast $K^+$ current by 4-aminopyridine.

<u>Dr. Galvan:</u> Dr. Dubois, is the fast current similar to the transient outward (A-current) observed in molluscan neurons?

<u>Dr. Dubois:</u> The fast current in frog myelinated nerve fibres resembles the transient outward (A-current) in molluscan neurons. It is blocked by 4-aminopyridine and it is inactivated during depolarization. However, in contrast to the A-current the fast current is not inactivated at the resting potential level (-70 mV) and its inactivation time constant is in the order of several seconds.

<u>Dr. Meves:</u> Is the ionic selectivity of the fast and the slow $K^+$ channel identical? What is the permeability of the slow channel for $NH_4$, for instance?

<u>Dr. Dubois:</u> The fast $K^+$-current represents about 80% of the total $K^+$-current. Thus, the ionic selectivity of the fast channel is very similar to the ionic selectivity of the whole population of $K^+$-channels as described by Hille (1973). I do not know whether slow channels are permeable to $NH_4$. I have studied the permeability of slow channels to the alkali cations ($Li^+$, $Na^+$, $K^+$, $Rb^+$, $Cs^+$). The results suggest that the selectivity of slow channels is similar to that of fast channels (i.e. $pK^+ >$ $pRb^+ \gg pNa^+$, $pLi^+$, $pCs^+$). However, it was observed that the relative selectivity $pRb^+/pK^+$ of slow channels depends on the concentration of these cations in the external solution.

<u>Dr. Ulbricht:</u> Have you computed action potentials with your slow channel data and do they fit your 4-aminopyridine or TEA results?

<u>Dr. Dubois:</u> No, I have not computed action potentials with the slow channel data. I think that at the present time it is difficult to compute action potentials with fast and slow $K^+$-currents because the fast current is composed of two components whose voltage and time dependencies are not completely described.

<u>Dr. McArdle:</u> Is the repetitive firing with 4-aminopyridine which Dr. Pichon described due solely to depolarization?

<u>Dr. Pichon:</u> If the membrane potential is maintained near its resting level by current injection, repetitive activity may appear if the 4-aminopyridine concentration is sufficient. Under normal experimental conditions, however, spontaneous activity is due to drug induced slow membrane depolarization and to membrane hyperexcitability.

<u>Dr. Meves:</u> What is the pH dependence of the 4-aminopyridine effect?

<u>Dr. Pichon:</u> This point has not been studied systematically. We have made a few experiments with modified extracellular pH and the effects were much smaller than expected if one assumes that the number of active molecules depends on the difference between pH and pK. This result is in agreement with the observation of Yeh and coworkers (1976) who found that 3-aminopyridine and 2-aminopyridine, the pK of which

## Discussion

are clearly different from that of 4-aminopyridine, are nearly equipotent to 4-aminopyridine. One explanation might be that the pH at the $K^+$ channel is not the same as in the bulk solution. Another explanation, which is based on measurements in monolayers, is that the pK values are modified at the membrane-water interface.

Dr. Bergman: It is a short comment I would like to make in connection with the question of Dr. Meves about pH. In our laboratory, J. Tanguy recently performed some experiments on the node of Ranvier with 4-aminopyridine to know how selective can be the blockade of the K channel by this molecule. She found that the addition of 1mM 4-aminopyridine to the normal Ringer solution induces a significant decrease of the Na current recorded under voltage clamp conditions, a further and more complete investigation revealed that this effect has to be attributed to alterations of the Ringer's pH.

Dr. Bergmann: Dr. Llinas, if both $Na^+$ and $K^+$ transport is blocked, is the amount of $Ca^{2+}$ transported sufficient to explain the observed current? Was $Ca^{2+}$ transport measured by isotope technique?

Dr. Llinás: Because in the absence of $Na^+$ from the extracellular medium one can see a clear inward current which disappears if $Ca^{2+}$ is removed I feel that necessary and sufficient evidence is available to assert that the inward current is carried by $Ca^{2+}$.

Dr. Molgo: Are there differences between TEA and 4-aminopyridine concerning calcium inactivation when gNa is blocked? When you applied two depolarizing current pulses to TTX treated nerve terminals did you see differences in calcium inactivation?

Dr. Llinás: We do not see $Ca^{2+}$ current inactivation with our pulses, probably because the pulses are too short. Two pulses appear to produce facilitation without an increase in the $Ca^{2+}$ current for the second pulse.

Dr. Yanagisawa: Is there in nerve terminals a mechanism, like in skeletal muscle, whereby $Ca^{2+}$ entry releases further $Ca^{2+}$? Is the $Ca^{2+}$ which enters the terminal sufficient to release the neurotransmitter?

Dr. Llinás: No, the $Ca^{2+}$ current itself is not sufficient to release transmitter. If EGTA is injected intracellularly into the terminal, $Ca^{2+}$ enters but does not generate transmitter release.

Dr. Shimahara: Did you observe changes in intracellular pH in the presence of 4-aminopyridine?

Dr. Llinás: No, we have sofar not attempted such experiments.

Dr. Pichon: What is the value for the $Ca^{2+}$ current (and $Ca^{2+}$ conductance) compared to that expected from the $Ca^{2+}$ permeability of $Na^+$ channels?

Dr. Llinás: We have not determined single channel conductances. However, experiments in invertebrates suggest that $Ca^{2+}$ channel conductances are two orders of magnitudes smaller than for the $Na^+$ channel.

# Aminopyridines and Synaptic Transmission

*Chairman:* S. Thesleff

# General Principles of Synaptic Transmission

S. Thesleff

Department of Pharmacology, University of Lund, Lund, Sweden

ABSTRACT

At motor nerve terminals three types of transmitter release are present. One mechanism is located at specialized sites, the "active zones" in the nerve terminal membrane. All nerve impulse-evoked transmitter release, as well as a majority of spontaneous quantal transmitter release, originate from this site. The amount of transmitter liberated is correlated to the amount of calcium entry into the nerve terminal. Due to low chloride and other leak conductances in the nerve terminal membrane, blockade of outward potassium currents by drugs like the aminopyridines greatly increase the inward calcium flux and thereby the amount of transmitter liberated. Botulinal neurotoxins selectively block this mechanism for transmitter release.

A second type of release occurs also as quantal, probably vesicular, release of acetylcholine but from sites presumably different from the "active zones". This release is unaffected by transmembrane calcium fluxes and accounts normally only for the presence of a small population of spontaneous sub- and giant miniature endplate potentials. Under certain experimental conditions aminopyridines and some related compounds enhance this type of release and induce the appearance of a large number of giant miniature endplate potentials. Botulinal neurotoxins fail to affect this type of transmitter release.

A third type of transmitter release consists of molecular leakage of acetylcholine from the nerve terminal cytoplasm into the extracellular medium. It is believed to be one of the mechanisms by which the nerve exerts a neurotrophic influence on its target organ. Aminopyridines have no known effect on this type of transmitter release.

KEYWORDS

Trasmitter release, facilitation of transmitter release, aminopyridines, giant miniature endplate potentials, properties of nerve terminals.

At this session of the symposium we will learn that aminopyridines and certain other drugs enormously enhance synaptic transmission by increasing the amount of transmitter released by nerve impulses. To understand their mode of action I should like to summarize some main physiological principles of synaptic transmitter release with emphasis on those mechanisms upon which the aminopyridines seem to act.

A large part of our understanding of synaptic transmission comes from studies of cholinergic synapses and I will use the motor nerve terminal as a model for describing synaptic transmission. I am well aware that other types of synapses may differ in various aspects from the endplate but, in general, the functional principles are similar.

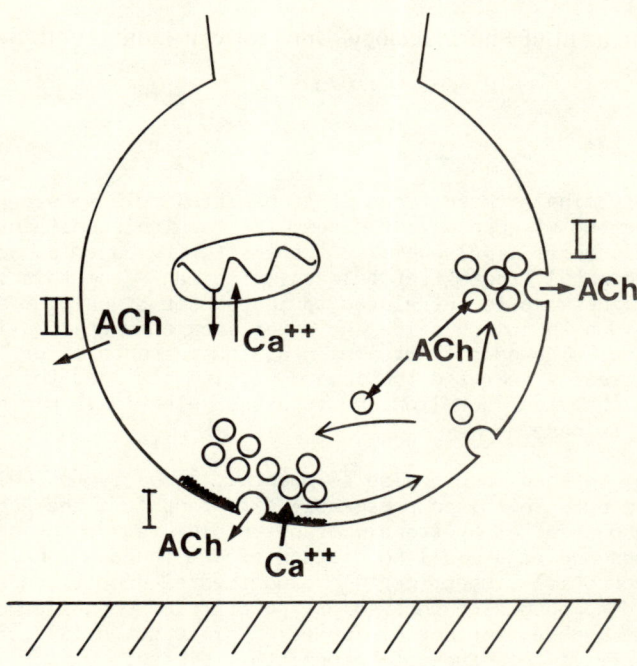

Fig. 1. A schematic model of a motor nerve terminal showing the three (I - III) proposed mechanisms for acetylcholine release. For explanation, see text.

Figure 1 is a schematic model of a cholinergic synapse showing three distinct mechanisms for acetylcholine release. The first mechanism (I) is located at specialized sites, the so-called "active zones", in the nerve terminal membrane which are opposite to the crests of the postsynaptic folds which have the highest density of cholinergic receptors. All nerve impulse-evoked transmitter release comes from this site. The nerve terminal depolarization produced by the nerve action potential opens voltage-sentitive calcium channels, probably located in the "active zones". The resulting massive influx of calcium ions, along its electrochemical gradient, allows a synchronous exocytosis of a large number of synaptic vesicles and thereby produces the postsynaptic endplate potential. The amount of transmitter released is correlated to the amount of calcium that enters the nerve terminal and this in turn is determined by how long the preterminal calcium channels remains open. This mechanism is greatly enhanced by the aminopyridines which, as will be pointed out, greatly prolong the period of calcium entry and thereby the amount of transmitter released. The "active zones" are also the sites for a large portion of the spontaneous quantal vesicular transmitter release which is recorded as miniature endplate potentials in the postsynaptic membrane. The frequency of miniature endplate potentials is accelerated by nerve terminal depolarization, for instance, by high extracellular potassium concentrations and it is similarly affected by alterations in the extracellular calcium concentration. Botulinal and tetanus neurotoxins seem selectively to block the type I kind of transmitter release by reducing its calcium sensitivity (Cull-Candy, Lundh and Thesleff, 1976; Thesleff, 1981).

The second type of release (II) occurs as quantal, probably vesicular, release from highly dispersed sites in the nerve terminal, presumably outside of the "active zones" (Thesleff, 1981). This release is unaffected by nerve terminal depolarization and transmembrane calcium fluxes and seems, under normal conditions, to account for the small population of sub- and giant miniature endplate potentials seen at neuromuscular junctions. Under certain experimental conditions aminopyridines and aminopyridine related compounds enhance this type of release and induce the appearance of a large number of giant miniature endplate potentials (Molgó and Thesleff, 1981a). Botulinum or tetanus poisoning fail to affect the type II release and spontaneous quantal transmitter release observed at poisoned junctions comes from that type of release (Thesleff, 1981).

A third type of transmitter release (III) consists of passive molecular leakage of acetylcholine molecules from the nerve terminal cytoplasm into the extracellular medium. This type of release accounts for more than 90% of total transmitter release under resting conditions. Little is known about the mechanisms which control this type of diffusion of acetylcholine or its physiological importance but it is believed to be related to neurotrophic activity i.e. to be a mechanism by which the nerve exerts a long-term control of the biochemical properties of the postsynaptic membrane including its receptor density and sensitivity (Mathers and Thesleff, 1978; Thesleff and Sellin, 1980). Aminopyridines have no known effect on this type of release.

How can aminopyridines so dramatically augment the type I kind of nerve impulse evoked transmitter release? I should like to suggest that it depends upon certain unique electrophysiological properties of the presynaptic nerve terminal membrane. Let me illustrate this by showing some results from experiments carried out by Molgó and myself on frog motor nerve terminals (Molgó and Thesleff, 1981b). To obtain information about the electric membrane properties of motor nerve terminals we have examined how brief depolarizing or hyperpolarizing current pulses to the preterminal axon affect the efficacy of a subsequent depolarization to release transmitter. The experiments were made in the presence of tetrodotoxin (TTX) to block sodium channels. Under these conditions a depolarizing current pulse of 2-8 ms duration and 1-10 µA strength caused the release of transmitter, the amplitude of the endplate potential being graded with current (Fig. 2A). A preceding condi-

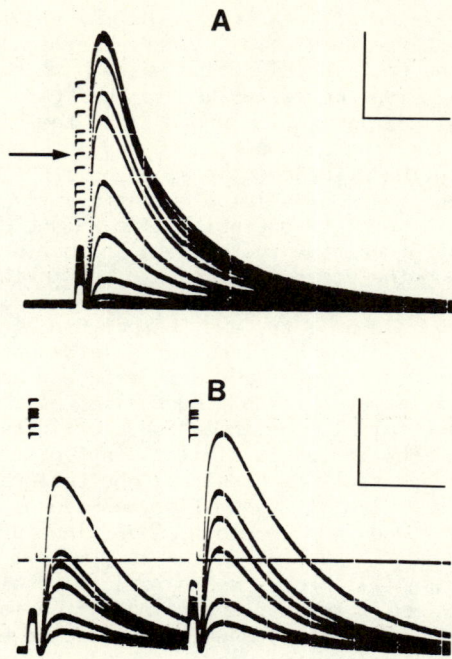

Fig. 2. A – End-plate potentials induced by depolarizing current pulses (indicated by an arrow) of 4 ms duration and intensities between 2.05 to 5.15 µA to the motor nerve. Each stimulus was applied every 30 s to avoid transmitter depletion from influencing the results. Tetrodotoxin 1 µM and neostigmine 3 µM. Temp. 3°C. Resting membrane potential – 80 mV. Calibration 20 mV, 40 ms and 2 µA.
B – Same end-plate as in A showing end-plate potentials triggered by twin depolarizing current pulses of 4 ms duration at different intensities (between 3 and 3.8 µA). Note facilitation of the response to the second pulse. The interval between the pulses was 70 ms. Calibration and experimental conditions as in A. (From Molgó and Thesleff, 1981 b).

tioning depolarizing current pulse had a short-lasting and intensity-graded facilitatory effect on release as shown in Fig. 2B. A preceding hyperpolarizing current pulse of similar duration produced, on the other hand, a pronounced inhibition of release the inhibition lasting up to 100 ms (Fig. 3). When sodium channels are blocked by TTX inward ionic currents, causing transmitter release, are carried by calcium ions, as discussed by Katz and Miledi (1967). Under these conditions a brief depolarizing current pulse to the terminal caused only a slight and graded facilitation of transmitter release while hyperpolarizing pulses produced inhibition lasting for one hundred ms. It suggests that electrotonic spread of hyperpolarizing but not of depolarizing current has a long-lasting effect on transmitter release and that therefore current rectification is prominent in the nerve terminal membrane.

When in addition potassium channels were blocked by 3,4-diaminopyridine or tetraethylammonium a depolarizing current pulse of suprathreshold strength triggered

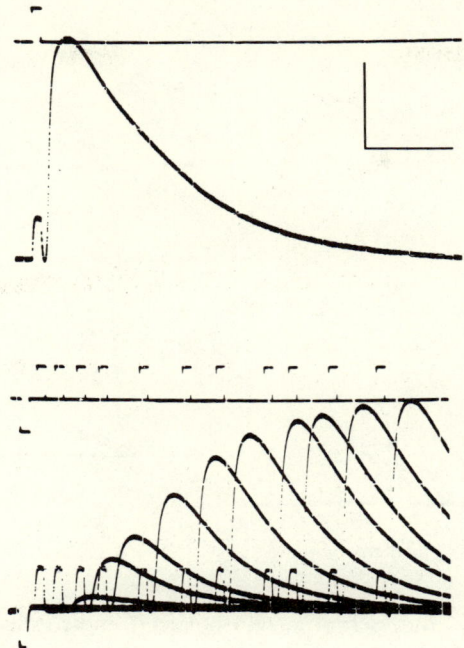

Fig. 3. Upper record: End-plate potential evoked by a depolarizing current pulse of 4.2 µA and 4 ms duration (upper tracing). Calibration 20 mV, 40 ms and 10 µA. Temp. 3°C. Resting membrane potential - 80 mV.
Lower record: Same end-plate showing the inhibition by a hyperpolarizing current prepulse of 4 ms; 4.2 µA of end-plate potentials caused by subsequent depolarizing pulses of the same duration and strength. The interval between pulses was varied between 3 and 160 ms. Tetrodotoxin 1 µM and neostigmine 3 µM. (From Molgó and Thesleff, 1981 b).

a regenerative influx of calcium and thereby a massive release of transmitter as shown in Fig. 4. Under this condition a subthreshold depolarizing prepulse caused facilitation of transmitter release in an almost all-or-none manner as shown in Fig. 5. Facilitation lasted as long as 50 ms which indicates that most of the rectifying outward current in the nerve terminal is carried by potassium ions and that chloride or "leak" conductances are small.

These findings are in marked contrast to the nerve axon where blockade of potassium channels causes only a slight reduction in the outward current, the main outward current being carried by leak conductances which rapidly repolarize the membrane. Thus, it appears that voltage dependent sodium, calcium and potassium conductances combined with low leak conductances and therefore a high specific membrane resistance characterize the presynaptic nerve terminal while large leak conductance and therefore a low specific membrane resistance is typical of the axon.

With a high specific membrane resistance, blockade of potassium channels drasti-

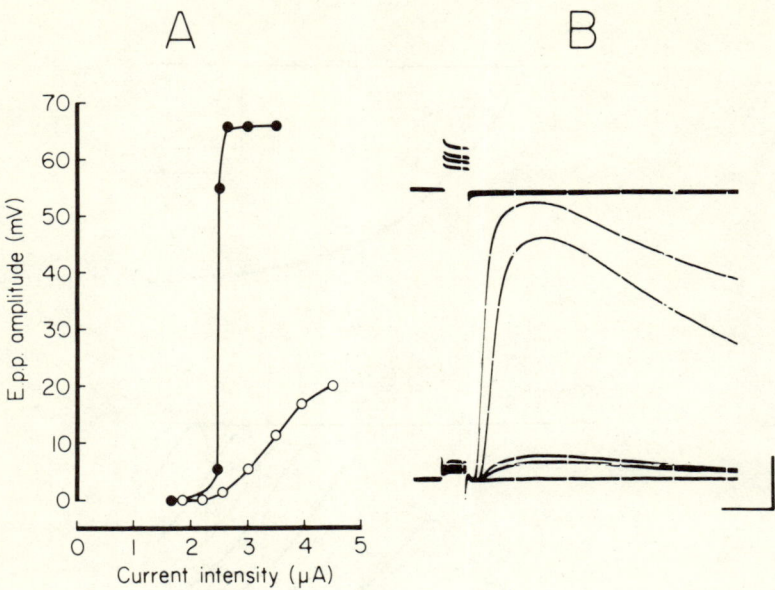

Fig. 4. A - The relationship between end-plate potential amplitude and the strength of current pulses of 4 ms duration applied to the preterminal axon before (o) and in the presence of 3,4-diaminopyridine (100 µM) (●). Data obtained from the same end-plate. Tetrodotoxin 1 µM. Resting membrane potential - 82 mV, temp. 3.5°C.
B - End-plate potentials evoked by depolarizing current pulses of 5 ms duration at intensities between 0.9 and 1.6 µA (upper tracing). 3,4-diaminopyridine (5 µM) and tetrodotoxin (1 µM) present. Resting membrane potential - 70 mV, temp. 3.5°C. Note the almost all-or-none response to a small increment in current strength. Calibration 10 mV, 10 ms and 2 µA. (From Molgó and Thesleff, 1981 b).

cally prolongs the duration of action potential depolarization and this would explain the potent facilitatory effect on transmitter release by drugs like the aminopyridines. A prolongation of the action potential increases the amount of calcium that enters the terminal through its voltage-sensitive calcium channels and thereby the amount of transmitter released.

Thus, it appears that the aminopyridines augment transmitter release by blocking the only outward ionic current present in the nerve terminal membrane, i.e. the potassium channel. In addition it is possible that the drugs have a direct delaying action on inactivation of voltage-dependent calcium channels but experimental evidence for such a mode of action has so far not been obtained.

Finally, I should like to end my presentation by expressing my admiration for the pioneering studies carried out during the last 25 years by Professor P. Lechat and Dr. M. Lemeignan on the basic pharmacology of aminopyridines, for the courage of the Bulgarian scientists who introduced 4-aminopyridine into the clinic and

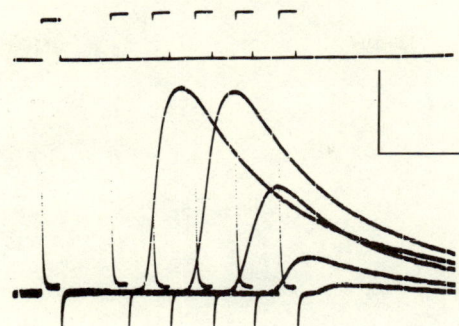

Fig. 5. Facilitatory influence of a subthreshold depolarizing current pulse (4 ms; 4.75 µA) on transmitter release by a second subthreshold pulse of same duration but higher intensity (5.3 µA). Note that the facilitation of the end-plate potentials decreases when the interval between the pulses is increased. The intervals between the two pulses is respectively 12; 22; 32; 41; and 51 ms. Tetrodotoxin 1 µM; 3,4-diaminopyridine 20 µM. Temp. 2.5°C. Calibration is 20 mV, 20 ms and 10 µA. Resting membrane potential - 68 mV. (From Molgó and Thesleff, 1981 b).

for my old friend Professor F.F. Foldes whose studies in humans laid the basis for their subsequent further clinical trials. Professor Foldes is also the person who introduced me to this interesting class of drugs.

REFERENCES

Cull-Candy, S.G., H. Lundh and S. Thesleff (1976). J. Physiol. (London), 260, 177-203.
Katz, B. and R. Miledi (1967). J. Physiol. (London), 192, 407-436.
Mathers, D.A. and S. Thesleff (1978). J. Physiol. (London), 282, 105-114.
Molgó, J. and S. Thesleff (1981a). Proc. Roy. Soc., Accepted for publication.
Molgó, J. and S. Thesleff (1981b). Acta Physiol. Scand., Accepted for publication.
Thesleff, S. (1981). Neurophysiologic aspects of botulinum poisoning. In G.E. Lewis (Ed.), Biochemical Aspects of Botulism, Academic Press, New York.
Thesleff, S. and L.C. Sellin (1980). T.I.N.S. May, 122-126.

# Effects of Aminopyridines on Neuromuscular Transmission

## J. Molgo

Institut de Pharmacologie, Laboratoire Associé du C.N.R.S. n° 206,
15, rue de l'Ecole de Médecine, 75006 Paris, France

### ABSTRACT

In this chapter the effects of the isomeric mono and diaminopyridines are documented in an attempt to understand the mechanism underlying their action at the neuromuscular junction.

### KEYWORDS

Aminopyridines ; neuromuscular junction ; spontaneous transmitter release ; evoked transmitter release ; motor nerve terminals ; botulinum toxin ; antibiotics ; facilitation ; depression ; end-plate currents ; potassium conductance.

### INTRODUCTION

The potent neuromuscular effects of the isomeric monoaminopyridines were first reported by Fastier and McDowall (1958) who found that 2,3 and 4-aminopyridine (AP) potentiated directly and indirectly elicited muscle twitch in isolated mammalian neuromuscular preparations. The facilitatory effect of 4-AP on neuromuscular transmission was confirmed by Kapff (1959). Later on Vohra and Pradhan (1964) briefly reported that 3,4-diaminopyridine (3,4-DAP) increased indirectly elicited twitches and reversed the neuromuscular blockade produced by (+)-tubocurarine. Furthermore, they reported that in frog muscles treated with 3,4-DAP spontaneous twitching was followed by contractures which could be antagonized by (+)-tubocurarine.
The antagonistic action of 4-AP on some neuromuscular blocking agents was studied by Lemeignan and Lechat (1967) and by Sobek and co-workers (1968). These authors showed that 4-AP was able to restore neurally-evoked contractions previously blocked by (+)-tubocurarine or gallamine *in vivo* and *in vitro* but did not restore depressed contractions produced by succinylcholine or decamethonium. Furthermore, they confirmed the previous work of Shaw and Bentley (1953) showing that 4-AP was devoid of anticholinesterase activity in the range of concentrations studied. These observations raised the possibility that 4-AP may have effects on motor nerve endings, on the post-junctional membrane or on both sites. Subsequent experiments showed that 4-AP in micromolar concentrations produced a dose-dependent increase in the amplitude of neurally evoked end-plate potentials (EPPs) in frog neuromuscular junctions previously blocked by (+)-tubocurarine and a decrease in the failure rate in junctions in which the normal release of transmitter has been reduced by a low calcium/high magnesium medium. Since no significant effects were detected in the resting membrane potential or in the amplitude of spontaneous miniature end-plate potentials

(MEPPs) the increase in EPP amplitude produced by 4-AP was attributed to an increase in the average number of transmitter quanta released by each presynaptic action potential (Molgo and co-workers, 1975). These observations have been subsequently confirmed in a variety of neuromuscular preparations from both vertebrates and invertebrates (Bowman and co-workers, 1976; Foldes and co-workers, 1976, Schauf and co-workers, 1976; Lundh and co-workers, 1977a) and in other chemical synapses (for a recent review see Thesleff, 1980). It is worth mentioning that the ability of 4-AP to antagonize non depolarizing neuromuscular blocking agents has been exploited in anaesthetic practice in Bulgaria since 1973 as first reported by Paskov and co-workers (1973).

The goals of the present paper are twofold: a) to provide a brief review of current work on the effects of the aminopyridines at the neuromuscular junction of vertebrates and invertebrates and b) to discuss and define the possible mechanism(s) by which the aminopyridines induce changes in transmitter release from motor nerve terminals.

Details of the electrophysiological methodology employed in the present studies have been reported elsewhere (Molgo and co-workers, 1977).

## AMINOPYRIDINES ON VERTEBRATE NEUROMUSCULAR JUNCTIONS.

### Effects on evoked transmitter release and presynaptic events.

Potency. The main effect of the aminopyridines at the vertebrate neuromuscular junction is to greatly increase the release of acetylcholine evoked by nerve impulses. All the isomeric monoaminopyridines (4-AP; 3-AP; 2-AP) and diaminopyridines studied (3,4-DAP; 2,3-DAP; 2,6-DAP) have similar actions but differ in potency. 3,4-DAP and 4-AP are the most potent in enhancing neuromuscular transmission (Bowman and co-workers, 1976,1977; Harvey and Marshall, 1977a,b,c). As illustrated in Fig. 1, 4-AP and 3,4-DAP in micromolar concentrations increased the quantal content of the EPP in junctions in which the normal release of transmitter has been reduced by a low calcium/high magnesium medium. From the analysis of similar dose-response curves it was evident that 3,4-DAP was about 6-10 times more potent than 4-AP in increasing nerve-impulse evoked transmitter release in both frog and mammalian neuromuscular junctions (Molgo and co-workers, 1980a).

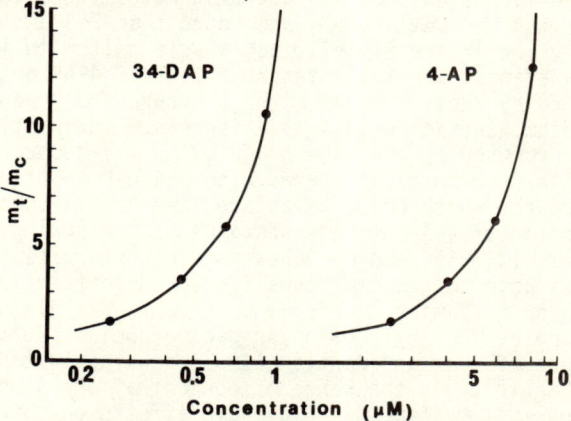

Fig. 1- Comparison of the relative potencies of 3,4-DAP and 4-AP to increase the quantal content ($m$) of the EPP. Ordinate scale: ratio between $m$ obtained in the presence of 3,4-DAP or 4-AP ($m_t$) and in its absence ($m_c$). Each dose response curve was made on a different frog end-plate bathed in Ringer solution containing 1 mM calcium and 10 mM magnesium.

Statistical parameters of release. According to the model proposed by del Castillo and Katz (1954), transmitter release occurs in the form of discrete units (quanta) and the number of quanta released ($m$) by the nerve terminal action potential is directly proportional to the stores of transmitter available ($n$) for release and the mean probability of release ($p$) for the quantal units. The analysis of amplitude frequency histograms of EPPs at the neuromuscular junction has revealed that transmitter release obeys binomial statistics (Wernig, 1975). When binomial statistics were applied during the action of 4-AP, it was reported that the drug increased the average number of quanta ($m$) released in response to nerve impulses at different frequencies by increasing the binomial parameter $n$, while $p$ remained almost unchanged (Lundh, 1979; Molgo and co-workers, 1979a). The physical meaning of $n$ and $p$ is at present not clear and many studies have attempted to find structural or functional analogues of these parameters. It has been suggested that $n$ represents the number of quanta available for release or the number of transmitter release sites and that the parameter $p$ is a compound probability both for the activation of the release sites and the probability of release for the available quanta (Zucker, 1973; Bennett and Florin, 1974; Wernig, 1975). In these terms the calculated increase in $n$ by 4-AP may indicate that on the average more release sites are active during the action of 4-AP than in the controls. In line with these findings, recent morphological studies in frog neuromuscular junctions that were quick-frozen after nerve stimulation have shown through freeze-fracture replicas of the active zones that 4-AP increased the number of dimples in the release sites, structures that have been interpreted to correspond to the sites of fusion between the synaptic vesicles and the axolemma (Heuser and co-workers, 1979).

Calcium dependence. It is well known the important role that calcium plays in the coupling between nerve terminal depolarization and transmitter release. The facilitatory action of 4-AP on evoked transmitter release requires the presence of calcium in the extracellular medium. When experiments were performed in the absence of calcium and in the presence of the chelating agents EDTA or EGTA, 4-AP failed to induce the release of transmitter by nerve impulses (Molgo and co-workers, 1977; Kim and co-workers, 1980a) or by an electrotonic depolarization of the nerve terminals (Illes and Thesleff, 1978). Therefore, it seems clear that 4-AP cannot substitute for calcium nor facilitate evoked transmitter release in its absence. Furthermore, the analysis of the relation between external calcium concentration and evoked transmitter release suggests that the cooperative requirements of calcium for the process of quantal acetylcholine release (Rahamimoff, 1976) are not affected in normal junctions either by 4-AP or by 3,4-DAP (Molgo and co-workers, 1977; 1980a).

Synaptic delay. After an action potential invades the motor nerve terminal there is a variable latency before a postsynaptic response occurs. It has been shown by Katz and Miledi (1965) that the main part of this synaptic delay is due to the process coupling nerve terminal depolarization to secretion of acetylcholine quanta. The time course of events following a spike consists of a brief period when no transmitter is secreted followed by a period during which quanta are released. Investigations dealing with the effects of 4-AP and 3,4-DAP have shown that both drugs increased the minimum synaptic delay as measured by extracellular focal recordings as the time elapsed between the peak of the terminal spike and the beginning of the postsynaptic current flow, in both frog and mammalian neuromuscular junctions (Molgo and co-workers, 1977, 1979b; Datyner and Gage, 1980). However, 4-AP has been shown to have no effect on the time course of transmitter secretion following an action potential and termed phasic secretion (Datyner and Gage, 1980). As shown in Fig. 2, 3,4-DAP reduced the late positive wave of the presynaptic action potential and increased the duration of the extracellularly recorded presynaptic spike indicating that the increase in synaptic delay may be in part related to the increase in the width of the presynaptic action potential. Thus, it appears that even though aminopyridines cause an increase in transmitter release and in minimum latency they do not affect the time course of transmitter secretion following the spike.

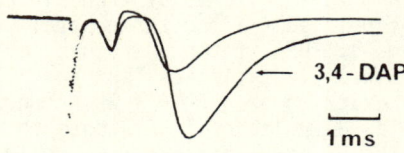

Fig. 2 - Changes in the configuration of the averaged presynaptic action potential and increase in the amplitude of extracellular end-plate current during the action of 3,4-DAP (1 µM). Each trace represents the averaged response to 126 suprathreshold stimuli (stimulation rate 0.5 Hz). Standard frog Ringer containing (+)-tubocurarine (4 µM).

Repetitive synaptic activity. 4-AP and 3,4-DAP not only enhanced the amount of transmitter released by nerve stimuli but also induced in high concentrations (100 µM - 1 mM) repetitive EPPs in response to a single nerve impulse (Lundh, 1978; Marshall and co-workers, 1979). The repetitive EPPs are induced by multiple action potentials in the motor nerve terminals as shown by extracellular focal recordings (Heuser and co-workers, 1979). During repetitive firing of the nerve terminal the successive presynaptic spikes released progressively less transmitter as revealed by the reduction in EPC amplitude (Fig. 3). Repetitive firing of the nerve terminals is more evident when the levels of calcium or of other divalent cations present in the extracellular medium is low. Raising the normal extracellular calcium concentration abolishes repetitive activity (Illes and Thesleff, 1978). This effect of calcium may be due to changes in the threshold for initiating an action potential in the nerve membrane (Frankenhaeuser, 1957).

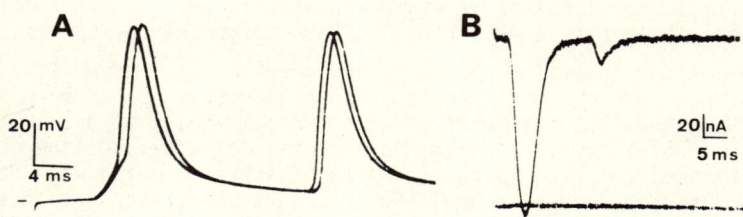

Fig. 3 - A) Repetitive action potentials in response to single nerve impulses. Intracellular recordings made in junctional areas of a frog neuromuscular junction, bathed in standard Ringer containing 100 µM 3,4-DAP in which excitation contraction was uncoupled by the use of the formamide method. B) Repetitive end-plate currents recorded at a holding membrane potential of -80 mV (lower tracing) during the action of 3,4-DAP (100 µM). Frog neuromuscular junction bathed in standard Ringer solution containing 7.5 µM (+)-tubocurarine. Excitation-contraction was uncoupled by the use of the glycerol method.

Spontaneous repetitive action potentials and autonomic activity has been observed with high concentrations of aminopyridines on different nerve structures of invertebrates and vertebrates (Pelhate and co-workers, 1972; Lemeignan, 1973; Hue and co-workers, 1976; Kirsch and Narahashi, 1978; Shapovalov and Shiriaev, 1978). This type of spontaneous activity when propagated to the motor nerve terminals probably induces a marked increase in transmitter output in the absence of nerve stimulation to give rise to strong contractures of the muscle (Vohra and Pradhan, 1964; Bowman and co-workers, 1976,1977; Harvey and Marshall, 1977a), which can be prevented by tetrodotoxin (TTX) as shown by Marshall and co-workers (1979).

Aminopyridines during repetitive nerve stimulation. Facilitation is a characteristic of many chemical synapses whereby the efficacy of synaptic transmission is increased following presynaptic activity. The effect of 4-AP has been investigated during repetitive nerve stimulation in order to gain more information about the mechanism of its presynaptic action. For this purpose, in some experiments, the motor nerve was stimulated with paired pulses of equal duration and intensity separated by different intervals, while in others by trains of stimuli at different frequencies. As shown in Fig. 4, facilitation, defined as $f = V-V_o/V_o$ (c.f. Mallart and Martin, 1967) where Vo and V are the amplitudes of the first and second EPPs produced by two action potentials, was found to be increased in magnitude by low concentrations of 4-AP (1-5 µM) when compared to controls. These results differ from those previously reported by Jacobs and Burley (1978) who found that the magnitude of facilitation at a given interval between pulses (30 msec) was not modified by low concentrations of 4-AP (5 µM). As illustrated in Fig. 4, facilitation of the second EPP decayed as the interval between the two EPPs increased. Altough 4-AP increased the magnitude of facilitation its rate of decay remained unaffected.

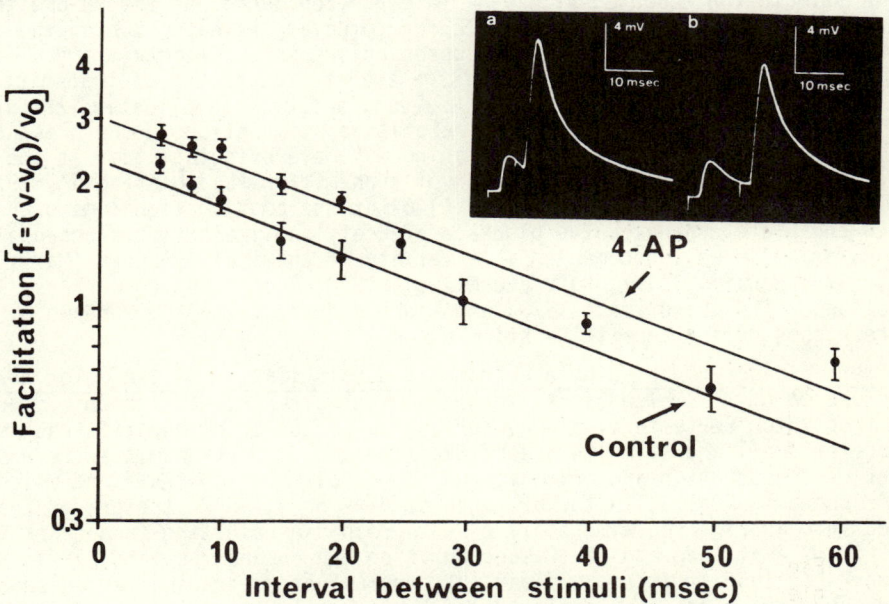

Fig. 4 - Magnitude and time course of facilitation of EPPs after a single conditioning stimulation under control conditions and during 4-AP (4 µM) treatment. Results obtained on the same frog junction bathed in standard Ringer containing (+)-tubocurarine (5 µM). Temperature 20°C. Each point is the mean ± S.E. of 10 measurements. Insert pairs of EPPs elicited at intervals of 5 msec (A) and 10 msec (B) in the presence of 4-AP.

With higher concentrations of 4-AP (10-50 µM), when pairs of stimuli were applied to curarized junctions, it was found that the second EPP of the pair was usually depressed at intervals interstimuli between 5 and 60 msec. Thus, instead of facilitation, a depression of the second response was always observed. It is worth noting that a similar depression was observed in curarized junctions when transmitter release was increased by elevating the extracellular calcium concentration to 6 or 8mM (Molgo, unpublished).

In mammalian junctions in which transmitter release was depressed by a low calcium/high magnesium medium, 4-AP has been reported to increase EPP amplitude in response to every successive stimulus during tetanic (100 Hz) nerve stimulation (Lundh, 1978). Similarly, in frog junctions in which the average quantal content of the EPP was small, 4-AP increased transmitter release during continual nerve stimulation at rates between 0.2 to 25 Hz (Molgo and co-workers, 1979a). These results obtained in junctions in which the normal release of transmitter has been depressed and in which probably large losses of transmitter do not occur, indicate that transmitter release can be well maintained during repetitive stimulation by an effective rate of transmitter mobilization from the stores to the release sites in the presence of 4-AP.

In contrast to the results obtained in junctions depressed by magnesium, when similar experiments were made in curarized junction, at nerve stimulation frequencies of 4 Hz at or above 50 Hz, only the first and sometimes also the second nerve impulse caused enhanced EPPs in the presence of 4-AP. The subsequent impulses evoked EPPs of either the same amplitude or of reduced size when compared to those recorded in the absence of the drug (Lundh, 1978; Illes and Thesleff, 1978; Molgo and co-workers, 1979a; Heuser and co-workers, 1979).

Thus, it is possible that the depression of the EPP amplitude during paired or tetanic nerve stimulation reported with 4-AP in curarized junctions may be due to a depletion of the transmitter pool available for immediate release, during the first response. Consistent with this idea are observations in the electric organ of Torpedo showing that the degree of depression was related to the amount of transmitter released (Dunant and co-workers, 1980). However, a factor complicating the interpretation of the rundown of the EPP during repetitive stimulation in the presence of 4-AP is the possibility that (+)-tubocurarine may have effects either at the presynaptic level impairing the mobilization of transmitter (see Glavinovic, 1979; Bowman, 1980; Magleby and co-workers, 1981) or at the postjunctional membrane blocking open end-plate channels. The blockade of acetylcholine-activated channels by (+)-tubocurarine is well documented in a variety of chemical synapses (Marty and co-workers, 1976; Manalis, 1977; Katz and Miledi, 1978; Ascher and co-workers, 1978, 1979; Colquhoun and co-workers, 1979) and might contribute to the rundown of the evoked responses during repetitive stimulation.

Transmitter release triggered by electrotonic depolarization of the motor nerve.

In the presence of TTX which blocks inward sodium currents, electrotonic depolarization of frog motor nerve terminals by current pulses of brief duration causes the appearance of small and stimulus graded EPP. The amount of transmitter released being dependent on the duration and intensity of the depolarization (Katz and Miledi, 1967, 1969). As shown in Fig. 5, in the presence of 4-AP or 3,4-DAP the graded EPP is converted into a triggered almost all or none response resulting in a giant EPP of about 50-70 mV amplitude and 50-80 msec duration (Lundh and Thesleff, 1977; Molgo and co-workers, 1980a). It seems clear that the amount of transmitter released contributed not only to the peak amplitude of the large EPP but also to their prolonged time course.

Similar large EPPs were also obtained when instead of using TTX, the preparations were exposed to high concentrations of calcium substituting the sodium content of the Ringer solution (Lundh and Thesleff, 1977; Lundh, 1978).

The large EPPs could be abolished in the absence of extracellular calcium but their calcium dependence was interpreted as being very low, since EPPs of approximately similar size could be generated in the presence of 0.2 to 20 mM external calcium concentration (Illes and Thesleff, 1978). However, it must be noted that as the EPP closely approached the limit set by the equilibrium potential for acetylcholine (about - 8 mV

-10 mV) variations in the EPP amplitude are difficult to detect. As reported by Illes and Thesleff (1978) manganese ions which are known to block the membrane permeability to calcium(Hagiwara and Byerly, 1981) completely abolished, when present in high concentrations the release of transmitter by an electrotonic current pulse. Furthermore, magnesium ions which compete with calcium and inhibit the liberation of acetylcholine by nerve impulses, failed even in concentrations as high as 32 mM to affect the size or the shape of the large EPPs. However, when the extracellular calcium concentration was reduced to 0.2 mM, 32 mM of magnesium blocked the all or none response and converted it into a stimulus graded EPP.

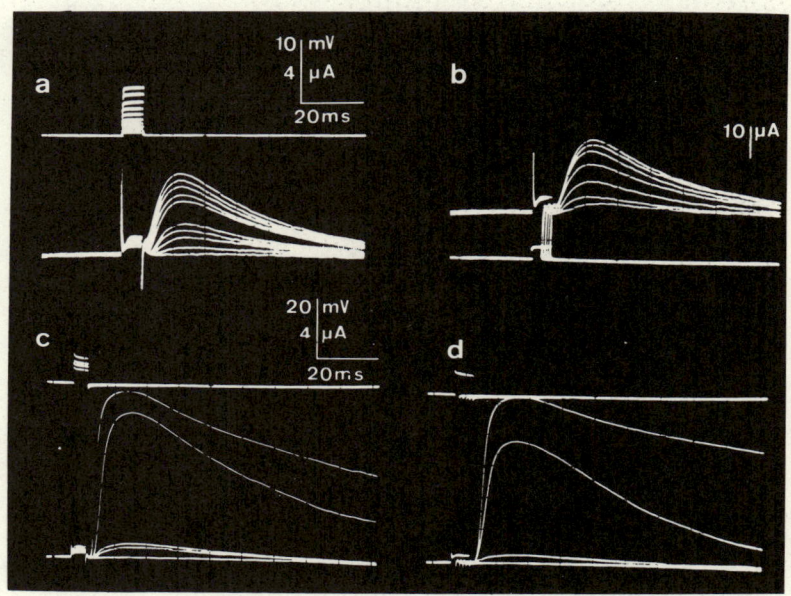

Fig. 5 - EPPs evoked by depolarizing current pulses applied to the preterminal of a frog neuromuscular junction bathed in standard Ringer containing 1 μM TTX before (a, b) and after 3,4-DAP (5 μM) treatment (c, d). Note the graded EPPs (a, b) and the almost all or none EPPs (c, d) in response to small increments in current intensity (a, c) or duration (b, d). Temperature 3.5°C. Resting membrane potential -70mV (Molgo and Thesleff unpublished).

Katz and Miledi (1979) have estimated by measuring end-plate currents (EPCs) and miniature end-plate currents (MEPCs), the number of quantal transmitter packets released from TTX-treated motor nerve terminals in response to brief depolarizing pulses either before or after 3,4-DAP treatment. By measuring this at a stable holding membrane potential these authors avoided the difficulties arising from non-linear summation of the voltage, which introduces uncertainty in estimating the quantal content of large EPPs. As shown by Katz and Miledi after 3,4-DAP (0.1-4 mM) treatment, transmitter release in response to a single stimulus was greatly increased. Estimations of the quantal content values during 3,4-DAP treatment based on the ratio between EPCs/MEPCs or from the ratio of the total charge (amplitude x duration) gave values between 1,000 and 46,200 quanta. Fig. 6 shows some examples of EPPs and EPCs obtained by electrotonic depolarization of TTX-treated motor nerve terminals during the action of 4-AP. As shown in these recordings the duration of

the EPPs or EPCs exceeded that of the MEPPs or MEPCs. This difference may reflect
the temporal dispersion of quanta due to the prolonged transmitter release during
the action of 4-AP.

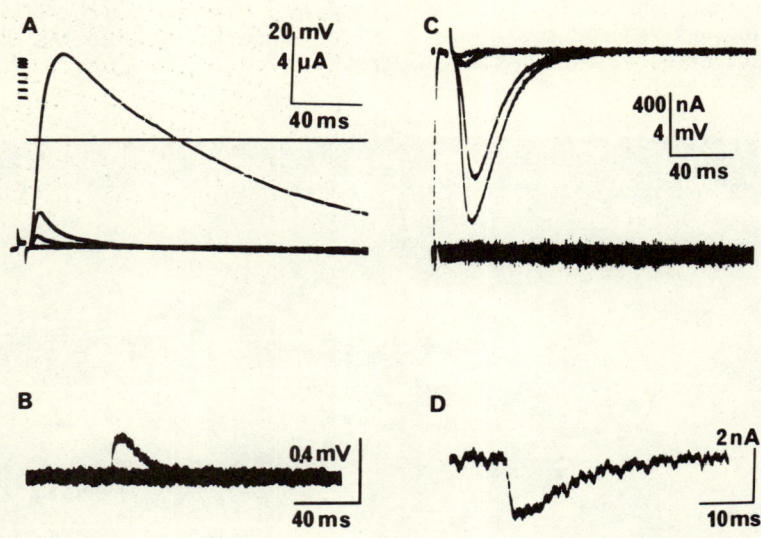

Fig. 6 - A. EPPs induced by depolarizing current pulses of
constant duration and increasing intensity (superimposed
tracing) applied to TTX-treated motor nerve terminals during
the action of 4-AP (1 mM). B. MEPP recorded on the same
end-plate before triggering the evoked responses. Resting
membrane potential -80 mV in A and B. C. EPCs recorded on
a different end-plate at a holding potential of -80 mV and
triggered by depolarizing current pulses of increasing
intensities (2 - 2.2 µA) applied to the TTX-treated motor
nerve terminals during the action of 3,4-DAP (100 µM).
D. MEPC recorded on the same junction as in C at a holding
potential of -80 mV.
In A, B, C and D, the frog neuromuscular junctions were
bathed in standard Ringer containing 1 µM TTX. Temperature
3°C.

One interesting effect observed during the action of 4-AP or 3,4-DAP was that
stimulation of TTX-treated motor nerve terminals with depolarizing currents, which
by itself caused little release of transmitter as judged by the magnitude of the
EPP evoked, when followed by an identical current pulse to the preceding one, facilitated in an all or none manner transmitter release as shown in Fig. 7. The facilitation of release may be due to the electrotonic properties which characterizes
the motor nerve terminals as discussed by Molgo and Thesleff (1981b). Alternatively,
the kinetics of the terminal voltage-sensitive calcium channels could be involved
i.e. the conditioning pulse may be altering the threshold for calcium influx, but
experimental evidence for such an action has so far not been obtained.

Reversal of antibiotic-induced neuromuscular blockade. The neuromuscular block produced by several antibiotics has been widely documented (see reviews by Corrado, 1963, Pittinger and Adamson, 1972 and Sanders and Sanders, 1979). Most of the experimental evidence indicates that both pre and postsynaptic mechanism are implicated in the neuromuscular block of the major group of antibiotics: the aminoglycosides, the polymyxins, the tetracyclines and the lincosamides. However, the relative contributions of both pre and postjunctional effects have not been quantitatively determined. Both 4-AP and 3,4-DAP through their selective action which increases evoked transmitter release have been reported to antagonize *in vitro* the neuromuscular block produced by the following aminoglycoside antibiotics: neomycin, amikacin, kanamycin, streptomycin and bekanamycin (Sobek and co-workers, 1968; Singh and co-workers, 1978a; Molgo and co-workers, 1979b; Maeno and Enomoto, 1980; Uchiyama and co-workers, 1981). Similarly 4-AP is an effective antagonist of the neuromuscular blockade produced by polymyxin B either *in vitro* (Singh and co-workers, 1978b; Durant and Lambert, 1981) or in anesthetized cats (Lee and co-workers, 1978). In contrast, the neuromuscular block produced by the tetracyclines or by some of the lincosamide antibiotics like clindamycin are not reversed by 3,4-DAP (Singh and co-workers, 1978b).
4-AP has also been shown to be effective in reversing the neuromuscular block produced by a combination of pancuronium and lincomycin in man (Booij and co-workers, 1978).
In conclusion, both 4-AP and 3,4-DAP antagonize the neuromuscular block produced by antibiotics which have magnesium-like prejunctional effects while they have little or no action when the predominant blocking action is postjunctional .

Antagonism of neurotoxins acting at the presynaptic level. The neurotoxic component of botulinum toxin which exists in several immunologically distinct forms (designated) A through G), inhibits the quantal release of acetylcholine from motor nerve terminals (for recent reviews see Thesleff, 1978; Howard and Gundersen, 1980; Sellin, 1981).
Experimental studies have shown that 4-AP is effective in overcoming the depression in transmitter release and to restore depressed neuromuscular transmission induced by botulinum toxin type A in mammalian and frog isolated neuromuscular preparations (Lundh and co-workers, 1977a; Tazieff-Depierre and co-workers, 1978; Simpson, 1978). Recent studies have shown that 3,4-DAP is about 6-7 times more potent than 4-AP in increasing evoked transmitter release in mammalian junctions poisoned with botulinum toxin type A (Molgo and co-workers, 1980a). The more marked effect of 3,4-DAP can be of clinical importance since 3,4-DAP has been reported to be less convulsant than 4-AP in laboratory animals (Lechat and co-workers, 1968). It is well known that botulinum toxin poisoned end-plates have a reduced sensitivity to extracellular calcium. The slope of the calcium dependence is about one third than at normal endplates (Cull Candy and co-workers, 1976a; Simpson, 1978). It is noteworthy that 4-AP restored the calcium dependence to approximately normal values (Lundh and co-workers, 1977a). The mechanism by which 4-AP affects the calcium dependence of the evoked transmitter release process is uncertain. This is not surprising since very little is known about the mechanism by which calcium initiates the release of transmitter at chemical synapses.
*In vivo*, 4-AP is particularly effective against botulinum toxin type A poisoning. The intravenous injection of 4-5 mg/kg 4-AP temporarily restored neuromuscular transmission in the rat from complete paralysis to normal as shown by measuring isometric twitches and tetanic tension in skeletal muscles indirectly stimulated. 4-AP was also effective in restoring muscle tone and general locomotor activity in rats that were dying after a lethal dose of the toxin, the effect lasting 1-2 hr (Thesleff and Lundh, 1979). In a recent outbreak of human type E botulism in England, 4-AP has been demonstrated to be of benefit in reducing the peripheral paralysis (Ball and co-workers, 1979). From the experimental and clinical studies, it appears that the aminopyridines may be useful antagonists of the paralytic effect of botulinum toxin. Since, as discussed by Sellin (1981), a likely treatment for

botulism might be the administration of a drug which increases transmitter release like 3,4-DAP or 4-AP plus an antitoxin.

Tetanus toxin strikingly resembles botulinum toxin in its neuromuscular paralyzing effect (Duchen and Tonge, 1973; Mellanby and Green, 1981). As with botulinum toxin, 4-AP temporarily restored neuromuscular transmission in the mouse phrenic-nerve hemidiaphragm preparation exposed to tetanus toxin in the organ bath. However, after development of complete paralysis, 4-AP was almost wholly inneffective in restoring neuromuscular transmission (Habermann and co-workers, 1980) as it has been reported for botulinum toxin (Simpson, 1978).

4-AP has also been reported to antagonize *in vitro* the neuromuscular block produced by crotoxin (Vital-Brazil and co-workers, 1979). This neurotoxin also inhibits the evoked release of acetylcholine from motor nerve terminals (Chang and Lee, 1977). In addition, Harvey and Marshall (1977b) and Kamenskaya and Thesleff (1979) have reported that aminopyridines improved neuromuscular transmission of nerve-muscle preparations partially blocked by β-bungarotoxin and taipoxin. However, this antagonistic effect of the aminopyridines was transient and followed by a complete neuromuscular blockade. In line with these findings, a recent study of Gundersen and co-workers (1981) using a gas chromatographic mass spectrometric assay for acetylcholine has shown that prior to the final inhibition by β-bungarotoxin of evoked transmitter release there was a significant increase of acetylcholine content in the rat diaphragm. However, 4-AP was inneffective in increasing acetylcholine output and failed to overcome the β-bungarotoxin-mediated blockade of transmitter release. In addition, Chang and Su (1980) have shown that 3,4-DAP markedly accelerates the time needed for β-bungarotoxin to inhibit neuromuscular transmission in isolated mouse diaphragm preparations. This suggests that the expected increase in calcium influx during the action of 3,4-DAP which probably leads to an increased transmitter output may increase the phospholipase activity of the toxin and consequently enhance its toxicity at the presynaptic level.

<u>4-aminopyridine on pathological conditions in which neuromuscular transmission is defective</u>. Human myasthenia gravis is a neuromuscular disease characterized by weakness and abnormal fatigability of skeletal muscle caused by an autoimmune response affecting the acetylcholine receptor protein complex at the end-plate (for recent reviews see Lindstrom and Dau, 1980; Vincent, 1980). A disease similar to human myasthenia can be produced in experimental animals by immunization with purified acetylcholine receptors. This has provided a model for studying both the complex pathological mechanism by which the autoimmune response impairs neuromuscular transmission and the basis for a rationale therapy.

In a recent electrophysiological study of neuromuscular transmission in rats immunized with acetylcholine receptors from Torpedo electric organ and in intercostal muscles taken at biopsy from patients with myasthenia gravis, Kim and co-workers (1980b) found that 4-AP dose-dependently increased EPP amplitude without altering spontaneous MEPP size. In addition, 4-AP reversed the postsynaptic block produced by low concentrations of (+)-tubocurarine, a drug known to be more effective in myasthenic than in normal muscles. The facilitatory action of 4-AP increases the safety margin of neuromuscular transmission in the myasthenic muscles so that even when the postsynaptic conductance change to acetylcholine presynaptically released is reduced in this condition , the increase in the quantal content of the EPP by 4-AP results in suprathreshold depolarization of the end-plate sufficient to trigger action potentials and restore muscle contraction in the diseased muscles. Consistent with these electrophysiological studies are the observations showing that 4-AP, when injected i.v. into rabbits with experimental autoimmune myasthenia, improved neuromuscular transmission as judged from electromyographic evidence (Heilbronn and co-workers, 1977). Similarly, repeated administration of 4-AP to patients with myasthenia gravis improved muscle strength as demonstrated by electrophysiological and clinical studies (Lundh and co-workers, 1979; Murray and Newson-Davis, 1981).

4-AP has also been tested in the myasthenic syndrome sometimes associated with bronchogenic carcinoma (Eaton-Lambert syndrome) a disorder of impaired transmitter release (Lambert and Elmqvist, 1971; Cull-Candy and co-workers, 1980) for which treatment is unsatisfactory. As shown by Sanders and co-workers (1980), 4-AP, in *in vitro* reversed the reduction in evoked transmitter release characterizing this pathological condition. Clinical studies have confirmed the effectiveness of 4-AP in improving neuromuscular transmission and the clinical state in patients with Eaton-Lambert syndrome (Lundh and co-workers, 1977b; Agoston and co-workers, 1978; Sanders and co-workers, 1980; Murray and Newson-Davis, 1981).

In conclusion, the results obtained with 4-AP in junctions affected by experimental autoimmune myasthenia, myasthenia gravis and Eaton-Lambert disorder indicate that the drug is effective in overcoming the defective neuromuscular transmission present in these diseases. Though presynaptic changes in myasthenia gravis or experimental autoimmune myasthenia do not seem to be the primary cause of the defect on neuromuscular transmission (Cull-Candy and co-workers, 1980; Alema and co-workers, 1981).

Antagonism of competitive neuromuscular blocking agents.
Experimental studies have shown that aminopyridines are effective antagonists of the block produced by (+)-tubocurarine, gallamine and pancuronium. In addition, the antagonistic effect of 4-AP as would be expected is greatly potentiated by small doses of anticholinesterase drugs such as neostigmine and pyridostigmine (Miller and co-workers, 1978). Among the aminopyridines studied, as far as we know only 4-AP has been used as a post-operative antagonist of muscle relaxants in clinical practice (Paskov and co-workers, 1973; Stoyanov and Vulchev, 1975; Stoyanov and co-workers, 1976; Miller and co-workers, 1979).

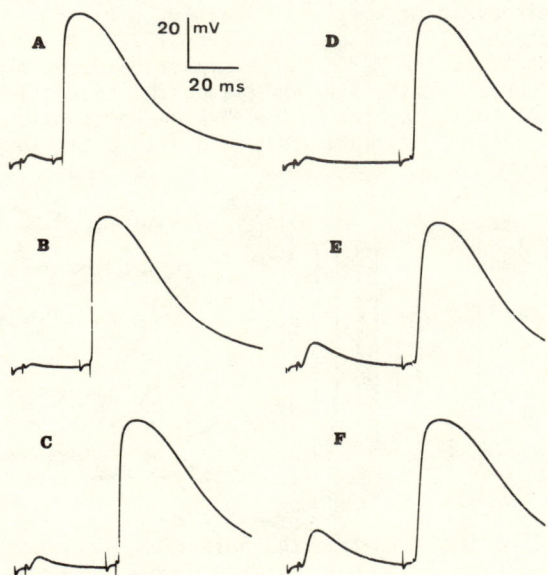

Fig. 7 - Facilitation of EPPs elicited by twin electrotonic depolarizing current pulses applied to TTX-treated motor nerve terminals during the action of 3,4-DAP (20μM). In A,B, C, EPPs were evoked at intervals of 12,23 and 32 msec. In D,E,F, at intervals of 42 msec. In D,E,F the stimulus intensity was increased gradually (pulses of 4 msec and 1.2, 1.3 and 1.4 μA, not shown). An interval of 2 min was allowed between the twin pulses. Calibration in A applies to all the recordings. Resting membrane potential -72 mV. Temperature 3°C. Frog neuromuscular junction bathed in standard Ringer containing 1 μM TTX.

Aminopyridines and spontaneous transmitter release.

Spontaneous quantal transmitter release at normal, depolarized and botulinum treated junctions. Studies of the actions of 4-AP or 3,4-DAP at frog end-plates have shown that both drugs in micromolar concentrations have no consistent effect on spontaneous quantal transmitter release as far as can be judged from MEPP frequency (Molgo and co-workers, 1977; Jacobs and Burley, 1978; Durant and Marshall, 1978). Although a gradual increase in the frequency of MEPPs after addition of 1 mM 4-AP with time has been reported (Marshall and co-workers, 1979) these effects are minor and not always reproducible in frog, unstimulated end-plates bathed in normal Ringer solution containing TTX to block sodium currents (Lemeignan and Molgo, unpublished). Similarly, 4-AP and 3,4-DAP failed to affect MEPP frequency in normal or botulinum toxin poisoned mammalian end-plates (Lundh,1978; Kim and co-workers, 1980a; Molgo and co-workers, 1980a). However, in the presence of ouabain a drug that has no effect on MEPP frequency in botulinum treated junctions (Cull-Candy and co-workers, 1976a), 4-AP was reported to produce bursts of high frequency MEPPs (Lundh and co-workers, 1977a). The mechanism of this action remains as yet unclear.
It is well known that depolarization of the motor nerve terminals either by focal currents or by increasing the potassium concentration in the extracellular medium, increases the frequency of MEPPs (del Castillo and Katz, 1954b; Liley, 1956). The increase in MEPP frequency produced by a raised potassium concentration presumably results from the opening of gated voltage-sensitive calcium channels allowing calcium influx which leads to an increase in both intraterminal calcium and transmitter output. Since the aminopyridines may act directly on voltage-sensitive calcium channels in the nerve terminals (Lundh and Thesleff, 1977) it was of interest to study if 4-AP or 3,4-DAP modifies the MEPP frequency activated by a maintained depolarization of the motor nerve terminals brought about by increasing the external potassium concentration. As shown in Fig. 8, 3,4-DAP had no consistent effect on MEPP frequency at frog end-plates depolarized by elevated potassium ions.

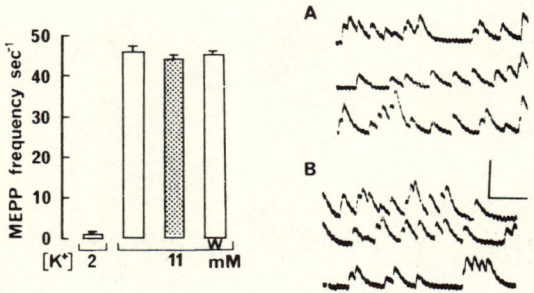

Fig. 8 - Effect of changing the potassium concentration in the medium from 2 to 11 mM on MEPP frequency (ordinate).Note that 100µM 3,4-DAP applied for 20 min (stippled column) had no further effect on the increase in MEPP frequency produced by raised potassium when compared to controls or after washing out the drug (W). Resting membrane potential remained unchanged after 3,4-DAP treatment in high potassium medium. Temperature was 20°C. The Ringer solution contained 1 mM calcium and 1µM TTX. The columns from left to right indicate the order in which the recordings were made.
A and B show examples of MEPPs recorded before (A) and after 100µM 3,4-DAP treatment (B) in a frog end-plate bathed in Ringer solution containing 1 mM calcium, 11 mM potassium and TTX (1µM). Temperature was 10°C. Calibration in B is 1 mV and 200 msec. and applies also to A.

It has also been reported that 4-AP (1 mM) has no effect on the increase in MEPP frequency in frog end-plates depolarized in elevated external $K^+$ and it does not modify the increase in MEPP rate produced in depolarized junctions by increasing external calcium concentration (Van der Kloot and Madden, 1981). Therefore, these results do not seem to support the hypothesis that aminopyridines have a direct effect on voltage-sensitive calcium channel kinetics.

Non quantal transmitter release. It is well known that only a small fraction of the spontaneous release of acetylcholine from resting motor nerve terminals is in the form of quanta. Most of the release occurs in the form of molecular acetylcholine efflux which depolarizes the end-plate by about 40 μV (see Katz and Miledi, 1977 for a discussion of non-quantal acetylcholine release). Recent studies of Gundersen and Jenden (1981) who used a gas chromatographic mass spectrometric assay for acetylcholine, have shown that 4-AP (100 μM) does not have a measurable effect on the resting output of acetylcholine from rat diaphragm preparations indicating that 4-AP in the concentrations used probably does not effect the molecular leakage of acetylcholine.

"Giant" MEPPs. 3,4-DAP in concentrations of about 1 mM has been reported to induce the appearance of a population of spontaneous MEPPs with larger than normal amplitude, the so called "giant MEPPs" (G-MEPPs), at frog end-plates treated with TTX (Durant and Marshall, 1978,1980; Katz and Miledi, 1979). Similar G-MEPPs were observed in the presence of 3,4-DAP and 4-AP (Fig. 9 ) following repetitive electrotonic stimulation of TTX-treated motor nerve terminals (Molgo and Thesleff, unpublished).

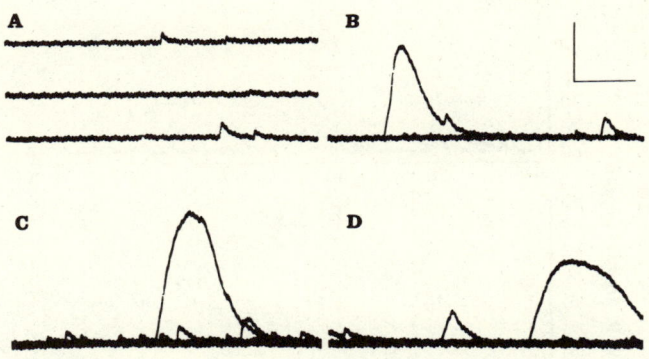

Fig.9 - Examples of intracellularly recorded MEPPs and G-MEPPs before (A) and after electrotonic stimulation (5 Hz for 2 min) of the motor nerve preterminal (B,C and D) of a frog neuromuscular junction bathed in Ringer solution containing 1 mM 4-AP and 1 μM TTX. Temperature was 3°C. Note that both time to peak and decay time of G-MEPPs (B, C,D) are prolonged compared with MEPPs. Resting membrane potential during recordings was -80 mV. Calibration in B is 1 mV and 200 msec and applies to A, C and D.

It seems quite probable that G-MEPPs such as those shown in Fig. 9, result from the interaction of large amounts of acetylcholine with the postsynaptic receptors since (+)-tubocurarine (5 μM) abolished all MEPPs including the G-MEPPs. In addition since the G-MEPPs were recorded in the presence of TTX, this seems to exclude the possibility that inward sodium currents may be involved in their generation. Furthermore, if the G-MEPPs result from the synchronous release of acetylcholine quanta it would be expected that by lowering the temperature of the bathing medium it would be possible to detect the individual quanta making up the G-MEPPs but as shown in Fig. 9, no obvious steps in the rising phase of the G-MEPPs were observed which could indicate temporal dispersion of quanta. G-MEPPs which have different electrophysiological properties than those characterizing normal MEPPs have also been reported with 4-aminoquinoline (Molgo and co-workers, 1980b; Molgo and Thesleff, 1981a). Altough several experimental procedures which drastically affect transmitter release are known to induce G-MEPPs (Katz and Miledi, 1969; Pécot-Dechavassine, 1970; Benoit and co-workers, 1973; Hawgood and Santana de Sa, 1979; Cull-Candy and co-workers, 1976a,b; Spira, 1976) their nature and functional significance remains for the moment quite obscure. G-MEPPs observed in the presence of acid pH, hypertonicity, vinblastine and repetitive stimulation have been attributed to the pluriquantal release of acetylcholine from large packets formed from the fusion of synaptic vesicles prior to exocytosis (Pécot-Dechavassine and Couteaux, 1972a,b; Pécot-Dechavassine, 1976) or from oversized vesicles formed during vesicle membrane recycling (Heuser, 1974). It is not possible at present to state whether similar morphological correlates account for the G-MEPPs observed with the aminopyridines and related compounds.

Spontaneous MEPPs after nerve stimulation. The aminopyridines have also been reported to have interesting effects on MEPP frequency during and after repetitive nerve stimulation. As described by many investigators high frequency stimulation of the motor nerve (10-100 Hz) increases the frequency of MEPPs during the period of tetanic stimulation and after its cessation. These increases in MEPP frequency were further accelerated by the aminopyridines studied. As shown by Lev-Tov and Rahamimoff (1980) 3-AP (5 mM) greatly increased the frequency of MEPPs during and after tetanic stimulation (50 Hz for 40 sec) provided there is an inward electrochemical calcium gradient.

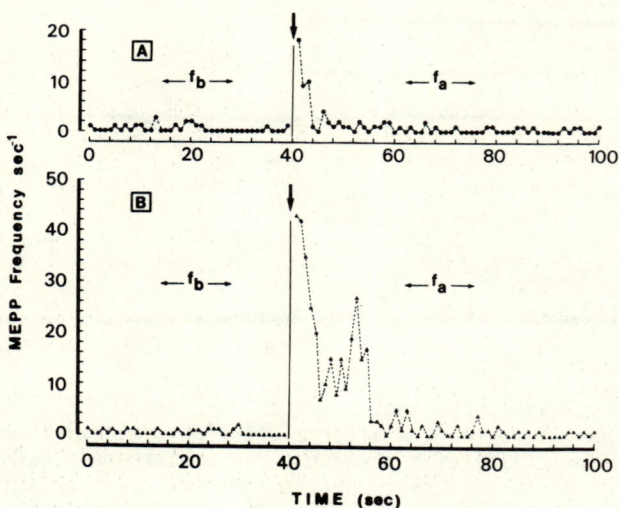

Fig. 10- Time course of the potentiation of MEPP frequency produced by a single electrotonic depolarization of the preterminal of a neuromuscular junction bathed in strontium-Ringer containing TTX (1 µM) before(A) and after 4-AP (20µM) treatment(B). $f_b$ denotes MEPP frequency before stimulation. $f_a$ denotes the frequency of MEPPs after applying an electrotonic current pulse of 4 msec duration and 2 µA intensity (indicated by an arrow)either before or after 4-AP treatment Temperature was 6°C. Each circle or triangle indicates data collected per second.

Similarly 4-AP (10-50µM) increased the frequency of MEPPs appearing after nerve stimulation at low rates (0.2-4 Hz) in frog end-plates in which the extracellular calcium has been substituted by strontium (Molgo and Guerrero, unpublished). In addition as shown in a representative experiment (Fig. 10) 4-AP markedly increased the frequency of MEPPs when single electrotonic depolarizations were applied to TTX-treated motor nerve terminals and prolonged the post-stimulation decay of the MEPP frequency. The aminopyridine-induced increase in MEPP frequency during and after repetitive nerve stimulation or after a single electrotonic depolarization of the motor nerve terminals may be related to an augmented influx of the activating cation mediating transmitter release. Since under conditions in which the extracellular calcium concentration is probably less than the intracellular concentration (reversed calcium gradient) it has been reported that 3-AP supresses the tetanic potentiation of MEPPs (Lev-Tov and Rahamimoff, 1980).

## AMINOPYRIDINES ON INVERTEBRATE NEUROMUSCULAR JUNCTIONS.

The effects of some of the isomeric monoaminopyridines have also been studied on different neuromuscular junctions of invertebrates by using electrophysiological techniques. The results obtained at the lobster neuromuscular junction showed that 2-AP (1 mM) increased the amplitude of both neurally elicited excitatory and inhibitory post-synaptic potentials without altering either the resting membrane potential or the equilibrium potential at either synapse.

Moreover, in the excitatory synapse 2-AP did not affect the average miniature excitatory junctional potential amplitude or frequency but increased by approximately a factor of 3 the quantal content of the evoked potentials, indicating that the drug increased the amount of excitatory transmitter released. Although no direct evaluations of the quantal content of the inhibitory evoked responses could be performed it is likely that 2-AP also increased the release of transmitter at the inhibitory terminal (Schauf and co-workers, 1976).

4-AP (10 µM-10 mM) has also been reported to increase the amplitude of the excitatory post-synaptic currents at the locust neuromuscular junction probably by increasing the release of transmitter (Anwyl, 1977). Similarly, the amplitude of the excitatory junctional potentials evoked by pre-synaptic stimulation at frequencies of 1 and 10 Hz were increased by 4-AP (25 µM) at the crayfish neuromuscular junction (Zucker and Lara-Estrella, 1979).

A detailed analysis of the effects of 4-AP at the neuromuscular junction of *Drosophila larvae* made by Jan and co-workers (1977) has shown that the drug greatly increased the quantal content of the evoked junctional potentials without altering their calcium dependence. Moreover, 4-AP (4-8 mM) did not modify the amplitude or frequency of the spontaneous miniature excitatory junctional potentials but markedly increased their frequency after stimulation. Junctions treated with 4-AP also showed a prolonged increase of calcium conductance after nerve stimulation since iontophoresis of calcium at the nerve terminal as late as 30 msec after nerve stimulation could still induce transmitter release. The duration of the calcium conductance increase was dependent on 4-AP concentration and was insensitive to tetrodotoxin but could be suppressed at any time by applying a hyperpolarizing current pulse of sufficient strength.

In recent years there has been increasing evidence that l-glutamate is the most likely candidate for the excitatory transmitter at the arthropod neuromuscular junction (Gerschenfeld, 1973; Usherwood and Cull-Candy, 1975; Jan and Jan, 1976). It therefore seems reasonable to conclude that the aminopyridines enhance neurally evoked transmitter release not only at the vertebrate neuromuscular junction where acetylcholine is the transmitter, but also in invertebrate neuromuscular synapses where the excitatory transmitter is l-glutamate and possibly in those where aminobutyrate (GABA) is the inhibitory transmitter.

Aminopyridines at the postsynaptic level.

Resting membrane potential. None of the isomeric mono or diaminopyridines in the concentrations used (1 µM - 8 mM) exert any direct effect on the resting membrane potential from a variety of isolated skeletal muscle fibres from vertebrates and invertebrates suggesting that the resting potassium permeability is unaffected.

End-plate currents. When neurally elicited EPCs were recorded under controlled membrane potential, 4-AP, in low concentrations increased EPC amplitude without affecting its time course (Molgo and co-workers, 1977). Neither did the drug affect the time constant of the decay phase of EPCs in junctions treated with (+)-tubocurarine, a drug known to shorten the duration of the falling phase of the EPCs (Mallart and Molgo, 1978; Katz and Miledi, 1979). Furthermore, although 4-AP markedly increased the amplitude of EPCs recorded from lobeline or polymyxin-B treated junctions, the drug did not affect the shortened EPC duration observed with both treatments which is believed to be due to the blockade of conductance through the acetylcholine-activated channels of the end-plate (Lambert and co-workers, 1980; Durant and Lambert, 1981).

Analysis of the time course of EPCs elicited by electrotonic depolarization of TTX-treated motor nerve terminals has shown that when transmitter release is greatly potentiated by 4-AP or 3,4-DAP, the time course of the EPCs becomes dependent on the amount of transmitter released (see fig. 6; Katz and Miledi, 1979; Molgo and Thesleff, unpublished). These observations suggest that the time course of the falling phase of the EPCs varies with the amount of transmitter released from the motor nerve terminals and with the concentration of acetylcholine in the synaptic cleft. Although 4-AP and 3,4-DAP markedly increased the current flow in the postsynaptic membrane in response to nerve stimulation or to an electrotonic depolarization neither of the drugs caused any alteration in the equilibrium potential for acetylcholine i.e. the membrane potential at which acetylcholine presynaptically released did not elicit a net flow of current (Fig. 11) indicating that both drugs do not block the potassium conductance activated by transmitter action.

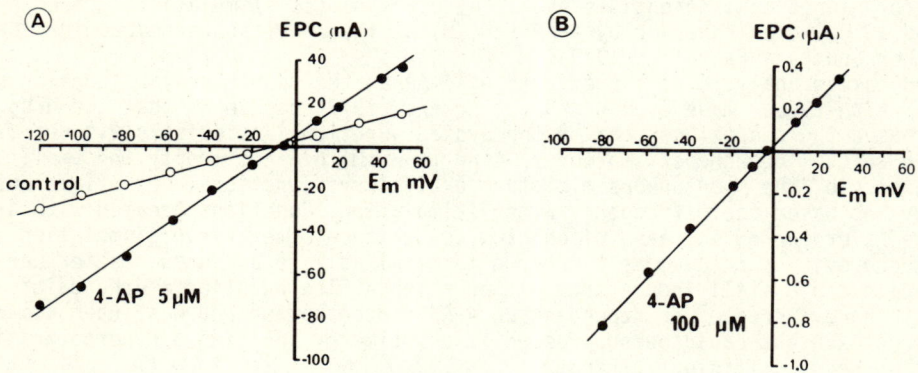

Fig. 11 - Current-voltage relationship for peak amplitude of EPCs recorded at frog end-plates. In A, EPCs were evoked by nerve stimulation and (+)-tubocurarine (5µM) was present before and after 4-AP (5µM) treatment on the same end-plate. Temperature 21°C. In B, EPCs were evoked by current pulses of 4 msec duration with constant intensities (3µA) applied to TTX-treated motor nerve preterminal during 4-AP action. The interval between step changes in potential (Em) was 60 sec. Temperature 4°C.

Action potentials. 4-AP and 3,4-DAP slow the repolarizing phase without altering the rate of rise and the overshoot of directly and indirectly elicited action potentials in a variety of skeletal muscle membranes (Molgo and co-workers, 1975; Lundh and co-workers, 1977; Horn and co-workers, 1979; Durant and Marshall, 1980; Kim and co-workers, 1980). The aminopyridine-induced potassium channel blockade account for the prolongation of the repolarizing phase of the muscle action potential and might play an important role in the enhancement of muscle contractility (see Thesleff, 1980).

MECHANISM OF ACTION.

It is widely accepted in chemical synapses that when an action potential invades the nerve terminal, the large change in potential causes an influx of calcium and the subsequent release of transmitter. From the experimental evidence considered so far, it seems likely that the aminopyridines act at some stage in the transmitter release process related to the entry of calcium into the terminal. How can aminopyridines enhance calcium entry and hence transmitter release evoked by nerve impulses? The facilitatory effect of the aminopyridines on transmitter release evoked by nerve impulses has been related to the ability of these drugs to block the potassium channels of the spike in nerve membranes(Molgo and co-workers,1977). In fact there is quite good evidence that the mono and diaminopyridines both prolong the repolarizing phase of the action potential and block the voltage-dependent potassium channels in cockroach axons (Pelhate and co-workers, 1974), squid giant axons (Yeh and co-workers, 1976a,b; Meves and Pichon, 1977; Kirsch and Narahashi, 1978), presynaptic terminals of the squid stellate ganglion (Llinas and co-workers, 1976a,b), frog myelinated nerve fibres (Ulbricht and Wagner, 1976; Dubois unpublished) and mammalian non-myelinated or myelinated nerve fibres (Bostock and co-workers, 1981). Furthermore, there is strongly suggestive evidence that the aminopyridines also block the potassium conductance in the unmyelinated motor nerve terminals as may be inferred from the increase in the width of the presynaptic action potential at the frog neuromuscular junction (see Fig. 2). Thus the facilitatory effect of the aminopyridines can be explained by assuming that the prolongation of the presynaptic action potential in the nerve terminal increases the influx of calcium and thereby the amount of transmitter released in response to nerve impulses.

It is well known that voltage-sensitive calcium channels exist in the presynaptic membrane of the motor nerve terminals and that the calcium current flowing through these channels mediates evoked transmitter release (Katz and Miledi, 1969). Furthermore, the calcium current entering the motor nerve terminals upon depolarization is probably under normal conditions prevented from becoming regenerative by an opposing efflux of potassium that both the aminopyridines and tetraethylammonium can block. Thus, it would be expected that by suppressing the potassium current that normally opposes the inward calcium current this would allow the calcium current to become regenerative. Direct evidence for such a calcium current has been obtained by Llinas and co-workers (1976b; 1981a,b) at the giant synapse of the squid following pharmacological blockade of both sodium and potassium conductances with TTX and the aminopyridines (3 or 4-AP). Under these conditions presynaptic depolarization can generate calcium spikes in the terminal and evoke the release of transmitter (Llinas and co-workers, 1976a). Similarly, at frog end-plates in which sodium and potassium conductances havebeen blocked by TTX and aminopyridines respectively, electrotonic depolarization of the motor nerve terminals probably also initiates regenerative calcium spikes which lead to a massive and prolonged release of transmitter (see Fig. 5 and 6), as previously shown by Katz and Miledi (1969) for tetraethylammonium, a well known potassium channel blocking agent.

In most of the nerve membranes studied, the blockade of potassium channels by the aminopyridines has been shown to be both time and voltage-dependent. The block being removed by repetitive pulsing or by long lasting depolarizations (Yeh and co-workers, 1976a,b; Ulbricht and Wagner, 1976; Llinas and co-workers, 1976a; Meves and Pichon, 1977; Kirsch and Narahashi, 1978). In addition the blockade of the potassium conductance by the aminopyridines in unmyelinated squid axons differs in many respects from that produced by tetraethylammonium as discussed by Yeh and co-workers (1976b). However, it is worth noting that the facilitatory action of the aminopyridines and tetraethylammonium is rather similar in terms of their effects on transmitter release evoked by nerve stimuli or by an electrotonic depolarization of TTX-treated motor nerve terminals (Lundh and Thesleff, 1977; Katz and Miledi, 1979; Molgo and co-workers 1980a; Molgo and Thesleff, 1981b) suggesting that the aminopyridine-induced blockade of potassium channels at the unmyelinated motor nerve terminals differs from that reported in unmyelinated axons. Consistent with this idea are observations showing that the aminopyridines increase transmitter release in depressed junctions during repetitive nerve stimulation, which indicates that the blockade of potassium channels in the presynaptic nerve terminal is not time-dependent as it has been reported in unmyelinated axons. Since if repetitive pulsing had effectively removed the blockade of potassium channels induced by the aminopyridines, then it would be expected that transmitter release would be reduced during repetitive nerve stimulation. However, no such an effect was observed (Lundh, 1978; Molgo and co-workers, 1979a). Furthermore, although the reason is not at present completely clear, it is obvious that the electrotonic properties which characterize the presynaptic motor nerve terminals differ from those of the axon (Molgo and Thesleff, 1981b) and may explain the facilitatory effects of aminopyridines during paired electrotonic depolarization of TTX-treated motor nerve terminals (see Fig. 7). In addition, these observations suggest that the aminopyridine-induced potassium channel blockade of the motor nerve terminals is not voltage-dependent as it has been reported in axonal membranes. Therefore, it is conceivable that the potassium conductance system of the motor nerve terminals may involve processes substantially different from those evident in unmyelinated axons.

An alternative explanation of the effect of aminopyridines on the motor nerve terminal membrane has been proposed by Lundh and Thesleff (1977). They hypothesized that 4-AP might act directly on voltage-dependent calcium channels in the nerve terminal membrane increasing the influx of calcium associated with an action potential and the subsequent release of transmitter. This hypothesis that aminopyridines may have a direct effect on calcium conductance was tested in studies at frog motor nerve terminals using the frequency of MEPPs as a measure of calcium influx (see Fig. 8). However, the results of these experiments together with those recently reported by Van der Kloot and Madden (1981) do not seem to give support to this hypothesis, though the evidence is obviously quite indirect. Direct evidence that aminopyridines do not modify the voltage-dependent calcium conductance at the squid presynaptic terminal will be provided by Llinas and co-workers in this Symposium. It is worth mentioning that no evidence has been obtained indicating that the aminopyridines may trigger calcium release from intraterminal stores nor that these drugs may have direct effects on the cooperative requirements for calcium in the release process at both invertebrate and vertebrate neuromuscular junctions.

In conclusion, it appears well established that aminopyridines facilitate neuromuscular transmission by a predominant presynaptic action. The ability of aminopyridines to block the potassium conductance in the motor nerve terminal and hence lengthen the presynaptic action potential seems to be the primary action of these drugs which contributes to the enhanced calcium influx and consequently to the increase in evoked transmitter release. Although increasingly electrophysiological, biochemical and morphological information has become available on the effects of aminopyridines at the neuromuscular junction, we must be aware that a better understanding of the mechanism of transmitter release should lead to a better knowledge of the mode of action of these drugs; conversely we may learn probably more on the mechanisms which regulate transmitter release from further work on the mode of action of aminopyridines.

ACKNOWLEDGEMENTS

I would like to thank Mrs M. Lemeignan with whom I have worked during the past several years for many helpful discussions and comments, Mrs J. Josso and Mrs N. Letteron for expert technical and photographic assistance, Mrs C. Angeli for typing the manuscript, Professor P. Lechat for his continual interest concerning this work and to the C.N.R.S. for support.

REFERENCES

Agoston, S., P. van Weerden and A.Broekert (1978). Br. J. Anaesth. 50, 383-385.
Alema, S., S.G. Cull-Candy, R. Miledi and A. Trautmann (1981). J. Physiol.(London) 311, 251-266.
Anwyl, R. (1977). J. Physiol. (London) 273, 389-404.
Ascher, P., A. Marty and T.O. Neild (1978). J. Physiol. (London) 278, 207-235.
Ascher, P., W.A. Large and H.P. Rang (1979). J. Physiol. (London) 295, 139-170.
Ball, A.P., R.B. Hopkinson, I.D. Farrell, J.G.P. Hutchinson, R. Paul, R.D.S. Watson, A.J.F. Page, R.G.F. Parker, C.W. Edwards, M. Snow, D.K. Scott, A. Leone-Ganado, A. Hastings, A.C. Ghosh and R.J. Gilbert (1979). Quart. J. Med. New Series 48, 473-491.
Bennett, M.R. and T. Florin (1974). J. Physiol. (London) 238, 93-107.
Benoit P.H., M.L. Audibert-Benoit and M. Peyrot (1973).Arch. Ital. Biol. 111,323-335.
Booij, L.H.D.J., R.D. Miller and J.F. Crul (1978). Anesth. Analg. 57, 316-321.
Booij, L.H.D.J., F. Van der Pol, J.F. Crul and R.D. Miller (1980). Anesth. Analg. 59, 31-34.
Bostock, H., T.A. Sears and R.M. Sherratt (1981). J. Physiol. (London) 313, 301-315.
Bowman, W.C., A.L. Harvey and I.G. Marshall (1976). J. Pharm. Pharmacol. 88, 79P.
Bowman, W.C., A.L. Harvey and I.G. Marshall (1977). Naunyn-Schmiedeberg's Arch. Pharmacol. 297, 99-103.
Bowman, W.C. (1980). Anesth. Analg. 59, 935-943.
Chang, C.C. and J.D. Lee (1977). Naunyn-Schmiedeberg's Arch. Pharmacol. 296, 159-168.
Chang C.C. and M.J. Su (1980). Toxicon 18, 481-484.
Colquhoun, D., F. Dreyer and R.E. Sheridan (1979). J. Physiol. (London) 293, 247-284.
Corrado, A.P. (1963). Anesth. Analg. 42, 1-5.
Cull-Candy, S.G., H. Lundh and S. Thesleff (1976a). J. Physiol. (London) 260, 177-203.
Cull-Candy, S.G., J. Fohlman, D. Gustavsson, R. Lüllmann-Rauch and S. Thesleff (1976b) Neuroscience 1, 175-180.
Cull-Candy, S.G., R. Miledi and A. Trautmann (1979). J. Physiol. (London) 287, 247-265.
Cull-Candy, S.G., R. Miledi, A. Trautmann and O.D. Uchitel (1980). J. Physiol.(London) 299, 621-638.
Datyner, N.B. and P. Gage (1980). J. Physiol. (London) 303, 299-314.
del Castillo, J. and B. Katz (1954a). J. Physiol. (London) 124, 560-573.
del Castillo, J. and B. Katz (1954b). J. Physiol. (London) 124, 586-604.
Duchen, L.W. and D.A. Tonge (1973). J. Physiol. (London) 228, 157-172.
Dunant, Y., L. Eder and L. Servetiadis-Hirt (1980). J. Physiol. (London) 298, 185-203.
Durant, N.N. and I.G. Marshall (1978). J. Physiol. (London) 280, 21P
Durant, N.N. and I.G. Marshall (1980). Eur. J. Pharmacol. 67, 201-208.
Durant, N.N. and J.J. Lambert (1981). Br. J. Pharmacol. 72, 41-47.
Fastier, F.N. and M.A. Mc Dowall (1958). Aust. J. exp. Biol. 36, 365-372.
Foldes, F.F., G. Braak, H. van Wezel, R. Huynen, S. Agoston and J.F. Crul (1976). American Society of Anesthesiology. Abstract of Proceedings pp. 561-562.
Frankenhaeuser, B. (1957). J. Physiol. (London) 137, 245-260.
Gerschenfeld, H.M. (1973). Physiol. Rev. 53, 1-119.
Glavinovic, M.I. (1979). J. Physiol. (London) 290, 499-506.
Gundersen, C.B. and D.J. Jenden (1981). Br. J. Pharmac. 72, 461-470.
Gundersen, C.B., D.J. Jenden and M.W. Newton (1981). J. Physiol. (London) 310, 13-35.

Habermann, E., F. Dreyer and H. Bigalke (1980). Naunyn-Schmiedeberg's Arch. Pharmacol. 311, 33-40.
Hagiwara, S. and L. Byerly (1981). Ann. Rev. Neurosci. 4, 69-125.
Harvey,A.L.and I.G. Marshall (1977a). Comp. Biochem. Physiol. 58C, 161-165.
Harvey, A.L. and I.G. Marshall (1977b). Eur. J. Pharmacol. 44, 303-309.
Harvey, A.L. and I.G. Marshall (1977c). Naunyn-Schmiedeberg's Arch. Pharmacol. 299, 53-60.
Hawgood, B.J. and S. Santana de Sa (1979). Neuroscience 4, 293-303.
Heilbronn, E., C. Mattsson and E. Stalberg (1977). Excerpta Medica International Congress (Abstr.) Series n°427, p. 105.
Heuser,J.E.(1974). J. Physiol. (London) 239, 106-108P.
Heuser, J.E., T.S. Reese, M.J. Jan, L. Jan and L. Evans (1979). J. Cell. Biol. 81, 275-300.
Horn, A.S., J.J. Lambert and I.G. Marshall (1979). Br. J. Pharmacol. 65, 53-62.
Howard, B.D. and C.B. Gundersen (1980). Ann. Rev. Pharmacol. Toxicol. 20, 307-336.
Hue, B., M. Pelhate, J.J. Callec and J. Chanelet (1976). J. exp. Biol. 65, 517-527.
Illes, P. and S. Thesleff (1978). Br. J. Pharmacol. 64, 623-629.
Jacobs, R.S. and E.S. Burley (1978). Neuropharmacology 17, 439-444.
Jan, L.Y. and Y.N. Jan (1976). J. Physiol. (London) 262, 215-236.
Jan, Y.N., L.Y. Jan and M.J.D. Dennis (1977). Proc. R. Soc. (London) B, 198,87-108.
Kamenskaya, M.A. and S. Thesleff (1979). Toxicon 17, Suppl.1, P80.
Kapff, J. (1959). Arch. Exper. Path. Pharmacol. 236, 149-152.
Katz, B. and R. Miledi (1965). Proc.Roy.Soc. (London) B 161, 483-495.
Katz, B. and R. Miledi (1967). Proc. Roy. Soc. (London) B 167, 23-38.
Katz, B. and R. Miledi (1969). J. Physiol. (London) 203, 689-706.
Katz, B. and R. Miledi (1977). Proc. Roy. Soc. (London) B 197, 285-297.
Katz, B. and R. Miledi (1978). Proc. Roy. Soc. (London) B 203, 119-133.
Katz, B. and R. Miledi (1979). Proc. Roy. Soc. (London) B 205, 369-378.
Kim, Y.I., M.M. Goldner and D.B. Sanders (1980a). Muscle and Nerve 3, 105-111.
Kim, Y.L., M.M. Goldner and D.B. Sanders (1980b). Muscle and Nerve 3, 112-119.
Kirsch, G.E. and T. Narahashi (1978). Biophys. J. 22, 507-511.
Lambert, E.H. and D. Elmqvist (1971). Ann. N. Y. Acad. Sci. 183, 183-199.
Lambert, J.J., R.J. Volle and E.G. Henderson (1980). Proc. Natl. Acad. Sci. (USA) 77, 5003-5007.
Lechat, P., G. Deysson, M. Lemeignan and M. Adolphe (1968). Ann. Pharmac. Fr. 26, 345-349.
Lee, C., A.J.C. de Silva and R.L. Katz (1978). Anesthesiology 49, 256-259.
Lemeignan, M. and P. Lechat (1967). C. R. Acad. Sci. (Paris) Ser.D 264, 169-172.
Lemeignan, M. (1973). Neuropharmacology 12, 641-651.
Lev-Tov, A. and Rahamimoff, R. (1980). J. Physiol. (London) 309, 247-273.
Liley, A.W. (1956). J. Physiol. (London) 134, 427-443.
Lindstrom, J. and P. Dau (1980). Ann. Rev. Pharmacol. Toxicol. 20, 337-362.
Llinás, R., K. Walton and V. Bohr (1976a). Biophys. J. 16, 83-86.
Llinás, R., Steinberg, I.Z. and K. Walton (1976b). Proc. Natl. Acad. Sci. USA 73, 2918-2922.
Llinás, R., I.Z. Steinberg and K. Walton (1981a). Biophys. J. 33, 289-322.
Llinás, R., I.Z. Steinberg and K. Walton (1981b). Biophys. J. 33, 323-352.
Lundh, H. (1978). Brain Res. 153, 307-318.
Lundh, H. (1979). Acta Pharmacol. Toxicol. 44, 343-346.
Lundh, H., S. Leander and S. Thesleff (1977a). J. Neurol. Sci. 32, 29-43.
Lundh, H., O. Nilsson and I. Rosen (1977b). J. Neurol. Neurosurg. Psychiat. 40, 1109-1112.
Lundh, H. and S. Thesleff (1977). Eur. J. Pharmacol. 42, 411-412.
Lundh, H., O. Nilsson and I. Rosen (1979). J. Neurol. Neurosurg. Psychiat. 42, 171-175.
Maeno, T. and K. Enomoto (1980). Proc. Japan Acad. 56B, 486-491.
Magleby, K.L., B.S. Pallotta and D.A. Terrar (1981). J. Physiol. (London) 312, 97-113.

Mallart, A. and A.R. Martin (1967). J. Physiol. (London) 193, 679-694.
Mallart, A. and J. Molgo (1978). J. Physiol. (London) 276, 343-352.
Manalis, R.S. (1977). Nature 267, 366-367.
Marshall, I.G., J.J. Lambert and N.N. Durant (1979). Eur. J. Pharmacol. 54, 9-14.
Marty, A., T. Neild and P. Ascher (1976). Nature 261, 501-503.
Mellanby, J. and J. Green (1981). Neuroscience 6, 281-300.
Meves, H. and Y. Pichon (1977). J. Physiol. (London) 268, 511-532.
Miller, R.D., P.A.F. Dennissen, F. van der Pol, S. Agoston, L.H.D.J. Booij and J.F. Crul (1978). J. Pharm. Pharmacol. 30, 699-702.
Miller, R.D., Booij, L.H.D.J., Agoston, S. and J.F. Crul (1979). Anesthesiology 50, 416-420.
Molgo, J., M. Lemeignan and P. Lechat (1975). C. R. Acad. Sci. (Paris) Ser. D 281, 1637-1639.
Molgo, J., M. Lemeignan and P. Lechat (1977). J. Pharmacol. exp. Ther. 203, 653-663.
Molgo, J., M. Lemeignan and P. Lechat (1979a). Eur. J. Pharmacol. 53, 307-311.
Molgo, J., M. Lemeignan, T. Uchiyama and P. Lechat (1979b). Eur. J. Pharmacol. 57, 93-97.
Molgo, J., H. Lundh and S. Thesleff (1980a). Eur. J. Pharmacol. 61, 25-34.
Molgo, J., M. Lemeignan, P. Lechat and S. Thesleff (1980b). Neurosci. Lett. Suppl.5, S-367.
Molgo, J. and S. Thesleff (1981a). Proc. Roy. Soc. (London) B, (accepted for publication).
Molgo, J. and S. Thesleff (1981b). Acta Physiol. Scand.,(accepted for publication.
Murray, N.M.F. and J. Newsom-Davis (1981). Neurology 31, 265-271.
Paskov, D.S., E.A. Stoyanov and V.V. Mitzov (1973). Eksp. Khir. Anaesthesiol. 18, 48-52.
Pécot-Dechavassine, M. (1970). C. R. Acad. Sci. (Paris) Ser. D 271, 674-677.
Pécot-Dechavassine, M. (1976). J. Physiol. (London) 261, 31-48.
Pécot-Dechavassine, M. and R. Couteaux (1972a). C. R. Acad. Sci. (Paris) Ser. D 275, 983-986.
Pécot-Dechavassine, M. and R. Couteaux (1972b). International Symposium on Cholinergic transmission of the nerve impulse. INSERM, Paris pp. 177-185.
Pécot-Dechavassine, M. and R. Couteaux (1975). C. R. Acad. Sci. (Paris) Ser.D 280, 1099-1101.
Pelhate, M., B. Hue and J. Chanelet (1972). C. R. Soc. Biol. 166, 1598-1605.
Pelhate, M., B. Hue, Y. Pichon and J. Chanelet (1974). C. R. Acad. Sci. (Paris) Ser. D 278, 2807-2809.
Pittinger, C.B. and R. Adamson (1972). Ann. Rev. Pharmacol. 12, 169-184.
Rahamimoff, R. (1976). In S. Thesleff (Ed.), Motor inervation of muscle, Academic Press, New York pp. 117-149.
Sanders, W.E. and C.C. Sanders (1979). Ann. Rev. Pharmacol. Toxicol. 19, 53-83.
Sanders, D.B., Y.I. Kim, J.F. Howard and C.A. Goetsch (1980). J. Neurol. Neurosurg. Psychiat. 43, 978-985.
Schauf, C.L., C.A. Colton, J.S. Colton and F.A. Davis (1976). J. Pharmacol. exp. Ther. 197, 414-425.
Shapovalov, A.I. and B.I. Shiriaev (1978). Experientia 34, 67-68.
Shaw, F.H. and G.A. Bentley (1953). Aust. J. exp. Biol. 31, 573-576.
Sellin, L.C. (1981). Medical Biology 59, 11-20.
Simpson, L.L. (1978). J. Pharmacol. exp. Ther. 206, 661-669.
Singh, Y.N., I.G. Marshall and A.L. Harvey (1978a). Br. J. Anaesth. 50, 109-117.
Singh, Y.N., I.G. Marshall and A.L. Harvey (1978b). J. Pharm. Pharmacol. 30, 249-250.
Sobek, V., M. Lemeignan, G. Streichenberger, J.M. Benoist, A. Goguel and P. Lechat (1968). Arch. int. Pharmacodyn. 171, 356-368.
Spira, M.E., M. Klein, B. Hochner, Y. Yarom and M. Castel (1976). Neuroscience 1, 117-124.

Stoyanov, E. and P. Vulchev (1975). Medico-Biologic Information 5, 21-33.
Stoyanov, E., P. Vulchev, M. Shturbova and M. Marinova (1976). Anaesth. Resus. Inter. Ther. 4, 139-142.
Tazieff-Depierre, F., P. Métézeau and G. Wunderer (1978). C. R. Acad. Sci. (Paris) Ser.D 286, 655-658.
Thesleff, S. (1978). In Y. Cohen (Ed.), Advances in Pharmacology and Therapeutics Vol.9, Pergamon Press, Oxford, pp. 291-299.
Thesleff, S. and H. Lundh (1979). In B. Cecarelly and F. Clementi (Eds.), Advances in Cytopharmacology, Vol. 3, Academic Press, New York, pp. 35-43.
Thesleff, S. (1980). Neuroscience 5, 1413-1419.
Uchiyama, T., J. Molgo and M. Lemeignan (1981). Eur. J. Pharmacol. 72, 271-280.
Ulbricht, W. and H.H. Wagner (1976). Pflügers Arch. 367, 77-87.
Usherwood, P.N.R. and S.G. Cull-Candy (1975). In P.N.R. Usherwood (Ed.), Insect Muscle, Academic Press, New York, pp. 207-280.
Van der Kloot, W. and K.S. Madden (1981). Brain Res. 210, 467-470.
Vincent, A. (1980). Physiol. Rev. 60, 756-824.
Vital Brazil, O., M.D. Fontana and N.F. Heluany (1979). Toxicon 17, Suppl. 1, 16.
Vohra, M.M. and S.N. Pradhan (1964). Arch. int. Pharmacodyn. 150, 413-424.
Wernig, A. (1975). J. Physiol. (London) 244, 207-221.
Yeh, J.Z., G.S. Oxford, C.H. Wu and T. Narahashi (1976a). J. Gen. Physiol. 68, 519-535.
Yeh, J.Z., G.S. Oxford, C.H. Wu and T. Narahashi (1976b). Biophys. J. 16, 77-81.
Zucker, R.S. (1973). J. Physiol. (London) 229, 787-810.
Zucker, R.S. and L.O. Lara-Estrella (1979). Nature 278, 57-59.

# Effects of 4-Aminopyridine on Transmission in Excitatory and Inhibitory Synapses in the Spinal Cord

E. Jankowska

Department of Physiology, University of Göteborg, Box 33031,
Göteborg, Sweden

ABSTRACT

A survey of effects of 4-aminopyridine (4-AP) on synaptic transmission in the cat spinal cord (Jankowska, Lundberg, Rudomin and Syková, 1977) was made with a twofold aim: (i) to compare effects of 4-AP on excitatory and inhibitory synapses in various spinal pathways and (ii) to test these effects under conditions closest to clinical conditions, allowing comparison of effects of systemic and of local or in vitro applications. 4-AP has been found to facilitate all tested excitatory as well as inhibitory responses. It enhanced monosynaptic and polysynaptic excitation and disynaptic and polysynaptic inhibition of motoneurones, excitation of ascending tract cells and presynaptic depolarization of primary afferents; these synaptic actions were evoked by different types of afferents and various descending systems and were mediated via different interneuronal systems. In the case of the disynaptic inhibitory reflexes the evidence has been obtained that 4-AP may enhance both the excitation of the interposed interneurones and the inhibitory effects exerted by these interneurones on the motoneurones.

The described effects were evoked by 4-AP in doses up to 1 mg/kg. They appeared within the first minute of the injection, reached maximum after about 10-15 min and remained stable during at least several hours.

In an analysis of action of 4-AP on primary afferents and motoneurones no indications have been found of its direct effects on excitability of fibres or cells to electrical stimuli. No systematic changes in membrane potential of motoneurones, nor in duration of action potentials of these neurones or of primary afferents were seen. The study leads to the conclusion that small doses of 4-AP enhance various spinal reflexes primarily due to facilitation of synaptic transmission.

KEYWORDS

4-aminopyridine; synaptic transmission; spinal cord; spinal reflexes; inhibitory synapses.

## INTRODUCTION

When we took up the study of actions of 4-AP in the central nervous system (Jankowska, Lundberg, Rudomin and Syková, 1977 and in press) it was after only the first attempts had been made to apply it clinically, as an analeptic and anticurarising agent (Paskow, Stojanov and Micov, 1973; see Thesleff, 1980). Enhancement of synaptic transmission by 4-AP had then been established but primarily for excitatory synapses (Chanelet and Lemeignan, 1969; Saade, Chanelet and Longchampt, 1971; Lemeignan, 1972, 1973) and inhibition appeared to be either depressed or showed no consistent changes (Lemeignan, 1970, 1973). Since such an assymetry in actions of 4-AP might be of serious consequence for its more general use, these observations called for a reinvestigation. It appeared also important to make a survey of 4-AP effects under conditions close to clinical conditions. Our study was thus made after systemic (intravenous) application of 4-AP, previous data having been obtained mainly after local direct or intra-arterial injections (Chanelet and Lemeignan, 1969; Lemeignan, 1972, 1973).

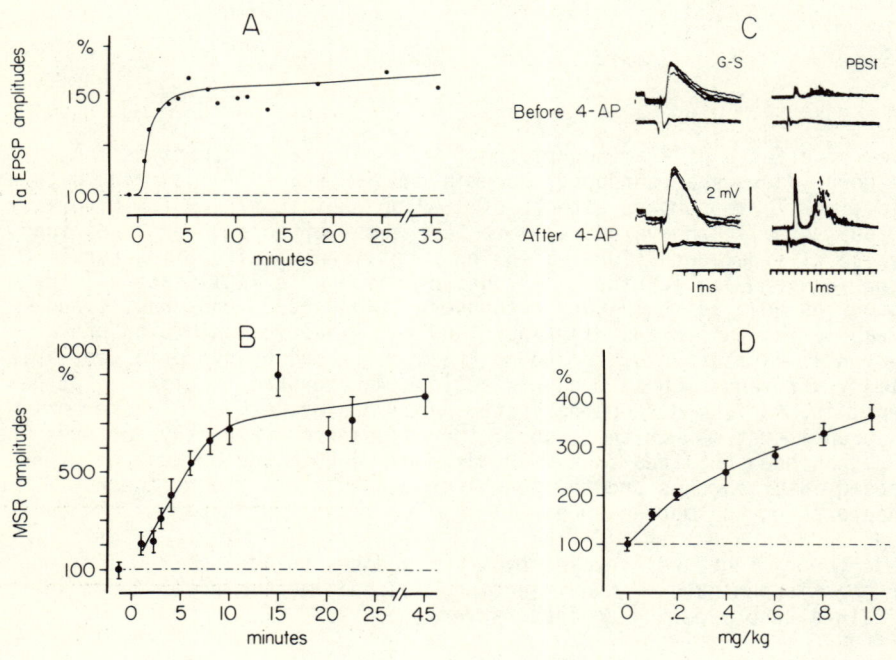

Fig. 1. Increase in amplitude of monosynaptic EPSPs (A) and of monosynaptic reflexes (B, D) after i.v. injection of 4-AP. Diagrams in A and B illustrate development of effects of 4-AP (1 mg/kg) as a function of time and that in D as a function of dose; the data in D are for effects found 30 min after each successively added 0.1-0.2 mg/kg of 4-AP. Sample records of EPSPs evoked in a triceps surae (G-S, stimulus twice threshold) motoneurone and of monosynaptic responses evoked from posterior biceps-semitendinosus (PBSt, stimulus three times threshold) are in C; lower row records were obtained after injection of 1 mg/kg 4-AP. The same dose was used in other illustrated experiments.

## MATERIAL AND METHODS

The experiments were made on 16 cats under chloralose anaesthesia (50-70 mg/kg) supplemented with pentobarbital sodium (Nembutal, Abbott, about 2 mg/kg/hour) and on 2 unanaesthetized decerebrate cats. The effects of 4-AP were investigated on synaptic actions on spinal motoneurones, spino-cerebellar tract cells and primary afferents. The synaptic actions were evoked by electrical stimulation of peripheral nerves, spinal roots and descending tract fibres. In addition, observations were made on a number of reflexes (e.g. neck, labyrinthine, crossed extension) in decerebrate cats and on membrane properties of motoneurones and primary afferents.

4-AP was injected intravenously as a solution of 1 mg per ml of 0.9 % sodium chloride in doses of 0.1-1.0 mg/kg; these doses are estimated to give 2-20 µM concentration of 4-AP in the body fluids, considering the total volume of the latter to be about 50 % of the body weight.

## DOSAGE AND TIME COURSE OF EFFECTS OF 4-AP

Since previous observations on cats were made with local injections of 4-AP we had first to establish the optimal doses of the intravenously applied 4-AP; its actions on monosynaptic EPSPs recorded in motoneurones and on monosynaptic reflexes were used for this purpose.

Fig. 1 D shows that dosages as low as 0.1-0.2 mg/kg had a clear facilitatory effect on the monosynaptic reflexes and that the amplitude of these reflexes grew with increasing doses of 4-AP. However, starting with doses about 1 mg/kg dorsal root reflexes became greatly enhanced modyfying the synaptic input to motoneurones and resulting in an increase in variability of amplitudes of monosynaptic reflexes. The effects of larger doses of 4-AP thus could not be quantified and 1 mg/kg was the maximal dose used. The effects of 4-AP appeared within the first few minutes, reached maximum within 10-15 min, as illustrated in Fig. 1 A and B, and remained practically unchanged during several hours.

Table 1. Synaptic actions found to be enhanced by 4-AP

| Tested synaptic actions | In |
|---|---|
| Excitation<br>monosynaptic from group Ia muscle afferents<br>polysynaptic from group II and III muscle afferents<br>monosynaptic from descending tracts<br><br>Inhibition<br>disynaptic from recurrent axon collaterals<br>disynaptic from group Ia muscle afferents<br>disynaptic from group Ib muscle afferents<br>polysynaptic from group II and III muscle afferents<br>polysynaptic from cutaneous afferents | motoneurones |
| Excitation: from group Ia and Ib muscle afferents<br>          from cutaneous afferents | ascending<br>tract cells |
| Presynaptic depolarization from various afferents | terminals of<br>primary afferents |

## EFFECTS OF 4-AP ON EXCITATORY PATHWAYS

4-AP regularly increased responses in all tested (Table 1) excitatory pathways: to motoneurones as well as to ascending tract cells and to primary afferents, from muscle as well as from cutaneous afferents or descending tract fibres. Enhancement of responses evoked di- or polysynaptically was usually as pronounced as of those evoked monosynaptically, as illustrated by right-most sample records in Fig. 1 C.

## EFFECTS OF 4-AP ON INHIBITORY PATHWAYS

The tested inhibitory actions are listed in Table 1 and Fig. 2 shows that they could be almost doubled by 4-AP. Similar enhancement was found in the case of disynaptic pathways (from group I, cf. Fig. 2 A) and of polysynaptic pathways (from group II or III muscle afferents and cutaneous afferents). The weakest and limited in time but unquestionable effects were exerted on recurrent inhibition (cf. Fig. 2 B).

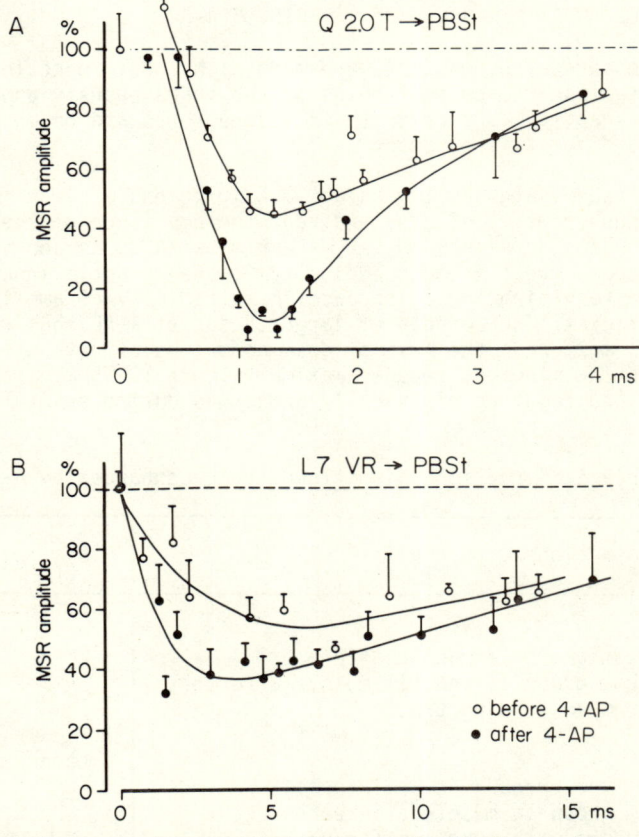

Fig. 2. Enhancement of inhibition by 4-AP. Upper diagram illustrates increase of reciprocal inhibition of knee flexors posterior biceps-semitendinosus (PBSt) by group I afferents of knee extensors quadriceps (Q); stimulus twice threshold. Lower diagram shows enhancement of the recurrent inhibition evoked by stimulation of L7 ventral root (VR; stimulus twice threshold). Both effects were tested on monosynaptic reflexes; the control values of the latter were normalized and taken as 100 %.

The observed facilitation of inhibition might have been due to enhancement of excitation of the inhibitory interneurones (black cell in the left diagram of Fig. 3) as well as of the action of these neurones on motoneurones. The following series of experiments was therefore made to find out the site of action of 4-AP. The reciprocal inhibition of knee flexors (posterior biceps-semitendinosus, PBSt) motoneurones was evoked by stimulation of Ia afferents of knee extensors

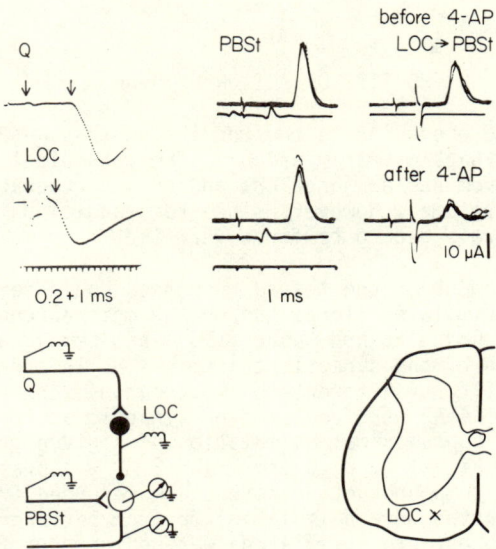

Fig. 3. Effects of 4-AP on transmission in inhibitory synapses. Diagrams show the pathway of the disynaptic reciprocal inhibition between antagonists and sites of stimulation and recording in different variants of experiments; the inhibitory interneurone is indicated in black. The records to the left are intracellular records from a posterior biceps-semitendinosus (PBSt) motoneurone showing IPSPs evoked by stimulation of quadriceps group Ia muscle spindle afferents (top) and of axons of the interposed interneurones (bottom); the latter IPSPs were evoked monosynaptically. Records in the middle are from L7 ventral root (top traces in each pair) and from the dorsal roots (bottom traces). They show test monosynaptic reflexes evoked from posterior biceps-semitendinosus. Two stimuli were used to evoke these test reflexes before and only one after 4-AP; its amplitude was adjusted so that it evoked the same size responses. Right records illustrate decrease of the test monosynaptic reflexes by conditioning intraspinal stimulation applied at site x in the diagram. The intraspinal stimuli (monitored in lower traces) were applied 0.2 msec before the arrival of the nerve impulses from PBSt. Note more pronounced inhibition after 4-AP.

(quadriceps, Q) and by stimulation of axons of the interposed interneurones. The latter run in the ventrolateral part of the ventral funiculus (Hultborn, Jankowska and Lindström, 1971; Jankowska and Roberts, 1972; Jankowska and

Lindström, 1972) and the intraspinal (local, Loc) stimulation sites were as indicated in the right diagram of Fig. 3. Intracellular records, exemplified in Fig. 3, left, showed that such intraspinal stimuli evoked monosynaptic IPSPs (with a latency of 0.6-0.8 msec, about 0.5 msec shorter than the latencies of IPSPs evoked by nerve stimulation). They also gave rise to depression of the monosynaptic reflexes (Fig. 3, right). Such a direct inhibition was clearly increased by 4-AP, as appears from a comparison of top and bottom records.

## CONTROL TESTS ON THE SITE OF ACTION OF 4-AP

The experiments described above led to the conclusion that 4-AP has a generalized facilitatory action on synaptic transmission in the cat spinal cord, comparable to its action on the neuromuscular junctions and on invertebrate synapses (cf. review of Molgo in this volume). However, since some additional factors might have contributed, their role had to be first verified.

Theoretically, an enhancement of the tested responses could be due to an increase in excitability of the stimulated fibres and/or the motoneurones, as already considered by Lemeignan, Chanelet and Saade (1969) and Lemeignan (1970, 1972), as well as to a facilitation of the synaptic transmission. In order to check whether 4-AP influenced excitability of afferents or motoneurones the following tests were made. The effects of 4-AP were analysed on synaptic actions evoked by submaximal as well as by supramaximal stimulation of a given group of afferents; for those illustrated in Fig. 1 A, B, C and D and 2 A, B supramaximal stimuli were used. Amplitudes of compound action potentials recorded from the dorsal roots (when peripheral nerves were stimulated) or from peripheral nerves (when terminals of afferent fibres were stimulated) were compared before and after 4-AP. Neither of these two tests indicated that the doses of 4-AP used increased excitability and, in consequence, numbers of the stimulated fibres. Furthermore, changes in the amplitude of EPSPs were examined with respect to changes in the membrane potential of the motoneurones, motoneurone excitability as defined by

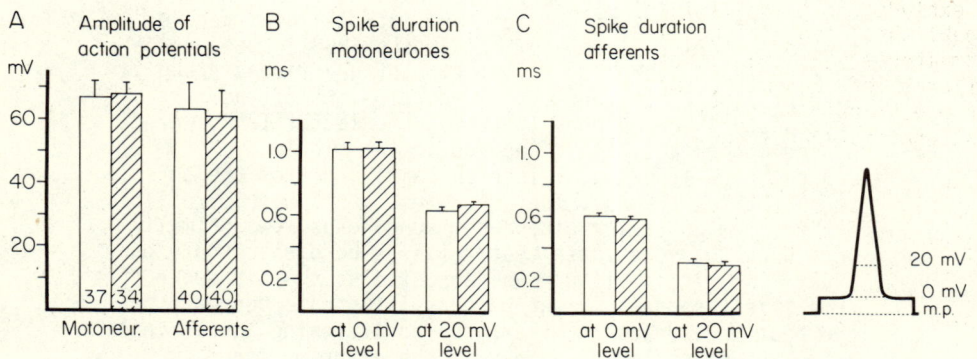

Fig. 4. Lack of effect of 4-AP (1 mg/kg) on duration of action potentials of motoneurones and primary afferents at a preterminal level. The numbers of the analysed cells and fibres are indicated in A where amplitudes of action potentials of the two samples are compared. The duration of the action potentials (± SE) was compared at 4 levels; at their foot and at 10, 20 and 30 mV level. Data for two of them are illustrated as indicated in the diagram.

threshold for firing by intracellularly applied electrical pulses, and time or space constants. By none of these tests could changes in motoneuronal responses be attributed to direct actions of 4-AP on the membrane.

A comparison of duration of action potentials of afferents impaled in the dorsal horn and of motoneurones, before and after injection of 1 mg/kg 4-AP, did not show any statistically significant increase ($p > 0.05$ in Student's t test), as illustrated in Fig. 4. Our observations are thus in agreement with observations of other authors on lack of effects of 4-AP on myelinated nerve fibres (Foster, Connors and Waxman, 1980; Kocsis and Waxman, 1980; Sherratt, Bastock and Sears, 1980). Our preparation did not allow a study of the unmyelinated terminal axonal branches; the duration of action potentials in these terminals might thus well be increased as in other unmyelinated fibres (Sherratt, Bostock and Sears, 1980; Foster, Connors and Waxman, 1980).

## COMMENTS ON THE USE OF 4-AP FOR CLINICAL PURPOSES AND IN STUDIES OF THE CENTRAL NERVOUS SYSTEM

Convulsive actions of 4-AP and the originally described stronger facilitation of excitatory then of inhibitory synaptic responses could raise some doubts on its wider applicability. It appears, however, that positive effects of 4-AP may be obtained already at concentrations subthreshold for convulsant actions, both in patients (see reviews of Folder, Lundh and Ball in this volume) and in experimental animals. Furthermore, the enhancement of excitation has as its counterpart an enhancement of inhibition although a comparison of effects of 4-AP on various excitatory and inhibitory spinal reflexes in anaesthetized animals does not allow an estimation of how well they are balanced. For this reason we checked effects of 4-AP also on reactions of non-anaesthetized, non-paralyzed decerebrate cats. These cats did not show any marked increase, or decrease, in the decerebrate rigidity by 4-AP, nor any conspicuous modification in neck, vestibular, righting or cross extension reflexes, indicating a generally similar degree of facilitation of transmission in various neuronal pathways. A certain modification in a relative strength of different reflex actions cannot, however, be excluded. E.g. preliminary observations (E. Jankowska and A. Lundberg, unpublished) suggest that 4-AP may enhance late flexion reflexes after L-DOPA to a greater extent than it enhances the associated depression of the early flexion reflexes (cf. Lundberg, 1979). The facilitation of transmission in pathways of the presynaptic inhibition may likewise be more pronounced than in pathways of postsynaptic inhibition or excitation.

In physiological experiments in which a quantitative estimation of various synaptic actions is not of prime importance, 4-AP has already found a place as a useful tool. By enhancing synaptic transmission in interneuronal pathways it has helped in disclosing otherwise difficult to detect weak polysynaptic actions (Fetz, Jankowska, Johannisson and Lipski, 1979; Jankowska, Johannisson and Lipski, 1981). It appeared also to activate depressed neuronal circuits involved in locomotor-like activity in spinal and decerebrate animals (Zangger, 1978; Russel and Zajac, 1979).

So far, there have been only two contra-indications for the experimental use of 4-AP. It appears to reduce to such an extent the subliminal fringe following submaximal stimuli (B. Alstermark, A. Lundberg and S. Sasaki, personal communication) that it may interfere with the use of the technique of spatial facilitation of various synaptic actions (Lundberg, 1975). Appearance of dorsal root reflexes may also hamper detection of some weak synaptic actions if they are being masked by larger actions of the discharging afferents. None of these complicating factors should, however, diminish the usefulness of 4-AP in other studies and in its clinical applications.

ACKNOWLEDGEMENT

The study was supported by the Swedish Medical Research Council (Project no. 94).

REFERENCES

Chanelet, J., et M. Lemeignan (1969). Effet d'une application microrégionale de 4-aminopyridine au niveau de la moelle lombaire du chat. C.R. Soc. Biol., 163, 365-372.
Fetz, E., E. Jankowska, T. Johannisson, and J. Lipski (1979). Autogenetic inhibition of motoneurones by impulses in group Ia muscle spindle afferents. J. Physiol., 293, 173-195.
Foster, R.E., B.W. Connors, and S.G. Waxman (1980). Development of conduction in rat optic nerve: Physiological and pharmacological observations correlated with myelination. Soc. for Neuroscience. 10th Ann. Meeting, 291.
Hultborn, H., E. Jankowska, and S. Lindström (1971). Recurrent inhibition of interneurones monosynaptically activated from group Ia afferents. J. Physiol. (Lond.), 215, 613-636.
Jankowska, E., T. Johannisson, and J. Lipski (1981). Common interneurones in reflex pathways from group Ia and Ib afferents of ankle extensors in the cat. J. Physiol. (Lond.), 310, 381-402.
Jankowska, E., and S. Lindström (1972). Morphology of interneurones mediating Ia reciprocal inhibition of motoneurones in the spinal cord of the cat. J. Physiol. (Lond.), 226, 805-823.
Jankowska, E., A. Lundberg, P. Rudomin, and E. Syková (1977). Effects of 4-aminopyridine on transmission in excitatory and inhibitory synapses in the spinal cord. Brain Research, 136, 387-392.
Jankowska, E., and W.J. Roberts (1972). Synaptic actions of single interneurones mediating reciprocal Ia inhibition of motoneurones. J. Physiol. (Lond.), 222, 623-642.
Kocsis, J.D., and S.G. Waxman (1980). Absence of potassium conductance in central myelinated axons. Nature, 287, 348-349.
Lemeignan, M. (1970). Étude du mécanisme de l'action convulsivante de l'amino-4-pyridine. Thèse. Faculté des Sciences de Paris.
Lemeignan, M. (1972). Analysis of the action of 4-aminopyridine on the cat lumbar spinal cord. I. Modification of the afferent volley, the monosynaptic discharge amplitude and the polysynaptic evoked responses. Neuropharmacology, 11, 551-558.
Lemeignan, M. (1973). Analysis of the effects of 4-aminopyridine on the lumbar spinal cord of the cat. II. Modifications of certain spinal inhibitory phenomena, post-tetanic potentiation and dorsal root potentials. Neuropharmacology, 12, 641-651.
Lemeignan, M., J. Chanelet, et N.E. Saade (1969). Étude de l'action d'un convulsivant spécial (la 4-aminopyridine) sur les nervs de vertebrés. C.R. Soc. de Biologie (Paris), 163, 359-372.
Lundberg, A. (1975). The control of spinal mechanisms from the brain. In D.B. Tower (Ed.), The Nervous System, Vol. 1. Raven Press, New York, 253-265.
Lundberg, A. (1979). Multisensory control of spinal reflex pathways. Progress in Brain Res, 50, 11-28.
Paskov, P.S., Stojanov, E.A., and Micov, V.V. (1973). New anti-curare and analeptic drug Pimadin and its use in anaesthesia. Eksper. Khir. Anestesiol., 18, 48 (in Russian).

Russell, F., and E. Zajac (1979). Effects of stimulating Deiters' nucleus and medial longitudinal fasciculus on the timing of the fictive locomotor rhythm induced in cats by DOPA. Brain Research, 177, 588-592.

Saade, N.E., J. Chanelet, et P. Longchampt (1971). Differantes modes d'activation reflexe de la même préparation de grenouille spinale: leur facilitation par la 4-aminopyridine. C.R. Soc. Biol., 165, 784.

Sherratt, R.M., H. Bostock, and T.A. Sears (1980). Effects of 4-aminopyridine on normal and demyelinated mammalian nerve fibres. Nature, 283, 570-572.

Thesleff, S. (1980). Aminopyridines and synaptic transmission. Neuroscience, 5, 1413-1419.

Zangger, P. (1978). Fictive locomotion in curarized high spinal cats elicited with 4-aminopyridine and DOPA. Experientia (Basel), 34, 904.

# The Influence of 4-Aminopyridine on Parasympathetic Transmission

F. F. Foldes*, Y. Ohta*, Y. Shiwaku*, E. S. Vizi*,
J. J. Van Dijk** and K. Morita*

*Departments of Anesthesiology, Montefiore Hospital and Medical
Center and Albert Einstein College of Medicine,
Bronx, N.Y. 10467, USA
**Department of Anesthesiology, Catholic University Medical School,
Nijmegen, The Netherlands

ABSTRACT

The influence of 4-aminopyridine (4-APYR) on parasympathetic transmission was investigated on the myenteric plexus - longitudinal muscle preparation of the guinea-pig ileum. 4-APYR increased the force of contraction of the longitudinal muscle elicited by electrical field stimulation or by the addition of nicotine to the bath. It had little effect on the contraction caused by the addition of acetylcholine (ACh) to the bath. The decrease of the force of electrical, ACh or nicotine contraction caused by decreasing the [Ca] to $0.5 \times 10^{-3}$M was antagonized by 4-APYR. Inhibition of the electrical contraction by homatropine methylbromide, normorphine, enkephalins or l-epinephrine was antagonized by 4-APYR. Similarly, the inhibition of the nicotine contraction by normorphine was also antagonized by 4-APYR. The site of the antagonist effect of 4-APYR on the inhibition of the electrical and nicotine contraction by normorphine appears to be different from that of naloxone. 4-APYR increased both the spontaneous and stimulated ACh release and the volley output of ACh in this preparation and also antagonized the inhibition of ACh release caused by normorphine and [$\underline{d}$-Ala$^2$-]-Met$^5$- enkephalin. The facilitation of parasympathetic transmission, in this preparation, by 4-APYR can be explained by its effect on stimulated ACh release.

KEYWORDS

4-Aminopyridine; enkephalins, epinephrine; hexamethonium; histamine; homatropine methylbromide; naloxone; nicotine; normorphine; parasympathetic transmission, facilitation of by 4-aminopyridine; myenteric plexus.

INTRODUCTION

The mechanism of action of 4-aminopyridine (4-APYR) and its effect on neuromuscular and adrenergic transmission has been discussed by other participants in this symposium. In this presentation the effects of 4-APYR on parasympathetic transmission in the isolated myenteric plexus - longitudinal muscle preparation of the guinea-pig ileum (Paton and Vizi, 1969) will be discussed.

In this preparation there are two types of cholinergic receptors: a nicotinic receptor located on the ganglion cell and a muscarinic receptor on the muscle. Under physiological circumstances the acetylcholine (ACh) released from preganglionic parasympathetic nerve endings is adsorbed primarily to the nicotinic receptors, depolarizes the ganglia and causes the release of ACh from postganglionic nerve endings. The ACh released at this site is adsorbed to muscarinic receptors on the muscle and causes it to contract. ACh is also released without preganglionic stimulation by autogenous ganglionic activity (Cowie, Kosterlitz and Watt, 1968; Paton, Vizi and Zar, 1971). Depolarization of the ganglia by electrical field stimulation (Paton, 1963; Paton and Zar, 1965) or by the application of nicotine also cause postganglionic ACh release and contraction of the muscle.

In addition to the two cholinergic receptors two other inhibitory receptors are also present in the myenteric plexus - longitudinal muscle preparation. One of these has specific affinity for narcotic analgesics (Paton, 1957a; Schaumann, 1956, 1957) and enkephalins (Hughes, Smith and Kosterlitz, 1975; Foldes and co-workers, 1979) and the other for noradrenaline and adrenaline (Kosterlitz, Lydon and Watt, 1970; Paton and Vizi, 1969). Application of narcotics (Paton, 1957a; Van Dijk, J.J., DePol, F. and Foldes, F.F., 1976 Unpublished) or enkephalins (Hughes, Smith and Kosterlitz, 1975; Foldes and co-workers, 1979) inhibit electrically induced contractions of and decrease spontaneous and stimulated ACh release (Paton, 1957a; Schaumann, 1957; Waterfield and co-workers, 1977; Shiwaku, Y., Morita, K. and Foldes, F.F., 1979, Unpublished) from the myenteric plexus - longitudinal muscle preparation.

Investigation of the interaction of 4-APYR with agonists and antagonists of these 4 receptors was undertaken to obtain information on the sites and mechanisms of action of 4-APYR on parasympathetic transmission.

METHODS

All experiments were carried out on the myenteric plexus - longitudinal muscle preparation of the guinea-pig ileum (Paton and Vizi, 1969). In the first part of the study the influence of 4-APYR alone, or in combination with other compounds, on the contraction of the muscle elicited by exogenous ACh, nicotine or electrical stimulation, and for sake of comparison, by histamine was investigated. In the second part of the study the effect of 4-APYR alone, or in combination with other compounds, on the spontaneous and electrically induced ACh release was observed.

Electrical and Drug Induced Contraction

Longitudinal muscle strips of 5 to 6 cm length and 0.06 to 0.10 g weight were suspended in 3.5 to 4.0 ml organ baths filled with mammalian Krebs' solution (Krebs and Henseleit, 1932) containing $2 \times 10^{-5}$M choline and aerated with 95% $O_2$ - 5% $CO_2$ (Fig. 1.). Fluid changes were made by an overflow system from a reservoir. The temperature of the fluid in the double jacketed organ baths and reservoir were kept at 37°C by circulating water from a thermostatically controlled water bath. To eliminate the effect of endogenous histamine on contraction of the longitudinal muscle $1.25 \times 10^{-7}$M mepyramine was added to the Krebs' solution. Mepyramine was not used, however, when the effect of histamine on the muscle was observed. The distal end of the muscle strip, or occasionally the end of 2 strips in parallel, were fixed to the bottom of the organ bath. When the preparations were stimulated electrically the proximal end(s) of the muscle strip(s) were attached to an FT03 transducer and the isometric contractions were continuously recorded on a Grass 7D polygraph. Field stimulation, through platinum electrodes placed near the ends of the muscles, was used to elicit electrical contraction. Supramaximal, square wave stimuli of 1 msec duration were applied at 0.1 Hz (unless stated otherwise) from a Grass S88 stimulator. The potential difference between the electrodes was 15 V. $cm^{-1}$. After a 60 to 80 min equilibration period the resting tension of the muscles was adjusted to about 0.5 g. ACh, nicotine and histamine contraction of the muscle were elicited by adding the appropriate amounts of these agents in 0.1 to 0.4 ml volumes to the baths. In these experiments a soft spring of 1 cm.$g^{-1}$ to

0.33 cm.g$^{-1}$ compliance was interposed between the proximal end(s) of the muscle(s) and the transducer and the auxotonic contraction (Paton, 1957b) was recorded. With a single strand of muscle the weaker, with a double strand the stronger spring was used.

## Acetylcholine Assay

ACh was assayed either on a segment of guinea-pig ileum (Vizi, Foldes and Theunisson, 1975) or on a segment of isolated longitudinal muscle (Kosterlitz, Lydon and Watt, 1970). The longitudinal muscle was found to be somewhat less sensitive to ACh than the whole gut, but the variation between parallel determinations was less than with the earlier method.

## Experiments Performed

The experiments performed included observations on the effects of atropine, homatropine methylbromide[1], hexamethonium (C6) naloxone, l-epinephrine, 4-APYR and [Ca], singly or in various combinations, on ACh, nicotine, histamine and electrical contraction and on the spontaneous and stimulated release of ACh from the isolated myenteric plexus - longitudinal muscle preparation of the guinea-pig ileum.

## Compounds Used

Acetylcholine bromide (Eastman Organic Chemicals, Rochester, NY).
Choline Chloride; Nicotine; Hexamethonium bromide; d,l-Homatropine methylbromide; l-Epinephrine bitartrate (Sigma Chemical Co., St. Louis, MO).
4-Aminopyridine; Atropine sulfate (Aldrich Chemical Co., Milwaukee, WI).
Normorphine (Gift of Merck, Sharp & Dohme, West Point, PA).
Mepyramine maleate (Merck, Sharp & Dohme, West Point, PA).
Naloxone hydrochloride (Gift of Endo Laboratories, Garden City, NY)
Met[5]- and Leu[5]-Enkephalin (Miles Laboratories, Elkhart, ILL).
[d-Ala[2]]-Met[5]-Enkephalin (Beckman Instruments, Palo Alto, CA).
Histamine phosphate (Eli Lilly & Co., Indianapolis, IN).

All other compounds used were reagent grade or better.

## RESULTS

The observations made in this study will be presented under 4 headings: ACh Contraction; Nicotine Contraction; Electrical Contraction; and ACh Release.

## ACh Contraction

Homatropine, 2 to 5x10$^{-8}$M, shifted the log dose - response regression line to the right (Fig. 2.). The addition of C6 had no effect on the force of ACh contraction. Decreasing the [Ca] caused a similar, progressive decrease of the ACh and histamine contraction (Fig. 3.). This indicates that lowering the [Ca] decreases ACh contraction, not by influencing the interaction of ACh with the muscarinic receptors, but by decreasing the contractile force of the muscle. The ACh contraction was increased by less than 10% of control by 5x10$^{-6}$M 4-APYR. The decrease of the

---

[1]Because of the more rapid development of its maximal effect and faster dissipation on its effect after washout, in most experiments, instead of atropine, homatropine methylbromide was used. The ratio of the Ke of atropine (1.3x10$^{-10}$M) to that of homatropine methylbromide (8.1x10$^{-9}$M) is about 60. For sake of brevity homatropine methylbromide will be referred to as homatropine.

force of ACh contraction in a low Ca milieu was less than that of the electrical contraction and was antagonized by 4-APYR less effectively than the electrical contraction (Table 1).

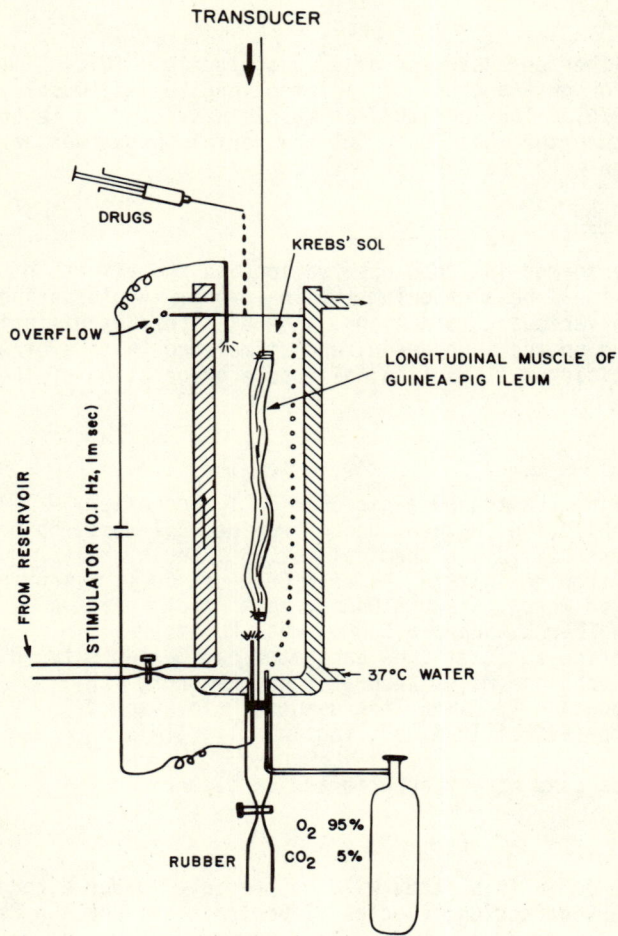

Fig. 1. Scheme of the experimental setup.

## Nicotine Contraction

In contrast to the ACh contraction the nicotine contraction was increased by about 30% by $5 \times 10^{-6}$M 4-APYR. Lowering the [Ca] to $0.5 \times 10^{-3}$M decreased the force of nicotine contraction. This decrease was antagonized by $5 \times 10^{-6}$M 4-APYR (see Table 1). The addition of $1 \times 10^{-5}$M C6 inhibited the nicotine contraction (Fig. 4.). $5 \times 10^{-6}$M 4-APYR antagonized the effects of C6. The addition of $1 \times 10^{-7}$M normorphine to the bath had a greater inhibitory effect on the nicotine than on the ACh contraction (Table 2). Naloxone, $1.5 \times 10^{-8}$M and $5 \times 10^{-6}$M 4-APYR both antagonized normorphine inhibition of the nicotine contraction (see Table 2).

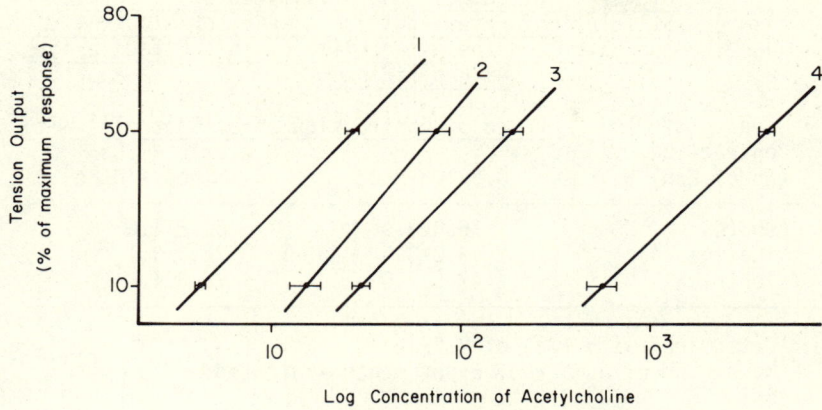

Fig.2. The influence of atropine, homatropine methylbromide on the acetylcholine (ACh) contraction of the longitudinal muscle of the guinea-pig ileum.
(1) ACh: (2) ACh + $2 \times 10^-$ M homatropine: (3) ACh + $5 \times 10^-$ M homatropine: (4) ACh + $2 \times 10^-$ M atropine.

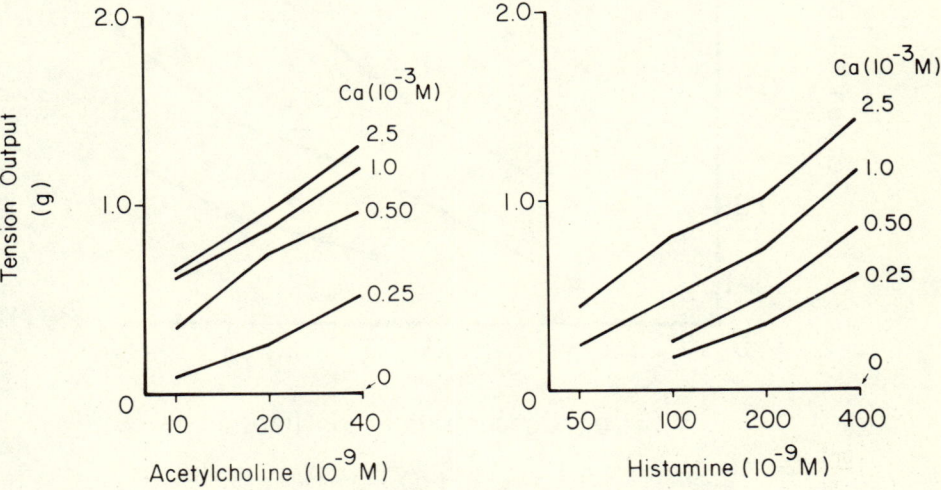

LOG CONCENTRATIONS

Fig. 3. The influence of [Ca] on the acetylcholine (ACh) and histamine contraction of the longitudinal muscle. Note that the effect of Ca on the ACh and histamine contraction are about the same. (For explanation see text.)

TABLE 1  The Effect of Low [Ca] on the Force of Contraction of the Longitudinal Muscle Elicited by Electrical Stimulation or the Addition of ACh or Nicotine to the Bath and the Antagonism of this Effect by 4-Aminopyridine.

| Type of Contraction (No of Exp) | Force of Contraction (% of Control[1]) With | |
|---|---|---|
| | $0.5 \times 10^{-3}$M Ca | $0.5 \times 10^{-3}$M Ca + 4-Aminopyridine[3] |
| ACh (4) | 76.0±0.9[2] | 80.8±1.0* |
| Nicotine (4) | 43.0±3.5 | 74.3±3.1† |
| Electrical (8) | 47.5±2.0 | 78.3±1.0† |

[1] Determined with [Ca] of $2.5 \times 10^{-3}$M.
[2] Mean ± SEM of number of experiments indicated.
[3] $5 \times 10^{-6}$M.
* and † indicate significance of the effects of 4-APYR at the the $p < 0.01$ and 0.001 levels respectively (paired $\underline{t}$ test).

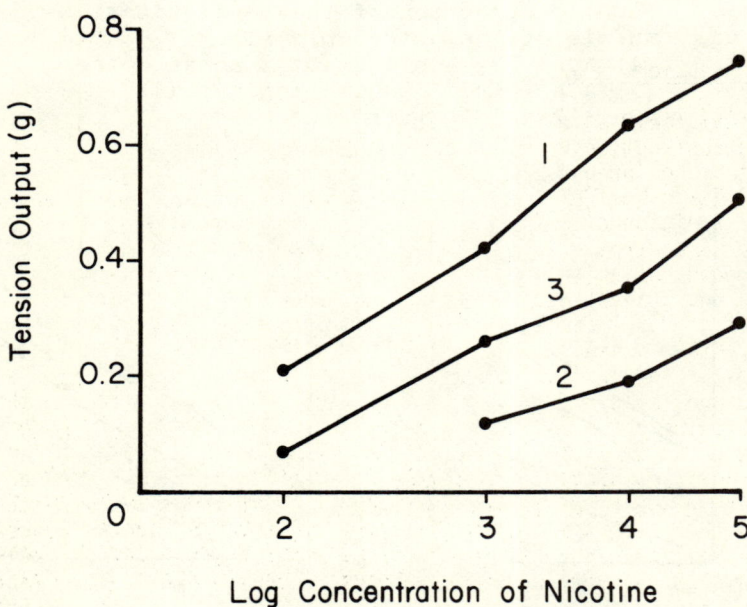

Fig. 4. The influence of hexamethonium (C6) and 4-aminopyridine (4-APYR) on the nicotine contraction of the longitudinal muscle. (1) Nicotine; (2) Nicotine + $1 \times 10^{-5}$M C6; (3) nicotine + $1 \times 10^{-5}$M C6 + $5 \times 10^{-6}$M 4-APYR.

TABLE 2  Comparison of the Antagonism of the Normorphine Induced Depression of the Nicotine and Electrical Contraction of the Longitudinal Muscle by Naloxone and 4-Aminopyridine.

| Type of Contraction | Force of Contraction (% of Control) With | | | |
|---|---|---|---|---|
| | Normorphine[3] | Naloxone[5] + Normorphine[3] | Normorphine[3] | 4-APYR[6] + Normorphine[3] |
| Nicotine | 22.5±3.0[4] | 77.8±3.9 | 23.6±6.3 | 87.2±8.4 |
| Electrical | 72.8±1.3* | 96.5±1.9 | 75.3±1.4* | 106.8±0.6 |

[1]Contraction produced by $5 \times 10^{-6}$M nicotine.
[2]Contraction produced by electrical field stimulation.
[3]$1 \times 10^{-7}$M.
[4]Mean ± SEM of 4 experiments.
[5]$1.5 \times 10^{-8}$M.
[6]$5 \times 10^{-6}$M.
*Indicates significant difference between the depression by normorphine of the nicotinic and electrical contraction at the $p < 0.01$ level (paired $t$ test).

### Electrical Contraction

During electrical field stimulation $5 \times 10^{-6}$M to $4 \times 10^{-5}$M 4-APYR dose relatedly increased muscle contraction by 10 to 40% of control. This effect of 4-APYR varied considerably from one preparation to the other. Decreasing the [Ca] from $2.5 \times 10^{-3}$M to $0.5 \times 10^{-3}$M significantly decreased the electrical contraction (see Table 1). The addition of $5 \times 10^{-6}$M 4-APYR to the bath returned the force of contraction close to control. The contraction was dose dependently inhibited by narcotics and enkephalins (Foldes and co-workers, 1979). This inhibition could be antagonized and prevented by 4-APYR or naloxone (Fig. 5.). The ID50 of normorphine, and that of Met[5]- and Leu[5]- enkephalin increased significantly in the presence of $4.25 \times 10^{-6}$M 4-APYR ($p < 0.01$ to $0.001$; paired $t$ test) resulting in dose ratios (DR) of 2.5 to 3.0 (Table 3). The increase of the ID50 in the presence of $1.5 \times 10^{-8}$M naloxone, however, was greater and the DR was twice higher than that obtained with $4.25 \times 10^{-6}$M 4-APYR. The antagonist effects of naloxone ($K_e = 2.7 \times 10^{-9}$M) and 4-APYR were additive but 4-APYR did not influence the $K_e$ of naloxone indicating that the two compounds act at different sites. The antagonist effect of 4-APYR was greater in the presence of higher than lower concentrations of normorphine (Fig. 6.). The electrical contraction was not influenced by C6 but it was dose dependently inhibited by homatropine. This inhibition could be antagonized by 4-APYR. The electrical contraction could be completely abolished by relatively high concentrations ($5 \times 10^{-7}$M) of homatropine or atropine ($5 \times 10^{-9}$M). Histamine contraction, however, remained unchanged in the presence of these homatropine and atropine concentrations. The inhibition of electrical contraction caused by epinephrine was also antagonized by 4-APYR (Fig. 7.).

### Influence of 4-APYR on ACh Release

The spontaneous ACh release and the ACh release elicited by electrical stimulation as well as the volley output of ACh was significantly increased by the addition of $4.25 \times 10^{-6}$M to $1 \times 10^{-4}$M 4-APYR (Table 4). Similarly the depression of ACh release caused by normorphine or [d-Ala[2]]-Met[5]- enkephalin of the spontaneous and stimulated ACh release was antagonized by 4-APYR (Fig. 8.).

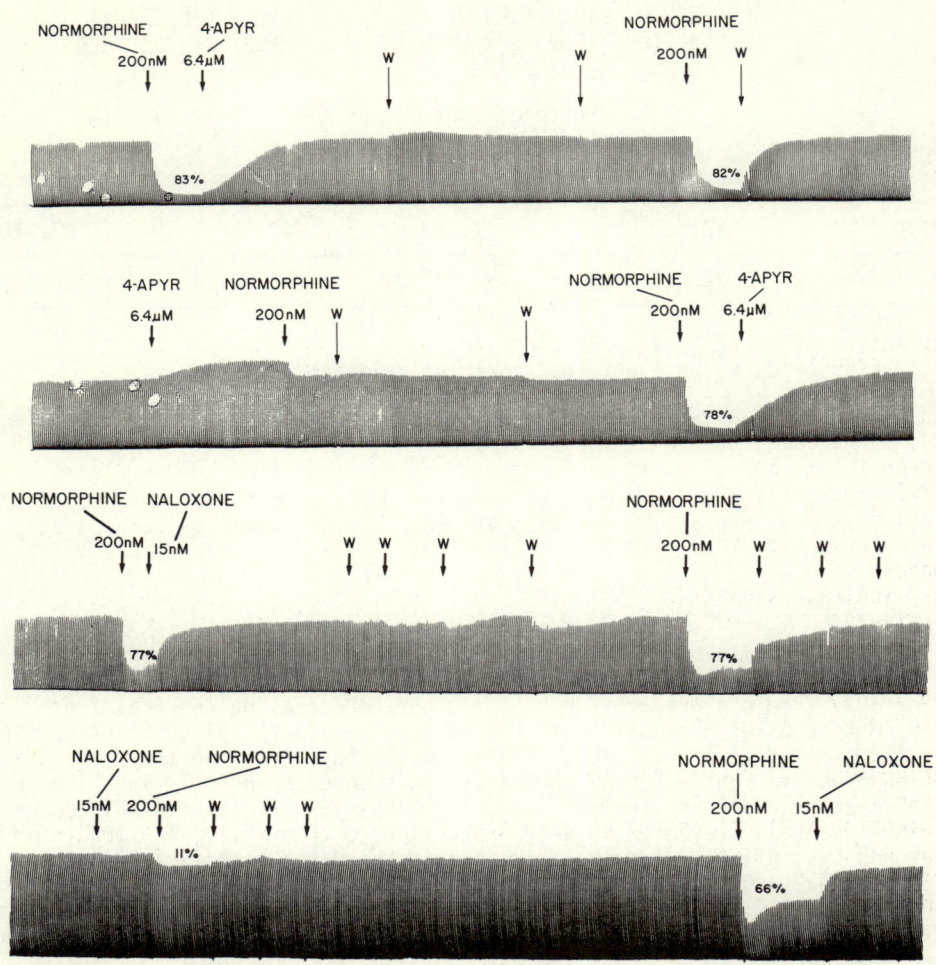

Fig. 5. Antagonism of the normorphine induced depression of the electrical contraction by $6.4 \times 10^{-6}$M 4-aminopyridine (4-APYR) or by $1.5 \times 10^{-8}$M naloxone.

DISCUSSION

The final step in parasympathetic transmission is the adsorption of ACh released at the postganglionic nerve terminals to muscarinic receptors located on the muscle. This can be prevented by muscarinic antagonists such as atropine or homatropine. Consequently contraction of the longitudinal muscle, whether initiated by presynaptic release of ACh under physiological circumstances, or under experimental conditions by the addition of nicotine or ACh to the organ bath or by electrical field stimulation, can be prevented by muscarinic antagonists. The influence of 4-APYR, however, on the contraction elicited by the addition of ACh or nicotine to the bath or by electrical stimulation is not the same. The contraction is increased by 4-APYR when it is elicited by nicotine or by electrical

TABLE 3  Antagonism by 4-APYR and Naloxone of the Inhibition of the Electrically Induced Twitch Tension of the Longitudinal Muscle Caused by Normorphine and Enkephalins.

| Compound | ID50[2] ($10^{-7}$M) | | | Dose Ratio[5] | |
| --- | --- | --- | --- | --- | --- |
| | Control | With 4-APYR[3] | With Naloxone[4] | With 4-APYR | With Naloxone |
| Normorphine | 0.95±0.12[1] (11) | 2.83±0.33* (4) | 5.90±0.97* (7) | 2.97 (4) | 8.21 (7) |
| Met[5]- Enkephalin | 1.19±0.09 (14) | 3.23±0.34† (6) | 7.35±0.90† (8) | 2.71 (6) | 6.17 (8) |
| Leu[5]- Enkephalin | 1.83±0.18 (13) | 4.89±0.58† (6) | 11.04±1.92* (7) | 2.67 (6) | 6.03 (7) |

[1]Mean ± SEM of number of experiments indicated in parenthesis.
[2]ID50 is the concentration that decreases the force of the electrically induced contraction to 50% of control.
[3]$4.25 \times 10^{-6}$M.
[4]$1.5 \times 10^{-8}$M.
[5]ID50 of compounds in presence of 4-APYR or naloxone divided by control ID50 of compounds.
* and † indicate significance (paired $t$ test) at the $p < 0.01$ and 0.001 levels respectively.

stimulation, but it remains unchanged when the contraction is caused by the addition of ACh to the bath.

Lowering the [Ca] caused greater decrease of the force of electrical or nicotine contraction than that of the ACh contraction and the decrease of the electrical and nicotine contraction was antagonized by 4-APYR more effectively than the decrease of the ACh contraction (see Table 1). The reason for this is that during electrical stimulation or after addition of nicotine to the bath, contraction of the muscle is elicited by ACh released at the postganglionic nerve terminal. The release of ACh is Ca-dependent and 4-APYR increases ACh release in the presence of both normal (see Table 4) and low [Ca] (Vizi, Van Dijk and Foldes, 1977). These findings indicate that the Ca requirements for the release of endogenous ACh are greater than that required for the contraction of the longitudinal muscle by exogenous ACh.

The influence of 4-APYR on the 3 types of contractions in the presence of compounds which are antagonists of muscarinic or nicotinic receptors or are narcotic agonists or antagonists or adrenergic agonists is also different. 4-APYR does not antagonize the effect of homatropine on ACh contraction, but it antagonizes its effect on the electrical contraction. Nicotine contraction is inhibited by C6 or normorphine. C6 competes with nicotine for the nicotinic receptors and inhibits nicotine induced depolarization. The inhibitory effect of normorphine, and presumably also that of other narcotics and enkephalins are probably more complex. It has been reported that normorphine hyperpolarizes the ganglia of the myenteric plexus (North and Tonini, 1977). This may render some of the ganglia resistant to depolarization by nicotine, decrease the postganglionic ACh release and thereby reduce the force of contraction of the muscle. The possibility, however, cannot be excluded that normorphine also inhibits ACh release directly at its release sites on the postganglionic nerve terminals. Naloxone would be expected to antagonize the effects of normorphine at both sites. It is conceivable,

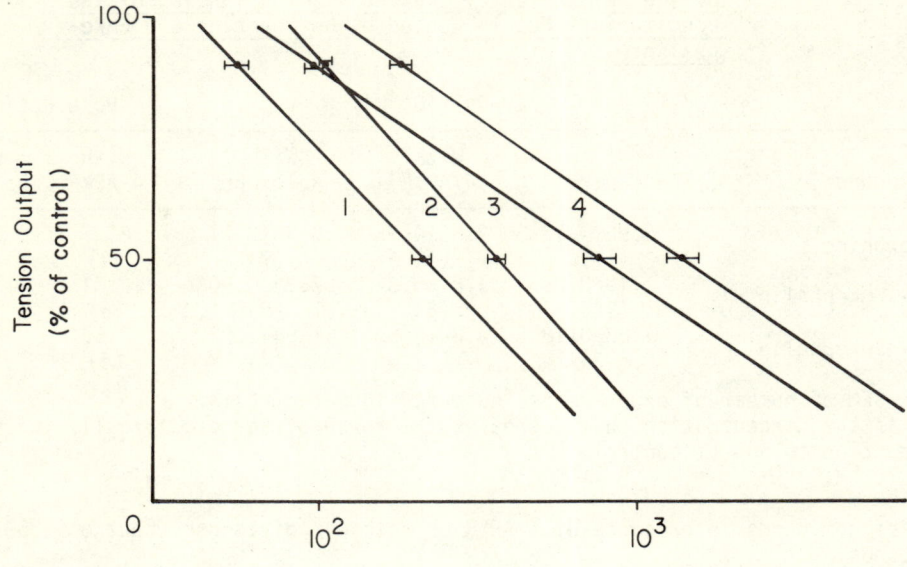

Fig. 6. The log dose - response regression lines of the normorphine induced depression of the electrical contraction with or without naloxone and 4-aminopyridine (4-APYR). (1) Normorphine; (2) Normorphine + $2 \times 10^{-9}$M naloxone; (3) Normorphine + $2 \times 10^{-6}$M 4-APYR; (4) Normorphine + $2 \times 10^{-9}$M naloxone + $2 \times 10^{-6}$M 4-APYR.

however, that 4-APYR only antagonizes the effects of normorphine at the Ca-dependent release site of ACh.

During electrical field stimulation, in all probability, the pre- and postganglionic nerve terminals and the ganglia themselves are all depolarized. The observation that blocking the nicotinic receptors by C6 has no effect on the force of isometric contraction of the muscle elicited by field stimulation indicates that depolarization of the preganglionic fibers and adsorption of the released ACh to nicotinic receptors have little effect on tension development during electrical stimulation in this preparation. In contrast decrease of the force of electrical contraction by narcotics, enkephalins or epinephrine, all of which inhibit postganglionic ACh release, indicates that ACh released from the postganglionic nerve terminals is all important for the development of contraction. In agreement with this the inhibition of electrical contraction by these compounds can be antagonized by 4-APYR, a compound that increases ACh release.

The fact that the ability of histamine to produce contraction at a time when electrical contraction is abolished by homatropine confirmed the earlier finding of Paton and Zar (1968) that the denervated longitudinal muscle itself does not respond to electrical stimulation.

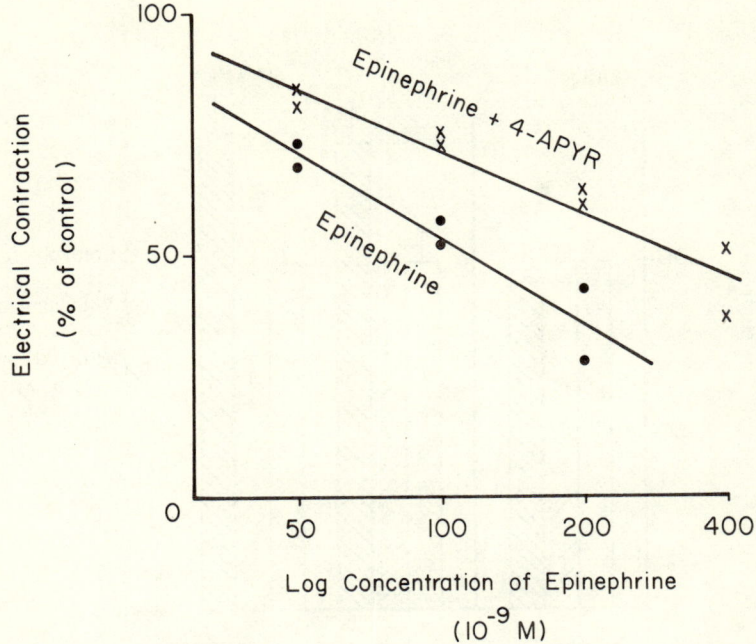

Fig. 7. Antagonism of the l-epinephrine induced depression of the electrical contraction of the longitudinal muscle by $5 \times 10^{-6}$M 4-aminopyridine (4-APYR).

TABLE 4  Influence of 4-Aminopyridine (4-APYR) on Acetylcholine (ACh) Release.

| 4-APYR (M) | Stimulation Rate (Hz) | ACh Release[2] Control | With 4-APYR | Volley Output of ACh[3] Control | With 4-APYR |
|---|---|---|---|---|---|
| $4.25 \times 10^{-6}$ | 0 | 663.3± 25.2 | 1215.5±187.5* | — | — |
|  | 5 | 3404.4±289.5 | 5003.0±602.9* | 7.6±1.5 | 10.8±1.6 |
| $1.00 \times 10^{-4}$ | 0 | 898.9±181.7 | 3944.9±278.9* | — | — |
|  | 0.5 | 1615.8±124.6 | 5011.9±285.7* | 23.4±2.2 | 35.6±2.8* |

[1]Mean ± SEM of 4 experiments.
[2]pmol.g tissue$^{-1}$. min$^{-1}$.
[3]pmol.g tissue$^{-1}$. volley; Calculated with the formula: (Stimulated ACh release.g tissue$^{-1}$. min$^{-1}$. - spontaneous ACh release.g tissue$^{-1}$.min$^{-1}$) X stimulation rate per min.
*Indicates significant difference from control at the $p < 0.01$ level (paired $\underline{t}$ test).

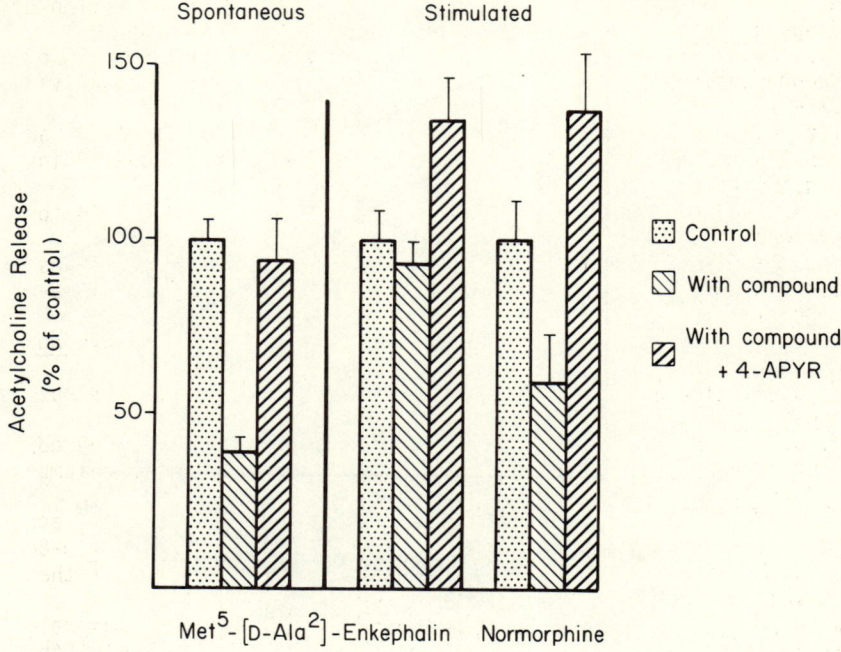

Fig. 8. Antagonism by 4-APYR of the depression of acetylcholine release caused by normorphine or by [d-Ala$^2$]-Met$^5$- enkephalin.

The inhibitory effect of adrenaline and noradrenaline on spontaneous and stimulated ACh release and on contraction of the longitudinal muscle by electrical stimulation has been attributed to effect of these amines on the ganglia (Paton and Vizi, 1969; Kosterlitz, Lydon and Watt, 1970). This effect is also antagonized by 4-APYR (see Fig. 8).

It follows from the above considerations, that although 4-APYR probably facilitates Ca-dependent ACh release from both pre- and postganglionic parasympathetic nerve terminals, from the functional point of view its postganglionic effect is of primary importance in this preparation. The facilitation by 4-APYR of the contraction of the longitudinal muscle elicited by electrical stimulation, and its antagonist effect on the inhibition of the nicotine contraction by C6 or normorphine, or that of the electrical contraction by narcotics, enkephalins and epinephrine are all compatible with this assumption.

In conclusion, 4-APYR facilitates transmission in the myenteric plexus - longitudinal muscle preparation of the guinea-pig ileum by increasing the Ca-dependent stimulated ACh release. 4-APYR will also antagonize the inhibitory effect of compounds (e.g., narcotics, enkephalins, epinephrine) which inhibit stimulated ACh release or compete with ACh (e.g., homatropine, atropine) for muscarinic receptors on the muscle. The effects of decreased ACh release caused by low [Ca] are also counteracted by 4-APYR.

## REFERENCES

Cowie, A. L., H. W. Kosterlitz, and A. J. Watt (1968). Mode of action of morphine-like drugs on autonomic neuro-effectors. Nature, 220, 1040-1042.

Hughes, J., T. W. Smith, and H. W. Kosterlitz (1975). Identification of two related pentopeptides from the brain with potent opiate agonist activity. Nature, 258, 577-579.

Kosterlitz, H.W., R. G. Lydon, and A. J. Watt (1970). The effects of adrenaline, noradrenaline on inhibitory and $\alpha$ and $\beta$ receptors in the longitudinal muscle of the guinea-pig ileum. Br. J. Pharmacol., 39, 398-413.

Krebs, H. A., and K. Henseleit (1932). Untersuchungen über die Harnstoffbildung im Tierkärper. Hoppe Seylers z. Physiol. Chem., 210, 33-66.

Paton, W. D. M. (1957a). The action of morphine and related substances on contraction and on acetylcholine output of coaxially stimulated guinea-pig ileum. Br. J. Pharmacol., 12, 119-127.

Paton, W. D. M. (1957b). A pendulum auxotonic lever. J. Physiol. (Lond.), 137, 35-36P.

Paton, W. D. M. (1963). Cholinergic transmission and acetylcholine output. Can. J. Biochem. Physiol., 41, 2637-2653.

Paton, W. D. M., and E. S. Vizi (1969). The inhibitory action of noradrenaline and adrenaline on acetylcholine output by guinea-pig longitudinal muscle strip. Br. J. Pharmacol., 35, 10-28.

Paton, W. D. M., E. S. Vizi, and M. A. Zar (1971). The mechanism of acetylcholine release from parasympathetic nerves. J. Physiol. (Lond.), 215, 819-848.

Paton, W. D. M., and M. A. Zar (1965). A denervated preparation of the longitudinal muscle of the guinea-pig ileum. J. Physiol. 179, 85-86F.

Paton, W. D. M., and M. A. Zar (1968). The origin of acetylcholine released from guinea-pig intestine and longitudinal muscle strip. J. Physiol. (Lond.), 194, 13-33.

Schaumann, W. (1956). Influence of atropine and morphine on the liberation of acetylcholine from the guinea-pig's intestine. Nature, 178, 1121-1122.

Schaumann, W. (1957). Inhibition by morphine of the release of acetylcholine from the intestine of the guinea-pig. Br. J. Pharmacol. 12, 115-118.

Vizi, E. S., J. Van Dijk, and F. F. Foldes (1977). The effect of 4-aminopyridine on acetylcholine release. J. Neural Transm., 41, 265-274.

Vizi, E. S., F. F. Foldes, J. Rich, and J. Knoll (1976). The structure-action relationship and kinetics of some naloxone and naltrexone derivatives. Pharmacology, 14, 76-85.

Vizi, E. S., F. F. Foldes, and J. Theunissen (1975). The Effects of Protoveratrine and Germines on the Release of Acetylcholine from the Auerbach Plexus of the Guinea-Pig Ileum. J. Neural Transm., 37, 43-60.

# DISCUSSION OF THE SECOND SESSION

Dr. Llinás: Dr. Thesleff, did you notice any change in synaptic delay following 4-aminopyridine?

Dr. Thesleff: Yes, we observed that 4-aminopyridine and 3,4-diaminopyridine increased the minimum synaptic delay.

Dr. Schiavone: I should like to ask Dr. Molgo if the increase in size and duration of the spontaneous "giant" miniature end-plate potentials seen in the presence of aminopyridines is partly due to the effects of these drugs at the postsynaptic membrane?

Dr. Molgo: I don't think that the amplitude and duration of the "giant" miniature end-plate potentials are related to postsynaptic effects of the aminopyridines, since in that case one would expect that also normal sized miniature end-plate potentials were affected in their size and duration. The larger than normal amplitude of the "giant" miniature end-plate potentials seems to be due to the release of large amounts of ACh by a mechanism different from the quantal release process responsible for the normal sized miniature end-plate potentials.

Dr. McArdle: Dr. Molgo, do extrajunctional (postjunctional) ACh receptors contribute to the prolonged time course of end-plate currents after 4-aminopyridine treatment?

Dr. Molgo: This is a very interesting question for which I can only give a speculative answer. During electrotonic depolarization of TTX-treated nerve terminals in the presence of aminopyridines, the amount of ACh released is so large that one may wonder if not end-plate cholinesterases become saturated. If that is the case, it is conceivable that ACh might activate not only junctional but also extrajunctional receptors during its diffusion.

Dr. Pichon: Following presynaptic stimulation Dr. Molgo has observed an increase in miniature end-plate potential frequency in the presence of 10 μM of 4-aminopyridine. Have you any evidence that the frequency increase oscillates as could be expected from the resonance properties of the membrane in the presence of TTX?

Dr. Molgo: From our experiments it is clear that 4-aminopyridine in the range of concentrations studied (10-50 μM) has no effect on spontaneous miniature end-plate potential frequency at the resting junctions. However, when the motor nerve is stimulated either by nerve impulses or by an electrotonic depolarization (preparation treated with TTX), the frequency of miniature end-plate potentials appearing after stimulation is markedly increased. The magnitude of the increase depends on $Ca^{2+}$ concentration, the rate of stimulation etc. The increase in frequency of miniature end-plate potentials showed some oscillations which were particularly evident when the frequency was low. However, the oscillations were not analysed in detail.

Dr. Pichon: I have another question, you mentioned that there is no voltage and time dependency of the effect of 3,4-diaminopyridine on presynaptic terminals. Is that also true for 4-aminopyridine and if that is so, what is your interpretation of this fact which contradicts results obtained on axonal membranes?

Dr. Molgo: The results that we have obtained with both 4-aminopyridine and 3,4-diaminopyridine are rather similar and suggest that at motor nerve terminals the blockade of the $K^+$ conductance is neither time nor voltage dependent. It is conceivable that the $K^+$ conductance system of motor nerve terminals has biophysical properties different from those characterizing axonal membranes.

Dr. Galvan: Dr. Jankowska, you mentioned that sometimes aminopyridines reduced IPSPs. Could you please enlarge on that?

Dr. Jankowska: We have never seen any depression of IPSPs in our experiments although it was reported previously. I would therefore attribute it to differences in the way of application of 4-aminopyridine, its concentration and/or a possible activation of neuronal systems with depressant actions on transmission in the tested pathways.

Dr. Edman: Dr. Foldes, the tissue you are using seems to offer an interesting possibility to investigate whether or not aminopyridines are able to directly affect the $Ca^{2+}$ inflow into the cell. Smooth muscles that are depolarized in an isotonic $K^+$ solution respond with a graded contracture as the $Ca^{2+}$ concentration is raised in the extracellular medium (Edman & Schild, J. Physiol., 1972). $Ca^{2+}$ apparently enters the cell and initiates contraction by activating the contractile system directly. It would therefore be of interest to see if aminopyridines alter this contractile response to $Ca^{2+}$ which would give us an indication as to whether the inflow of $Ca^{2+}$ into the cell is affected by this group of drugs. This point has been discussed in previous papers at this Symposium. Your preparation would be useful for looking into this question. Have you, or anybody else present, studied aminopyridine effects on $Ca^{2+}$-induced contractures of depolarized smooth muscle?

Dr. Foldes: No.

Dr. Glover: In response to Dr. Edman's question I perhaps could describe the effect of 4-aminopyridine on the responses of vascular smooth muscle to $Ca^{2+}$. When isolated arteries are perfused with $Ca^{2+}$-free, high $K^+$ solution they contract in response to injections of $Ca^{2+}$. When the $Na^+$ in the perfusate is completely replaced with $K^+$ and the arteries presumably are depolarized, the responses to $Ca^{2+}$ are not increased by 4-aminopyridine. However, when the $K^+$ concentration is 4 or 6 times normal, the responses to $Ca^{2+}$ are significantly increased by 4-aminopyridine ($10^{-4}$ M). This suggests that 4-aminopyridine increases the permeability to $Ca^{2+}$ in arteries which are not completely depolarized.

# Aminopyridines and the Release of Chemical Transmitters: Contrast with Apamin

*Chairman:* R. Couteaux

# Structure - Activity Relationships Amongst Aminopyridines

I. G. Marshall

Department of Physiology and Pharmacology, University of
Strathclyde, Glasgow G1 1XW, UK

## ABSTRACT

In this review the actions of a range of aminopyridine-like compounds are described on electrically excitable membranes, on the central nervous system, on neuromuscular transmission at skeletal muscle, on parasympathetic and sympathetic neuroeffector transmission and on cardiac muscle. Particular attention is paid to effects on electrically excitable membranes where the prime action of the drugs i.e. inhibition of potassium conductance, may be measured, and on neuromuscular transmission, which is the site of action of the drugs that has been exploited clinically. Examination of chemical structure and properties of a range of compounds indicates that several features are involved in their action, including lipid solubility which may determine access to sites of action, degree of ionization and nature of substituents on the pyridine nucleus which may determine affinity for sites of action.

## KEYWORDS

Aminopyridines; potassium conductance inhibition; convulsant action; analgesic action; neuromuscular facilitation; autonomic facilitation; positive inotropic action; ionization; lipid solubility; aminopyridine analogues.

## INTRODUCTION

In 1925 Dohrn demonstrated that 2-aminopyridine produced convulsant activity and subsequently Dingemanse and Wibaut (1928) showed that 3-aminopyridine (3-AP) produced convulsions in the frog. For the following twenty years the pharmacology of the aminopyridines received scant attention until the seminal work of Fastier and co-workers. After comparing the circulatory properties of 2-aminopyridine (2-AP) with those of various amidine derivatives (Fastier, 1948; Fastier and Reid, 1948), Fastier and McDowall (1958) went on to show that the three aminopyridines 2-AP, 3-AP and 4-aminopyridine (4-AP), when injected into anaesthetized cats, produced an increase in blood pressure, an increase in respiratory movement and twitching of the head and limbs. Further experiments showed that the aminopyridines produced vasoconstriction when injected into perfused rat hind-quarters, contracted the isolated rat ileum, increased the contractions of the isolated rat hemidiaphragm, and produced analgesia and convulsions in conscious mice. Essentially similar results were obtained by von Haxthausen

(1955). Thus early work on the aminopyridines showed that the compounds possessed effects on the central autonomic and somatic nervous systems.

In the past fifteen years there has been a great resurgence of interest in the actions of the aminopyridines catalysed by Lemeignan and Lechat's study of the anti-curare action of aminopyridines in 1967 and spurred by the use of 4-AP as an anti-curare drug by Bulgarian anaesthetists (Paskov, Stoyanov and Mitsov, 1973). The subject has been reviewed briefly by Thesleff (1980) and more comprehensively by Bowman and Savage (1981). Full details of the mechanisms of action and potential uses of aminopyridines can be found in these review articles and in other contributions to this symposium. In this article each main site of pharmacological action of aminopyridines will be considered in turn with a brief description of the mechanism of action at the site and details of the actions of the compounds that have been tested at the site.

## ACTIONS ON ELECTRICALLY EXCITABLE MEMBRANES

Aminopyridines prolong the repolarization phase of action potentials in both nerve and muscle fibres and voltage clamp studies have shown that this effect is due to an inhibition of the outward potassium current, with little or no effect on the inward sodium current. (Hue, Pelhate and Chanelet, 1973; Pelhate and Pichon, 1974; Pelhate and others, 1974; Meves and Pichon, 1975, 1977; Gillespie and Hutter, 1975; Gillespie, 1977; Yeh and others, 1976a and b; Llinás, Walton and Bohr, 1976, Kirsch and Narahashi, 1978; Molgo, 1978; Horn, Lambert and Marshall, 1979; Datyner and Gage, 1980).

Tetraethylammonium (TEA) has been known for several years to block potassium conductance (Armstrong and Binstock, 1965; Armstrong, 1966), but the action of aminopyridines is somewhat different when studied in squid axons (Yeh and others, 1976b). Thus aminopyridines are active whether applied externally or internally to membranes, whereas TEA is only effective on internal application. Aminopyridines, but not TEA, produce a small depolarization. Aminopyridine block is reduced by depolarization and by increased stimulation frequency. This indicates that the opening of potassium channels favours the removal of aminopyridine block, whereas such an opening enhances TEA block.

Yeh and others (1976b) found that 3-AP and 2-AP exhibited similar actions to those of 4-AP on the squid axon. 3-AP and 4-AP were equipotent, 1mM of each producing $93.8 \pm 2.2\%$ and $96.2 \pm 1.9\%$ block of potassium current measured at 0mV. 2-AP was less potent producing $74.8 \pm 2.7\%$ inhibition. These potencies were considered to be unrelated to the $pK_a$ values of the compounds (Yeh and others, 1976a), and certainly Meves and Pichon (1977) found that changing pH had no effect on the blocking potency of 4-AP.

In a later study, using the same techniques Kirsch and Narahashi (1978) showed that 3,4-diaminopyridine (3,4-DAP) was approximately fifty times more potent than 4-AP as a potassium channel blocker and that its mechanism of action was essentially similar. Several other aminopyridine analogues were tested by Kirsch and Narahashi (1978) who found that compounds lacking hydroxyl or amino substituents were inactive. Of the compounds they tested the rank order (most potent first) was as follows: 3,4-DAP, 4-AP, 2,3-DAP, 4-hydroxypyridine (4-OHP), 2,6-DAP, 3-OHP and 2-OHP. No potency values are quoted. One interesting apparent difference between 4-AP and 3,4-AP on the squid axon is that 4-AP was reported to be equally effective on either internal or external application (Yeh and others, 1976b; Meves and Pichon, 1977) whereas 3,4-DAP was much more potent on internal than on external application. This implies that 4-AP may be more lipid soluble than 3,4-DAP and hence have greater access to an intracellular site of action, although it presumably has less affinity for the site.

Very recent work on the cockroach giant axon (Pelhate and others, 1981) has shown that the pyridine nucleus itself is essentially ineffective in blocking potassium channels but that 4-AP and some of its analogues block potassium conductance in micromolar concentrations (Table 1). Of the compounds tested all but 9-aminoacridine (9-AA) blocked closed potassium channels. Thus in this study 9-AA appeared similar to TEA, although Yeh (1979) has shown similarities between 9-AA and both 4-AP and TEA. Both 9-AA and 4-aminoquinoline blocked sodium as well as potassium channels (Pelhate and others, 1981). The studies of Yeh and others (1976b), Kirsch and Narahashi (1978) and Pelhate and others (1981) are the only ones to have examined a range of compounds on potassium conductance but other aminopyridine analogues have been compared in isolation to 4-AP. Thus Fastier, Pelhate and Hue (1981) have shown that 5-methylthiouronium which was originally compared to 4-AP in 1958 by Fastier and McDowall can block potassium channels.

Other compounds related to the aminopyridines which have been shown to prolong muscle action potentials, although they have not yet been studied under voltage clamp conditions, are the quaternary analogue of 4-AP, 4-aminopyridine methiodide (4-APMI) (Horn, Lambert and Marshall, 1979) and 4-hydroxypyridine and 4-nitropyridine (Molgo and others, 1981). The pKa values of 4-AP and 3,4-DAP are around 9.18 and 9.08 respectively and those of 3-AP and 2-AP are 6.03 and 6.71 respectively. Thus at physiological pH (pH 7.4) most of the 4-AP and 3,4-DAP molecules will be protonated (98.36% and 97.95% respectively) whereas a lower number of 2-AP (16.95%) and 3-AP (4.09%) molecules will be charged. In broad terms it is tempting to relate protonation of the compounds to potency, but other factors such as size and ability to form hydrogen bonds must be important. Thus unsubstituted pyridine is ineffective and it has been suggested that the high potency of 3,4-DAP may be due to greater hydrogen bonding capacity compared to 4-AP (Kirsch and Narahashi, 1978).

Table 1 Effects of Aminopyridine Analogues on Potassium Conductance in Cockroach Giant Axon (from Pelhate and others (1981)

| Compound | Apparent Dissociation Constant (Kd)* |
|---|---|
| 3,4-diaminopyridine | $1.8 \times 10^{-5}$ M |
| 4-aminopyridine | $3 \times 10^{-5}$ M |
| 3-aminopyridine | $5 \times 10^{-5}$ M |
| 2-aminopyridine | $2 \times 10^{-4}$ M |
| 9-aminoacridine | $2.7 \times 10^{-4}$ M |
| 4-aminoquinoline | $3.7 \times 10^{-4}$ M |

*For 100 mV depolarization.

Almost all the reported central and peripheral actions of aminopyridines result from an inhibition of potassium conductance in electrically excitable membranes. Thus prolongation of action potentials in nerves leads to enhanced transmitter output giving rise to facilitated neuroeffector transmission. In addition aminopyridines enhance skeletal and possibly cardiac muscle contractility. It will be noted that in all the systems to be described the overall spectrum of potencies of the most commonly tested compounds, i.e. 4-AP, 3-AP, 2-AP and 3,4-DAP is remarkably similar providing further evidence that a common mechanism i.e. inhibition of potassium conductance is central to most of the actions of the aminopyridines.

## ACTIONS ON THE CENTRAL NERVOUS SYSTEM

As stated above, aminopyridines enhance evoked transmitter release from nerves. The initial evidence for this was from peripheral synapses (Molgo, Lemeignan and Lechat, 1975) but extensions of this type of work has shown that the compounds facilitate transmission and release at both excitatory and inhibitory synapses in the central nervous system (Saade, Chanelet and Lonchampt, 1971; Lemeignan, 1971, 1972, 1973; Jankowska and others, 1977; Galindo and Rudomin, 1978). The main results of this central facilitatory action are convulsions, respiratory stimulation and analgesia, the last presumably due to enhanced release of enkephalins.

Various workers have studied the convulsant activity of the aminopyridines as a broad indication of the central potency of the compounds. As the convulsions result in death, $LD_{50}$ values are generally used as a measure of activity of the compounds (Fastier and McDowall, 1958b). Convulsant potencies of a range of aminopyridines are shown in Table 2.

TABLE 2  $LD_{50}$ Values and Convulsant Activity of Aminopyridine Analogues

| Compound | $LD_{50}$ i.v. mg/kg | $LD_{50}$ s.c. mg/kg | Severity of convulsions (where stated) |
|---|---|---|---|
| 2-aminopyridine | 23 | 70<br>70+ | ++++ |
| 3-aminopyridine | 24 | 30<br>30+ | +++ |
| 4-aminopyridine | 7 | 5<br>5+ | ++++ |
| 3,4-diaminopyridine | 13<br>20* | 35* | +++ |
| 2,6-diaminopyridine | | 100x | |
| 3-methyl-2-aminopyridine | | 36x | |
| 4-methyl-2-aminopyridine | 39 | 100<br>80x | ++ |
| 5-methyl-2-aminopyridine | | 110x | |
| 6-methyl-2-aminopyridine | | 52x | |
| 4,6-dimethyl-2-aminopyridine | | 25x | |
| 2-dimethylaminopyridine | 182 | | Hyperexcitability – no convulsions |
| 2-methylaminopyridine | 270 | | |
| 2-aminomethylpyridine | 340 | | |
| 2-benzylaminopyridine | | | No convulsionsx at 200 mg/kg |
| 2,6-diacetylaminopyridine | | | |
| 5-chloro-2-aminopyridine | | | |

*Vohra and Pradhan (1964), + von Haxthausen (1955a), x Fastier and McDowall (1958b), remainder from Lechat and others (1968).

Interestingly, it can be seen from Table 2 that 3,4-DAP the most potent aminopyridine in blocking potassium conductance, and as will subsequently be shown, the most potent in enhancing peripheral synaptic transmission, was less potent than 4-AP in producing central effects and the convulsions were slower in onset (Harvey and Marshall, 1977) and less severe (Lechat and others, 1968) than those produced by 4-AP.

In addition to producing convulsions the 4-AP analogue 4-methyl-3-aminopyridine reduces sleeping time in barbiturate-treated animals (Abernethy and Fastier, 1958). 4-AP has been shown to enhance recovery from ketamine anaesthesia (Agoston and others, 1980) but not from phencyclidine anaesthesia (Agoston - cited by Bowman and Savage, 1981). Bowman and Savage (1981) suggest that the anaesthesia reversing action of 4-AP is due to inhibition of potassium conductance and explain the lack of action of 4-AP against phencyclidine in terms of the latter drug already blocking potassium channels (Tsai and others, 1980).

The analgesic activity of aminopyridines has been studied by von Haxthausen (1955b), Fastier and McDowall (1958b) and Bergmann and Elam (1980). The analgesic activity of the aminopyridines can be antagonized by the opiate antagonist nalorphine, but conversely 4-AP can in turn antagonize the respiratory depression caused by opiates (Shaw and Bentley, 1955) and the depression of isolated preparations caused by morphine (Stone, 1981; Henderson and Marshall - unpublished observation). The analgesic potency of aminopyridine analogues is shown in Table 3.

TABLE 3  Analgesic Potency of Aminopyridine Analogues[+]
(from Fastier and McDowall, 1958b)

| Compounds | Analgesic $ED_{50}$ (mg/kg) | Toxicity $LD_{50}$ (mg/kg) | Therapeutic Index |
|---|---|---|---|
| 2-aminopyridine | ca. 10 | 70 | 7 |
| 3-aminopyridine | 8 | 35 | 4.5 |
| 4-aminopyridine | 1 | 5 | 5 |
| 3-methyl-2-aminopyridine | 10 | 36 | 3.5 |
| 4-methyl-2-aminopyridine | 5.5 | 80 | 15 |
| 5-methyl-2-aminopyridine | ca. 35* | 110 | 3 |
| 6-methyl-2-aminopyridine | ca. 17 | 52 | 3 |
| 4,6-dimethyl-2-aminopyridine | 7.5 | 25 | 3 |

+Approximate values from Fastier and McDowall's data.   *Not dose-related.

Although 4-methyl-2-aminopyridine (4-Me-2-AP) had the greatest margin of safety, Fastier and McDowall (1958b) showed that its analgesic potency was only one-tenth of that of morphine. Again 4-AP, the most basic compound, was the most potent as an analgesic, but no clear relationship was seen between basicity and analgesic activity.

## EFFECTS ON NEUROMUSCULAR TRANSMISSION

The effects of the aminopyridines have been most widely studied on transmission at the skeletal muscle neuromuscular junction for the following reasons: 1) the site is easily accessible, 2) effects measured in vitro can be related to in vivo effects, 3) effects on transmitter release can be related to effects on muscle contractions 4) simple inexpensive preparations allow easy comparison of a large number of compounds 5) the actions of aminopyridines at this site have been exploited clinically leading to the use of 4-AP as an anti-curare agent and its proposed use in various disease states of the neuromuscular junction.

The effects of aminopyridines that are measured at the neuromuscular junction include augmentation of muscle twitch tension, generally in response to single shock stimulation of the motor nerve to the muscle, and reversal of neuromuscular block due to non-depolarizing neuromuscular blocking drugs such as tubocurarine. Both these effects are considered to be secondary to an increase in evoked release of acetylcholine.  Occasionally compounds have been compared on the release process although this type of experiment is technically difficult and hence not many compounds have been studied in this way.

After the initial observation that aminopyridines increased responses of the isolated rat hemi-diaphragm to both nerve stimulation and to direct muscle stimulation (Fastier and McDowall, 1958a), Lemeignan and Lechat (1967) and Bowman, Harvey and Marshall (1977) showed that 4-AP enhanced muscle contractions to nerve stimulation without increasing responses to injected or added acetylcholine.   The results of these simple experiments were taken to indicate that 4-AP had no postjunctional action, but probably increased acetylcholine output from the nerve. Electrophysiological studies and transmitter collection and assay studies confirmed that 4-AP increased acetylcholine release (Molgo, Lemeignan and Lechat, 1975, 1977, 1979; Lundh, Leander and Thesleff, 1976; Lundh, 1978, 1979; Lundh and Thesleff, 1977; Illes and Thesleff, 1978; Jacobs and Burley, 1978; Kim, Goldner and Sanders, 1980; Foldes and others, 1976). In particular, intracellular recording studies showed that 4-AP increased endplate potential amplitude in either magnesium or tubocurarine-paralysed nerve-muscle preparations by causing an increase in endplate potential quantal content.   Quantal content was increased not by increasing p, the probability of release, but by increasing n which is thought to reflect either the available store of transmitter or the number of release sites (Molgo, Lemeignan and Lechat, 1979; Lundh, 1979).   It is thought that inhibition of potassium conductance as described above leads to a prolongation of the nerve terminal action potential which in turn causes a prolongation of the open time of voltage-sensitive calcium channels in the nerve terminal membrane, allowing a greater than usual influx of calcium which leads to a greater release of acetylcholine.   If this is the case then the potencies of a range of compounds in enhancing neuromuscular transmission would be expected to relate to their potencies in blocking potassium conductance.   In general terms this is so.

In my own laboratory we have tested a wide range of aminopyridine analogues on the isolated chick biventer cervicis nerve-muscle preparation.   In this preparation compounds can be tested on the twitch responses of the focally innervated fibres to nerve stimulation and on the contractural responses of the multiply innervated fibres to added agonists such as acetylcholine and carbachol.   On this preparation it is possible to differentiate between compounds which facilitate transmission via inhibition of cholinesterase and those which act to increase transmitter output.   Augmenting effects on muscle contractility can also be studied in preparations stimulated directly in the presence of irreversible postjunctionally active snake toxins.

Initially we compared the actions of 2-AP, 3-AP and 4-AP (Bowman, Harvey and Marshall, 1977), followed by 3,4-DAP, 2,3-DAP and 2,6-DAP (Harvey and Marshall, 1977) and more recently 2,5-DAP (Harvey - personal communication).   All the compounds enhanced twitches in indirectly stimulated preparations and reversed tubocurarine-induced neuromuscular block. Except in the presence of 2,5-DAP responses to added agonists were unaffected.   The effects of the compounds on indirectly elicited twitches are shown in Fig. 1.

It can be seen from Fig. 1 that the descending order of potency of the compounds is 3,4-DAP⩾ 4-AP > 3-AP > 2-AP, with 2,6-DAP, 2,3-DAP and 2,5-DAP being very inactive.   At higher doses 2,5-DAP produced a blockade of both indirectly and directly elicited twitches. In a similar study on the rat hemidiaphragm preparation Savage (1979) showed that 3,4-DAP was slightly more potent than 4-AP in reversing tubocurarine-induced neuromuscular block.

Subsequent studies using electrophysiological recording techniques have confirmed that 3,4-DAP is the most potent of the aminopyridines tested so far in enhancing acetylcholine release (Durant

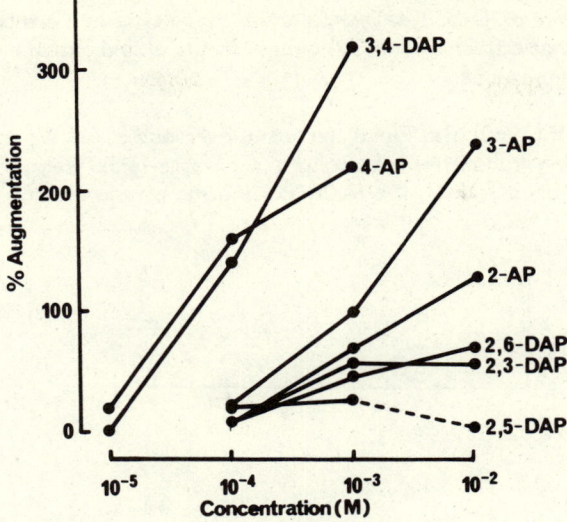

Fig. 1. Twitch augmentation produced by aminopyridines and diaminopyridines on the chick biventer cervicis muscle preparation.

and Marshall, 1978, 1980; Molgo, Lundh and Thesleff, 1980). 3,4-DAP was 6-7 times more potent than 4-AP in enhancing transmitter release both in the magnesium paralyzed mouse phrenic nerve-hemidiaphragm preparation and in the botulinum toxin-paralyzed rat extensor digitorum longus muscle preparation (Fig. 2). Indeed Katz and Miledi (1979) have shown in

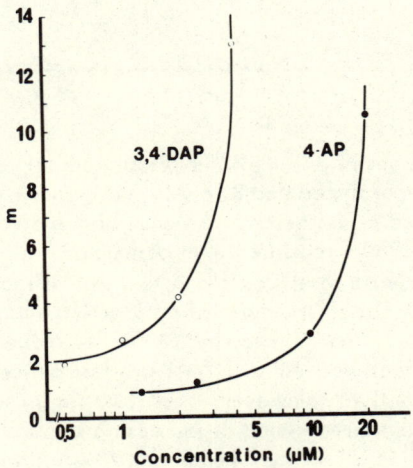

Fig. 2. Effects of 4-AP and 3,4-DAP on quantal content (m) in the magnesium-paralyzed mouse hemidiaphragm (from Molgo, Lundh and Thesleff, (1980) - reprinted with permission.

the frog that in the presence of 1mM 3,4-DAP, transmitter release in response to single shock nerve stimulation can increase from around 300 quanta in the absence of the drug to around ten thousand quanta in its presence.

Molgo, Lundh and Thesleff (1980) also found that both 4-AP and 3,4-DAP became considerably more effective at increasing transmitter release in a magnesium-paralysed preparation when the extracellular pH was raised from 7.4 to 9.0. Raising the pH alone had no significant effect on quantal content (Fig. 3).

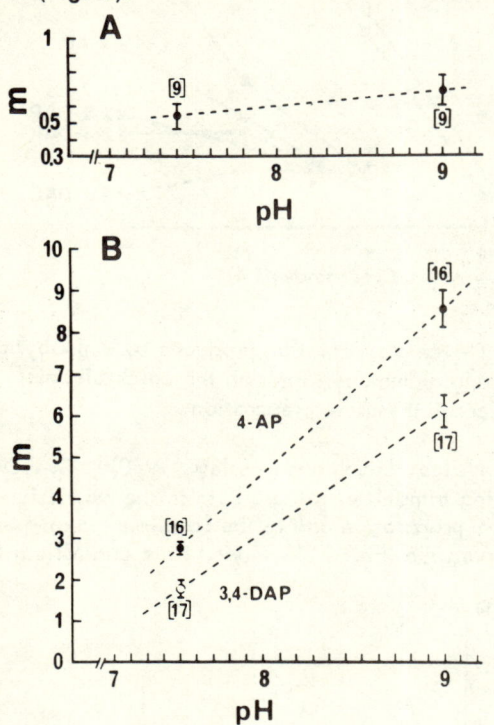

Fig. 3. Effects of changes in extracellular pH on quantal content in A) magnesium-paralyzed and B) 4-AP (5μM) and 3,4-DAP (0.5μM)-treated mouse hemidiaphragms (from Molgo, Lundh and Thesleff, 1980 - reprinted with permission.

This observation, taken together with results on the potency of aminopyridines with different $pK_a$ values may help shed some light on their site of action. As stated previously, the $pK_a$ values of 4-AP and 3,4-DAP are around 9.1 so that at pH 7.4 around 98% of the molecules will be protonated. As the less active 3-AP and 2-AP are less protonated it is possible that the protonated form is the most active. However, as will be shown subsequently, the quaternary analogue of 4-AP, 4-APMI, is extremely weak at increasing transmitter release (Horn, Lambert and Marshall, 1979). The findings of Molgo, Lundh and Thesleff on the pH dependency of 4-AP and 3,4-DAP may at least partially explain these apparently contradictory observations. With 4-AP and 3,4-DAP as the pH is increased, less of the compounds will be protonated with the result that at pH 9.0 39.8% and 45.4% respectively of the molecules will be in the more lipid-soluble non-ionized form. Molgo, Lundh and Thesleff (1980) suggested that at pH 9.0 the compounds would penetrate nerve terminals more effectively than at pH 7.4. Changes in extracellular pH have little or no effect on intracellular pH and hence once inside the terminal, the compounds would once again become largely protonated.

Despite the above observations, the finding that changes of pH have no effect on the potencies of the monoaminopyridines (Schauf and others, 1976; Meves and Pichon, 1977) makes it uncertain whether or not protonation of aminopyridines is a determining factor on potency.

Apart from the mono- and diaminopyridines several other aminopyridines have been tested, some in more detail than others, in attempts to find compounds with actions confined to the neuromuscular junction. Again, in our laboratory we have used the chick biventer cervicis muscle preparation as a primary screen. The formulae of the compounds tested on this preparation are shown in Figs. 4 a and b, and their potencies relative to the mono- and diaminopyridines on the same preparation are shown in Table 4.

Perhaps the compound of greatest interest was the quaternary analogue of 4-AP, (Horn, Lambert and Marshall, 1979). 4-APMI was about 10 - 30 times less potent than 4-AP in enhancing twitches of the indirectly stimulated chick biventer muscle preparation and was also less potent in reversing tubocurarine-induced neuromuscular blockade. In preparations in which the cholinesterase was inhibited both 4-AP and 3,4-DAP reversed tubocurarine-induced block, but 4-APMI was less effective than in the presence of functional cholinesterase. Taken together with the observation that responses to added acetylcholine were enhanced by 4-APMI these findings suggested that 4-APMI owed part of its facilitatory action to a 4-AP-like action and part to an anticholinesterase action. The weak effect of 4-APMI on transmitter release was shown by the compound producing only a slight increase in quantal content at a concentration

TABLE 4  Effects of Aminopyridine Analogues on the Indirectly Stimulated Chick Biventer Cervicis Nerve-Muscle Preparation

| Compound | Concentration required to produce 100% twitch augmentation | Effects on added acetylcholine | Other effects |
|---|---|---|---|
| 2-aminopyridine* | $2 \times 10^{-3}$M | 0 | - |
| 3-aminopyridine* | $10^{-3}$M | 0 | - |
| 4-aminopyridine* | $3 \times 10^{-3}$M | 0 | - |
| 3,4-diaminopyridine+ | $3 \times 10^{-3}$M | 0 | - |
| 2,3-diaminopyridine+ | 80% at $10^{-2}$M | 0 | - |
| 2,5-diaminopyridine° | 30% at $10^{-3}$M | Increase then dec. | Block at $10^{-3}$M |
| 2,6-diaminopyridine+ | 85% at $10^{-2}$M | 0 | - |
| 4-methyl-2-aminopyridine† | 50% at $10^{-2}$M | Increase | - |
| 4-aminopyridine methiodide× | $8 \times 10^{-4}$M | Increase | - |
| 4-dimethylaminopyridine | 53% at $3 \times 10^{-3}$M | Increase | - |
| 9-aminoacridine | 10% at $10^{-5}$M | Increase | - |
| 9-aminotetrahydroacridine | $10^{-4}$M | Increase | - |
| 4-aminobenzylpyridinium | 56% at $10^{-3}$M | Increase | Biphasic block |
| 4-pyridylpyridinium | - | - | Depolarizer |
| 4-AP C10 dimer | - | - | Non-depolarizer |
| 4-hydroxypyridine | 0 | 0 | - |

*Bowman, Harvey and Marshall (1977); †Harvey and Marshall (1977); ‡Kiloh, Harvey and Glover (1981); ×Horn, Lambert and Marshall (1979); °Harvey - personal communication.

one-hundred times that of 4-AP. The anticholinesterase activity of 4-APMI was confirmed both by inhibition of cholinesterase in chick muscle homogenates and by an observed prolongation of endplate potential time-course. Muscle action potential time course was also prolonged by both 4-AP and 4-APMI.

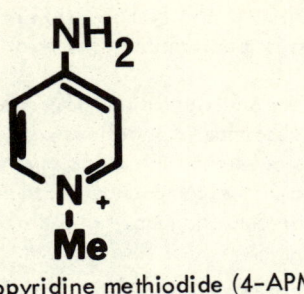
4-aminopyridine methiodide (4-APMI)

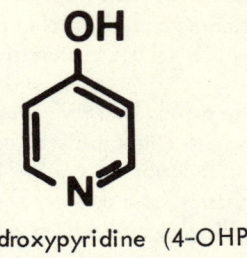
4-hydroxypyridine (4-OHP)

4-dimethylaminopyridine (4-DMAP)

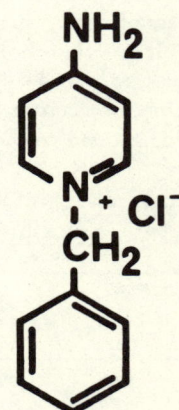
4-aminobenzyl pyridinium chloride (4-ABP)

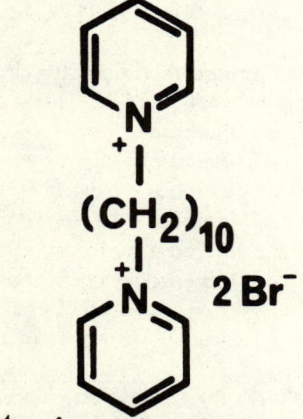
4-aminopyridine C10 dimer

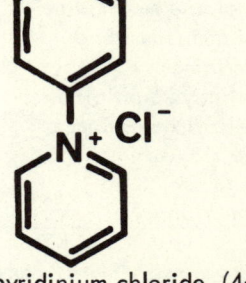
N-(4-pyridyl) pyridinium chloride (4-PPC)

Fig. 4a. Chemical formulae of aminopyridine analogues tested on chick biventer cervicis muscle preparation

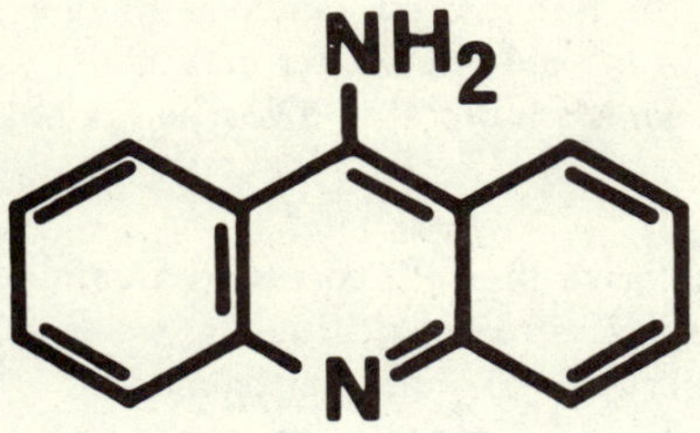

9-aminoacridine (9-AA)

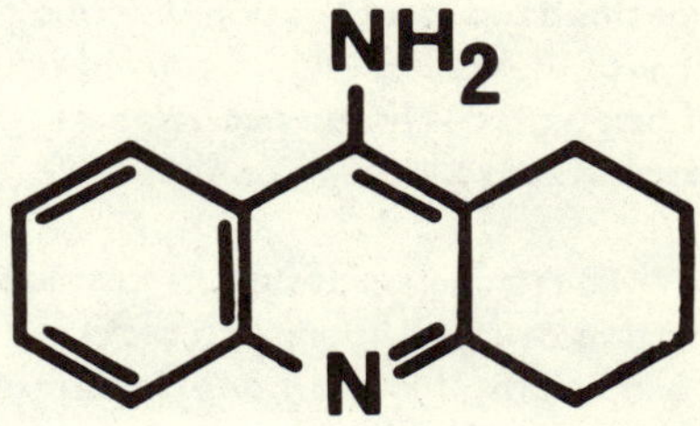

9-amino-1,2,3,4 tetrahydroacridine (9-ATHA)

Fig. 4b. Chemical formulae of aminopyridine analogues tested on chick biventer cervicis muscle preparation.

The relative lack of effect of the quaternary 4-APMI probably provides further evidence that the aminopyridines need to penetrate nerve terminals to exert their action. The anticholinesterase action of 4-APMI was rapid in onset and easily removed by washing, indicating that like edrophonium 4-APMI associates and dissociates rapidly with the enzyme receptor site, its structure allowing binding at the anionic site only.

Consideration of the structure of edrophonium also led us to examine the pharmacological activity of 4-hydroxypyridine (Lambert and Marshall - unpublished observations). Up to a concentration of $10^{-3}$M we were unable to show any activity on the chick biventer cervicis muscle, but subsequently Montoya and others (1981) and Molgo and others (1981) have shown that very high concentrations of 4-hydroxypyridine ($10^{-3}$ - $10^{-2}$M) increase transmitter release at the frog neuromuscular junction. 4-hydroxypyridine was approximately one thousand times less active than 4-AP (Montoya and others, 1981). 4-nitropyridine, studied in the same way, was around ten times more potent than 4-hydroxypyridine but had a lower maximum effect. Both compounds prolonged muscle action potentials and the authors considered that their action on transmitter release was a direct consequence of their inhibitory action on potassium conductance.

Amongst the other compounds we have tested, several, such as 4-APMI, enhanced responses to added acetylcholine and were almost inactive in reversing tubocurarine-induced neuromuscular block in the absence of functional cholinesterase. Agents with this type of action were 4-methyl-2-aminopyridine (Kiloh, Harvey and Glover, 1981), 4-dimethyl-2-aminopyridine, 9-aminoacridine and 9-aminotetrahydroacridine and it was concluded that all these compounds possessed mainly anticholinesterase activity.

N(4-pyridyl) pyridinium chloride produced contracture of the chick biventer cervicis muscle preparation indicating a depolarizing mechanism. This type of action has been confirmed in the anaesthetized cat (Agoston-personal communication). The bisquaternary decamethylene analogue of 4-AP (Fig. 4a) produced neuromuscular block in the chick biventer cervicis muscle associated with an abolition of responses to added agonists indicating a postjunctional non-depolarizing blocking action.

The final compound we tested, 4-aminobenzylpyridinium chloride (4-ABP) possessed a unique combination of facilitatory and blocking actions making its action rather difficult to categorize (Flavahan, Horn, Marshall and Schofield - unpublished observations). The compound was tested on the chick biventer cervicis muscle preparation and, with intracellular recording techniques, on the frog sartorius muscle preparation. In the chick muscle 4-ABP produced an initial twitch augmentation followed by a blockade of transmission. After washout only a partial recovery of transmission was observed.

The compound increased responses to acetylcholine and prolonged the time course of endplate potentials but did not increase quantal content, suggesting that the facilitatory effect of the compound was due to an anticholinesterase action. In addition, muscle action potentials were not affected by 4-ABP indicating that the compound had no 4-AP-like activity. 4-ABP depressed responses to added carbachol and abolished miniature endplate potential activity indicating a depression of postjunctional receptor sensitivity. The postjunctional blocking action of the compound was readily reversed by washing but prolonged exposure to the drug followed by washout led to the development of a secondary prejunctional block in which responses to carbachol and miniature endplate potential amplitude returned almost to control levels whereas twitches and quantal content remained low.

4-ABP is only poorly lipid soluble and hence the prejunctional blocking action is unlikely to be due to an intracellular action, despite very slow onset. It is possible that 4-ABP acts extracellularly to produce an essentially irreversible prejunctional block but that its rate of association with prejunctional sites is very slow.

Savage (1979) has tested a number of substances related to 4-AP for their ability to reverse tubocurarine-induced neuromuscular block in the rat hemidiaphragm. As stated previously, he showed that 3,4-DAP and 4-AP were the most potent compounds, 4-APMI was about seventy-five times less potent than 4-AP, 4-aminoquinaldine and 4-aminotetrahydroacridine were equipotent with 4-AP but the ceiling of their effects was much less than that of 4-AP, presumably because of a different mechanism of action. 4-Dimethylaminopyridine, 2-amino pyrimidine, 5-aminoquinoline and 3-aminoquinuclidine were inactive.

Most of the evidence from testing compounds at the neuromuscular junction indicates that facilitatory actions on transmission are closely related to inhibition of potassium conductance and that an intracellular site of action is probable. The requirements for new aminopyridine analogues to act on the neuromuscular junction will be discussed subsequently.

## EFFECTS ON PARASYMPATHETIC NEUROEFFECTOR TRANSMISSION

Fastier and McDowall (1958a) originally showed that aminopyridines produce a contractile effect in the isolated rat ileum. Vizi and others (1977) showed that 4-AP increased both spontaneous and evoked release of acetylcholine from the isolated guinea pig ileum. The effect of 4-AP, even on spontaneous release, was blocked by tetrodotoxin showing that the 4-AP-induced increase in spontaneous release could have been due to prolongation of the time course of reverberating action potentials in Auerbach's plexus. 2-AP was shown to be less effective than 4-AP. In a more comprehensive study Moritoki and others (1978) studied the effects of a range of aminopyridine analogues in producing contractions of the guinea pig ileum, in enhancing responses to nerve stimulation and in enhancing spontaneous release from the ileum. The results are summarized in Table 5.

TABLE 5  Effects of Aminopyridine Analogues on the Isolated Guinea Pig Ileum (from Moritoki and others, 1978).

| Compound | Concentration for 50% maximal contraction | Concentration for 100% increase in twitch tension | % increase in release at $10^{-3}$M |
| --- | --- | --- | --- |
| 2-aminopyridine | $2 \times 10^{-4}$M | $3 \times 10^{-6}$M | 480 |
| 3-aminopyridine | $9 \times 10^{-4}$M | $8 \times 10^{-5}$M | 240 |
| 4-aminopyridine | $3 \times 10^{-5}$M | $2 \times 10^{-7}$M | 960 |
| 3,4-diaminopyridine | $10^{-5}$M | - | 1130 |
| 2,3-diaminopyridine | $3 \times 10^{-4}$M | - | 430 |
| 2,6-diaminopyridine | ca $10^{-2}$M | - | 160 at $3 \times 10^{-3}$M |
| 2-amino-3-hydroxy pyridine | $8 \times 10^{-4}$M | - | 330 at $3 \times 10^{-3}$M |

Again the results are probably mainly due to inhibition of potassium conductance and again the order of potency is in broad agreement with order of potency on neuromuscular transmission and on potassium conductance.

## EFFECTS ON SYMPATHETIC NEUROEFFECTOR TRANSMISSION

As at other synapses, 4-AP has been shown to facilitate transmission at the postganglionic sympathetic neuroeffector junction by a prejunctional mechanism in which the release of the transmitter noradrenaline is increased (Johns and others, 1976; Leander, Arner and Johansson, 1977; Kirpekar, Kirpekar and Prat, 1977; Ito, Korenaga and Tajima, 1980). Johns and others (1976) tested a range of aminopyridine analogues on responses to transmural stimulation of the rabbit vas deferens. Responses were augmented by $10^{-5}$ and $10^{-4}$M 2-AP, 3-AP, 4-AP and 3,4-DAP, the order of potency being 3,4-DAP $\geqslant$ 4-AP $>$ 2-AP = 3-AP. At concentrations up to $10^{-4}$M pyridine, aniline, 4-dimethylaminopyridine, 4-aminomethylpyridine and 2-amino pyrimidine were without effect. The authors concluded that, in common with other systems, both a pyridine ring and an amino substituent were necessary for activity and that substitution on the amino group resulted in loss of activity.

It should be noted that 4-AP also augments transmission through sympathetic ganglia (Durant, Lee and Katz, 1980) but no analogues of 4-AP appear to have been studied at this site.

## EFFECTS ON CARDIAC MUSCLE

Almost all workers who have tested 4-AP on cardiac muscle have observed a positive inotropic effect but there is controversy over the exact mechanism involved. Aminopyridines are much less potent on the heart than on neuromuscular transmission and the effects produced by the large concentrations necessary may be due to noradrenaline release, to a direct action of the aminopyridines or to a rise in extracellular pH produced by the compounds (see Bowman and Savage, 1981 for full review of the pertinent literature). Part of the inotropic effect of 4-AP is undoubtedly due to noradrenaline release as the effect is blocked by propranolol (Yanagisawa and Taira, 1979; Woolmer, Wohlfart and Khan, 1979). In fact the entire action of 4-methyl-2-aminopyridine has been considered to be due to noradrenaline release (Schoepke and Shideman, 1961; Glover, 1979). Other studies have indicated that 4-AP prolongs the cardiac action potential (Frank, Flom and Ffrench-Mullen, 1978; Woolmer, Wohlfart and Khan, 1979; Freeman, 1979; Kenyon and Gibbons, 1979) and this prolongation is probably related to inhibition of potassium conductance. Rodger and Shahid (1981) have shown that effects of 4-AP on heart muscle can only be achieved at concentrations that raise the pH of the bathing fluid substantially and have shown that similar inotropic effects are produced by pH increases alone. However Kenyon and Gibbons (1979) did not measure tension in their experiments but recorded marked changes in action potentials and currents at pH's between 7.3 and 7.5.

It should be made clear that pH changes are only produced by very high concentrations of 4-AP in non-bicarbonate or phosphate buffered solutions. In bicarbonate buffered Kreb-Henseleit solution $10^{-2}$M 4-AP and 3,4-DAP produce only very small increases in pH. Hence pH increase is not likely to explain effects of low concentrations of aminopyridines on synaptic transmission.

## PRESENT AND POTENTIAL CLINICAL USES OF AMINOPYRIDINES

As stated previously, one of the main spurs for the recent work on aminopyridines has been the use of 4-aminopyridine (as the hydrochloride) as a reversal agent for non-depolarizing neuromuscular blocking agents by Bulgarian anaesthetists (Paskov, Stoyanov and Mitsov, 1973). In addition to reversing non-depolarizing blockers, aminopyridines have been shown to reverse neuromuscular block due to various groups of antibiotic drugs that are resistant to the reversing effects of the anticholinesterase agents; these include aminoglycosides, polymyxins, lincosamides and tetracyclines (Sobek and others, 1968; Singh, Harvey and Marshall, 1978; Lee, de Silva and Katz, 1978; Molgo and others, 1979).

Miller and others (1978, 1979) have shown that 4-AP potentiates the action of the anticholinerases neostigmine and pyridostigmine in reversing non-depolarizing neuromuscular block in both animals and man. Similar results in cats are seen with 3,4-DAP (Gandiha, Harvey and Marshall - unpublished observations). The advantages of such a combination of drugs is that it reduces the doses required of both the individual agents and reduces the need for atropine premedication. Initially we were hopeful that 4-aminopyridine methiodide would encompass both these mechanisms of action in one chemical but its facilitatory action proved extremely weak and short-lived when injected in vivo (Marshall - unpublished observation).

4-AP has also been tested and found to be effective in diseases affecting neuromuscular transmission including the Eaton-Lambert syndrome (Lundh, Nilsson and Rosen, 1977; Agoston and others, 1978), myasthenia gravis (Lundh, Nilsson and Rosen, 1979) and botulism (Ball and others, 1979).

Bostock, Sears and Sherratt (1981) have shown that voltage-dependent potassium channels do not occur at nodes of Ranvier in mammalian myelinated fibres, but that demyelination results in the appearance of potassium channels which are blocked by 4-AP and TEA. Thus 4-AP and TEA can overcome conduction block in demyelinated nerve fibres and it has been suggested that 4-AP be tested for alleviating the symptoms of multiple sclerosis.

In all the above conditions the main disadvantage of 4-AP is that in doses around those effective in enhancing nerve or neuromuscular transmission, the compound is likely to produce central effects resulting in convulsions. Thus, of the four patients poisoned by botulinum toxin and subsequently treated with 4-AP, two developed grand mal convulsions and had to be treated with diazepam (Ball and others, 1979). It is clear that a compound possessing similar peripheral effects to 4-AP but with less risk of central effects would be a potential improvement. Several studies have shown that 3,4-DAP is both a more potent peripheral facilitatory agent than 4-AP and a less potent convulsant agent. It may be that this compound is less efficient in penetrating the blood-brain barrier than 4-AP while possessing greater affinity than 4-AP for potassium channels. The results described previously for the difference in potencies of 4-AP and 3,4-DAP on internal and external application to the squid axon support the idea that 4-AP may be more lipid soluble and have better access to intracellular (and central) sites of action but that 3,4-DAP has much high affinity for the sites of action. There seems little rational reason for preferring 4-AP to 3,4-DAP either as a pharmacological tool or as a potential therapeutic agent.

Apart from 3,4-DAP none of the compounds so far tested shows significant improvement over 4-AP, suggesting that a different approach to selectively enhancing peripheral transmitter release, particularly acetylcholine release, may be necessary. From examination of a wide range of compounds it appears that aminopyridines have mainly an intracellular site of action and that they reach intracellular sites within nerve terminals by virtue of their lipid solubility. This, of course, also means that they will tend to reach potential central sites of action. Perhaps in future it will be possible to design compounds that reach such intracellular sites by one of the existing transport mechanisms in nerve terminals. It is unlikely that compounds small enough to pass through sodium channels will be effective in blocking potassium conductance but compounds based on calcium ionophores could be a possible approach. Another, more likely way of transporting charged compounds into cholinergic nerve terminals is via the choline transport mechanism. Indeed TEA is known to have affinity for this mechanism (Bhatnager and MacIntosh, 1967) and the substance triethylcholine which is taken up by the mechanism is known to increase transmitter release in the frog (Roberts, 1962), but unfortunately produces a presynaptic transmission failure in mammals (Bowman and Rand, 1961; Bowman, Hemsworth and Rand, 1962).

It is clear that future advances in this area will require the close co-operation of physiologists, pharmacologists and medicinal chemists.

## ACKNOWLEDGEMENT

The author would like to thank his colleagues and graduate students who have contributed to the work described particularly Prof. W.C. Bowman and Dr. A.L. Harvey for many invaluable discussions and access to their results, Dr. A.S. Horn for synthesizing many of the compounds described and Dr. S. Agoston for promoting collaboration between establishments. Many of the experiments were performed by Drs. N.N. Durant, J.J. Lambert, G.G. Schofield, Y.N. Singh, P. Teerapong, A. Gandiha and N. Flavahan. Thanks are also due to F. Henderson and A. Gibb for criticizing the manuscript and continuing the work on aminopyridines in my laboratory.

## REFERENCES

Abernethy, J.D. and F.N. Fastier (1958). Aust. J. Exp. Biol., 36, 487-490.
Agoston, S., P.J. Salt, W. Erdmann, J. Hilkemeijer, A. Bencini and D. Langrehr (1980). Br. J. Anaesth., 52, 367-370.

Agoston, S., T. van Weerden, P. Westra and A. Brockert (1978). Br. J. Anaesth., 50, 383-385.
Armstrong, C.M. (1966). J. Gen. Physiol., 50, 491-503.
Armstrong, C.M. and L. Binstock (1965). J. Gen. Physiol., 48, 859-872.
Ball, A.P., R.B. Hopkinson, I.D. Farrell, J.G.P. Hutchison, R. Paul, R.D.S. Watson, A.J.F. Page, R.G.F. Parker, C.W. Edwards, M. Snow, D.K. Scott, A. Leone-Ganado, A. Hastings, A.C. Ghosh and R.J. Gilbert (1979). Quart. J. Med., 48, 473-491.
Bergmann, F., and R. Elam (1980). Arch. Int. Pharmacodyn. Ther., 247, 275-282.
Bhatnager, S.P. and F.C. MacIntosh (1967). Can. J. Physiol. Pharmac., 45, 249-268.
Bostock, H., T.A. Sears and R.M. Sherratt (1981). J. Physiol. Lond., 313, 301-315.
Bowman, W.C., A.L. Harvey and I.G. Marshall (1977). Naunyn-Schmiedeberg's Arch. Pharmac., 297, 99-103.
Bowman, W.C., B.A. Hemsworth and M.J. Rand (1962). Br. J. Pharmac. Chemother., 19, 198-218.
Bowman, W.C. and M.J. Rand (1961). Br. J. Pharmac. Chemother., 17, 176-195.
Bowman, W.C. and A.O. Savage (1981). Rev. Pure Appl. Pharmac. Sci. (in press)
Datyner, N.B. and P.W. Gage (1980). J. Physiol. Lond., 303, 299-314.
Dingemanse, E. and J.P. Wibaut (1928). Naunyn-Schmiedeberg's Arch. Exp. Path. Pharmak., 132, 365-381.
Dohrn, M. (1925). Naunyn-Schmiedeberg's Arch. Exp. Path. Pharmak., 106, 10-11.
Durant, N.N., C. Lee and R.L. Katz (1980). Anesthesiology, 52, 381-384.
Durant, N.N. and I.G. Marshall (1978). J. Physiol. Lond., 280, 21P.
Durant, N.N. and I.G. Marshall (1980). Eur. J. Pharmac., 67, 201-208.
Fastier, F.N. (1948). Br. J. Pharmac. Chemother., 3, 198-204.
Fastier, F.N. and M.A. McDowall (1958a). Aust. J. Exp. Med. Sci., 36, 365-372.
Fastier, F.N. and M.A. McDowall (1958b). Aust. J. Exp. Biol. Med. Sci., 36, 491-498.
Fastier, F.N., M. Pelhate and B. Hue (1981). Abstracts 8th IUPHAR Congress Satellite Symposium - this meeting.
Fastier, F.N. and C.S.W. Reid (1948). Br. J. Pharmac. Chemother., 3, 205-210.
Foldes, F.F., S. Agoston, F. van der Pol. Y. Amaki, H. Nagashima and J.F. Crul (1976). American Society of Anesthesiology. Abstracts of Proceedings, 179-180.
Frank, M., L.L. Flom and J.M.H. Ffrench-Mullen (1978). Fed. Proc., 37, 863.
Freeman, S.E. (1979). J. Pharmac. Exp. Ther., 210, 7114.
Galindo, J. and P. Rudomin (1978). Neurosci. Letters, 10, 299-304.
Gillespie, J.I. (1977). J. Physiol. Lond., 273, 64P.
Gillespie, J.I. and O.F. Hutter (1975). J. Physiol. Lond., 252, 70-71P.
Glover, W.E. (1979). Proc. Aust. Physiol. Pharmac. Soc., 10, 243P.
Harvey, A.L. and I.G. Marshall (1977). Eur. J. Pharmac., 44, 303-309.
von Haxthausen, E. (1955a). Naunyn-Schmiedeberg's Arch. Exp. Path. Pharmak., 226, 163-171.
von Haxthausen, E. (1955b). Naunyn-Schmiedeberg's Arch. Exp. Path. Pharmak, 227, 234-238.
Horn, A.S., J.J. Lambert and I.G. Marshall (1979). Br. J. Pharmac., 65, 53-62.
Hue, B., M. Pelhate and J. Chanelet (1973). J. Physiol., Paris, 67, 346A.
Illes, P. and S. Thesleff (1978). Br. J. Pharmac., 64, 623-629.
Ito, Y., S. Korenaga and K. Tajima (1980). Br. J. Pharmac., 69, 453-460.
Jacobs, R.S. and E.S. Burley (1978). Neuropharmacology, 17, 439-444.
Jankowska, E., A. Lundberg, P. Rudomin and E. Sykova (1977). Brain Res., 136, 387-392.
Johns, A., D.S. Golko, P.A. Lanzon and D.M. Paton (1976). Eur. J. Pharmac., 38, 71-78.
Katz, B. and R. Miledi (1979). Proc. Roy. Soc. B.205, 369-378.
Kenyon, J.L. and W.R. Gibbons (1979). J. Gen. Physiol., 73, 139-157.

Kiloh, N., A.L. Harvey and W.E. Glover (1981). Eur. J. Pharmac., 70, 53-57.
Kim, Y.I., M.M. Goldner and D.B. Sanders (1980). Musc. Nerv., 3, 105-111.
Kirpekar, M., S.M. Kirpekar and J.C. Prat (1977). J. Physiol. Lond., 272, 517-528.
Kirsch, G.E. and T. Narahashi (1978). Biophys. J., 22, 507-512.
Leander, S., A. Arner and B. Johansson (1977). Eur. J. Pharmac., 46, 351-361.
Lechat, P., G. Deysson, M. Lemeignan and M. Adolphe (1968). Ann. Pharm. Fr., 26, 345-349.
Lee, C., A.J.C. de Silva and R.L. Katz (1978). Anesthesiology, 49, 256-259.
Lemeignan, M. (1971). Therapie, 26, 927-940.
Lemeignan, M. (1972). Neuropharmacology, 11, 551-558.
Lemeignan, M. (1973). Neuropharmacology, 12, 641-651.
Lemeignan, M. and Lechat, P. (1967). C.R. Acad. Sci. Paris, D., 264, 169-172.
Llinás, R., K. Walton and V. Bohr. (1976). Biophys. J., 16, 83-86.
Lundh, H. (1978). Brain Res., 153, 307-318.
Lundh, H. (1979). Acta. Pharmac. Toxicol., 44, 343-346.
Lundh, H., S. Leander and S. Thesleff (1977). J. Neurol. Sci., 32, 29-43.
Lundh, H., O. Nilsson and I. Rosen (1977). J. Neurol. Neurosurg. Psych., 40, 1109-1112.
Lundh, H., O. Nilsson and I. Rosen (1979). J. Neurol. Neurosurg. Psych., 42, 171-175.
Lundh, H., and S. Thesleff (1977). Eur. J. Pharmac., 42, 411-412.
Meves, H., and Y. Pichon (1975). J. Physiol. Lond., 251, 60-62P.
Meves, H., and Y. Pichon (1977). J. Physiol. Lond., 268, 511-532.
Miller, R.D., L.H.D.J. Booij, S. Agoston and J.F. Crul (1979). Anesthesiology, 50, 416-420.
Miller, R.D., P.A.F. Dennissen, F. van der Pol, S. Agoston, L.H.D.J. Booij and J.F. Crul (1978). J. Pharm. Pharmac., 30, 699-702.
Molgo, J. (1978). Experientia, 34, 1275-1276.
Molgo, J., M. Lemeignan and P. Lechat (1975). C.R. Acad. Sci. Paris. D., 281, 1637-1639.
Molgo, J., M. Lemeignan and P. Lechat (1977). J. Pharmac. Exp. Ther., 203, 653-663.
Molgo, J., M. Lemeignan and P. Lechat (1979). Eur. J. Pharmac., 53, 307-311.
Molgo, J., M. Lemeignan, T. Uchiyama and P. Lechat (1979). Eur. J. Pharmac., 57, 93-97.
Molgo, J., Lundh, H. and S. Thesleff (1980). Eur. J. Pharmac., 61, 25-34.
Molgo, J., G. Montoya, M. Lemeignan and P. Lechat (1981). C.R. Acad. Sci. Paris. (in press).
Montoya, G., J. Molgo, M. Lemeignan and P. Lechat (1981). Abstracts 8th IUPHAR Congress Satellite Symposium - this meeting.
Moritoki, H., M. Takei, N. Nakamoto and Y. Ishida (1978). Arch. Int. Pharmacodyn. Ther., 232, 28-41.
Paskov, D.S., E.A. Stoyanov and V.V. Mitsov (1973). Eksp. Khir. Anaestesiol., 18 43-52 (in Russian).
Pelhate, M., B. Hue, Y. Pichon and J. Chanelet (1974). C.R. Acad. Sci. Paris, D. 278, 2807-2809.
Pelhate, M., B. Hue, Y. Pichon and J. Chanelet (1981). Abstracts 8th IUPHAR Congress Satellite Symposium - this meeting.
Pelhate, M., and Y. Pichon (1974). J. Physiol. Lond., 242, 90-91P.
Roberts, D.V. (1962). J. Physiol. Lond., 160, 94-105.
Rodger, I.W. and M. Shahid (1981). Br. J. Pharmac., (in press).
Saade, N.Y., J. Chanelet and P. Lonchampt (1971). C.R. Acad. Sci. Paris. D. 165, 2069-2077.
Savage, A.O. (1979). Ph.D. thesis. Univ. Strathclyde.

Schauf, C.L., C.A. Colton, J.S. Colton and F.A. Davis (1976). J. Pharmac. Exp. Ther., 197, 414-425.
Schoepke, H.G. and F.E. Shideman (1961). J. Pharmac. Exp. Ther., 133, 171-179.
Shaw, F.H. and G. Bentley (1955). Aust. J. Biol., 33, 143-151.
Singh, Y.N., I.G. Marshall and A.L. Harvey (1978). J. Pharm. Pharmac., 30, 249-250.
Sobek, V., M. Lemeignan, G. Streichenberger, J.M. Benoist, A. Goguel and P. Lechat (1968). Arch. Int. Pharmacodyn. Ther., 171, 356-369.
Stone, T.W. (1981). Br. J. Pharmac., 73, 791-796.
Thesleff, S. (1980). Neuroscience, 5, 1413-1419.
Tsai, M-C., E.X. Albuquerque, R.S. Aronstam, A.T. Eldefrawi, M.E. Eldefrawi and D.J. Triggle (1980). Mol. Pharmac., 18, 159-166.
Vizi, E.S., J. van Dijk and F.F. Foldes (1977). J. Neur. Trans., 41, 265-274.
Vohra, M.M. and S.N. Pradhan (1964). Arch. Int. Pharmacodyn. Ther. 150, 413-424.
Wollmer, P., B. Wohlfart and R. Khan (1979). Acta Physiol. Scand. Suppl. 30.
Yanagisawa, T., K. Satoh and N. Taira (1978). Eur. J. Pharmac., 49, 189-192.
Yeh, J.Z. (1979). J. Gen. Physiol., 73, 1-21.
Yeh, J.Z., G.S. Oxford, C.H. Wu and T. Narahashi (1976a). Biophys. J., 16, 77-81.
Yeh, J.Z., G.S. Oxford, C.H. Wu and T. Narahashi (1976b). J. Gen. Physiol., 68, 519-535.

# Aminopyridine as a Tool to Investigate the Mechanism of Acetylcholine Release at the Nerve Electroplaque Junction

Y. Dunant, F. Clostre, G. J. Jones, F. Loctin and D. Muller

Département de Pharmacologie, Centre Médical Universitaire,
1211 Genève 4, Switzerland

ABSTRACT

Four-aminopyridine (4-AP) potentiates dramatically synaptic transmission in the cholinergic nerve-electroplaque junction of *Torpedo marmorata*. The postsynaptic electroplaque potential (e.p.p.) is increased in amplitude, and enormously in duration, exhibiting a rebound at about 300 ms after stimulus (giant e.p.p.). The giant e.p.p. area is dose dependent on 4-AP concentration from $10^{-6}$ to $10^{-4}$ M. Miniature e.p.p.s do not show significant changes on 4-AP treatment. The e.p.p. potentiation is due to a large increase in evoked acetylcholine (ACh) release, while resting ACh levels are *reduced* by 4-AP. ACh measured at short time intervals during the giant e.p.p. indicates release from the extravesicular ACh compartment, without transfer to the vesicular ACh; the late rebound appears associated with a late increase in intraterminal extravesicular ACh. Preliminary freeze-fracture studies of the presynaptic membrane during the giant e.p.p. indicate significant redistribution of intra-membrane particles during activity.

KEYWORDS

Synaptic transmission; acetylcholine release; aminopyridines; electric organ; (*Torpedo marmorata*).

INTRODUCTION

The electric organ of the marine fish *Torpedo marmorata* is a very suitable preparation for study of the action of aminopyridine on cholinergic synaptic transmission. This tissue has an extremely regular organisation and is provided with a profuse, purely cholinergic innervation (see Fessard, 1958). The electric organ is composed of a large number of prisms, arranged side by side. Each prism consists of approximately 500 superposed electroplaques, which are embryonically derived from muscle cells. However, unlike normal muscle fibres, the electroplaques are totally devoid of contractile material, and are not able to generate propagated and regenerative action potentials. It is possible with the electric organ to determine the amount of acetylcholine (ACh) which is contained in synaptic vesicles and also in the extravesicular pool of ACh; and these compartments can be analysed as a function of time during the course of nerve stimulation (see Israël, Dunant and Manaranche, 1979, for a review).

In the present study, we have used 4-aminopyridine (4-AP) as a tool for analysing in more detail the presynaptic mechanisms of synaptic transmission. The effects of 4-AP on transmission after a single impulse were first investigated electrophysiologically. Subsequently, the underlying biochemical changes were analysed at short time intervals using a rapid-freezing technique (Dunant, Jones and Loctin, 1981; Corthay, Dunant and Loctin, 1981). More recently, we have also used freeze-etching morphology to study the corresponding changes in the presynaptic membrane.

METHODS

A detailed account of the methods used in this study may be found in Dunant, Eder and Servetiadis-Hirt (1980), Dunant, Jones and Loctin (1981) and Corthay, Dunant and Loctin (1981).

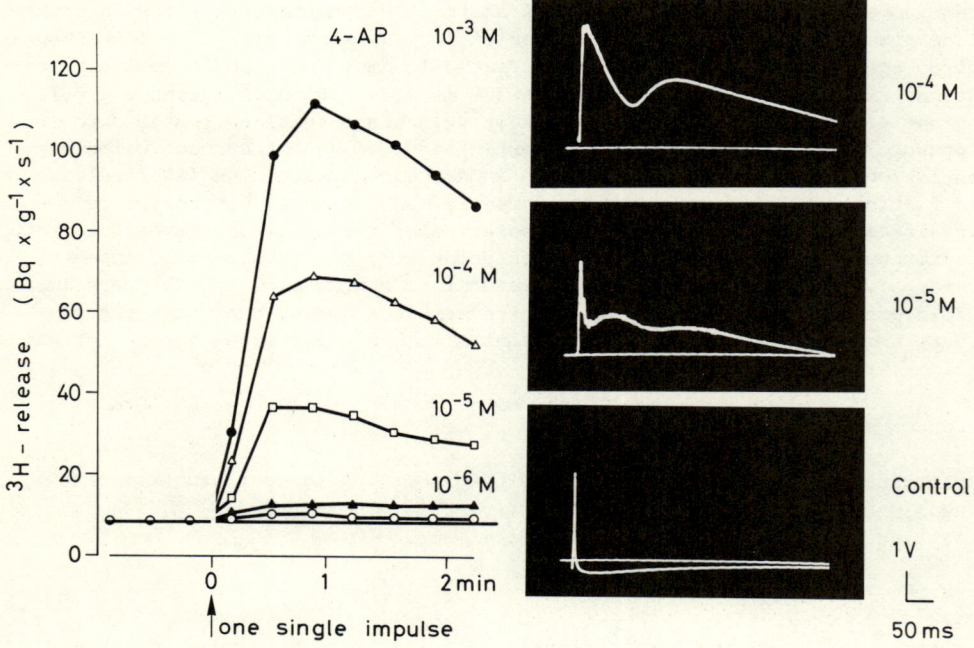

Fig. 1. ACh release and giant e.p.p.s at the *Torpedo* nerve-electroplaque junction, at different 4-AP concentrations. ACh release was measured by the overflow of radioactivity into the superfusion solution, after labelling the ACh stores with $^3$H-acetate. Controls, in the absence of 4-AP are shown as open circles. Mean values from two or three prisms. The electrical recordings are from one prism, before or after 4-AP.

## RESULTS AND DISCUSSION

### The 4-AP effect at the nerve-electroplaque junction

Isolated prisms of the *Torpedo* electric organ can be stimulated via their nerve, or by a field shock (which directly stimulates nerve endings). This produces a synchronised postsynaptic discharge, the electroplaque potential (e.p.p.), which can be recorded extracellularly, and which is similar in all respects to the end-plate potential of the neuromuscular junction. Four-aminopyridine has a dramatic potentiating effect on this e.p.p., producing an increase in amplitude, and much more significantly, a very large increase in duration. The resulting e.p.p. in this tissue is referred to as *the giant e.p.p.* (Figs. 1 and 3).

The giant e.p.p. consists of an initial peak and a late rebound. The initial peak last about 100 ms, and its amplitude is increased up to twice that of controls. The oscillation sometimes seen in the first 50 ms (Fig. 3) probably reflects re-excitation of the nerve terminals by the tissue discharge. The late rebound occurs about 300 ms after the stimulus, at room temperature, and has an amplitude lower than the initial peak. Temperature changes affect predominantly the late rebound of the giant e.p.p. Lowering the temperature to $10°C$ increases somewhat the duration of the initial peak, but greatly prolongs the time of the late rebound, and the overall duration of the giant e.p.p. then usually exceeds 1 s.

Although the general pattern of the giant e.p.p. is independent of 4-AP concentration at greater than $10^{-5}$ M, the giant e.p.p. size, as measured by its area, is dose-dependent over the range $10^{-6}$ to $10^{-4}$ M (Dunant and others, 1981). At $10^{-4}$ M, the e.p.p. area increases to 120 x the normal area. At $10^{-3}$ M the e.p.p. area becomes variable, indicating some other effects of the drug, possibly a curarising effect (see Heuser and others, 1979).

A single giant e.p.p. is best seen after a period of rest, since it greatly fatigues the nerve-electroplaque junctions. A second stimulus requires at least 3 s after the first to elicit a response. At this delay, however, the second response ressembles a normal e.p.p. - up to 10 s is required for recovery of the late rebound, and at least 10 to 15 min for full recovery of the giant e.p.p.

A prolongation of the *Torpedo* e.p.p. is also found after treatment with anticholinesterases (though these do not produce the characteristic late rebound found with 4-AP treatment). An anticholinesterase effect of 4-AP as a contribution to the production of the giant e.p.p. was ruled out by checking directly the effect of 4-AP on the cholinesterase of *Torpedo* electric organ homogenates. No inhibition was found for 4-AP up to $10^{-4}$ M.

### Miniature e.p.p.s

External microelectrodes were used to record spontaneous miniature e.p.p.s in the electroplaque tissue (Dunant and others, 1972). Miniature e.p.p.s recorded in the presence of 4-AP did not show any significant difference from controls, when their amplitude or shape was compared. There was, however, a definite tendency for the m.e.p.p.s to appear periodically in bursts in the presence of 4-AP, particularly at temperatures above $20°C$. In addition, a large and long-lasting potential was occasionally recorded with 4-AP, probably due to spontaneous firing of the pre-terminal fibre.

A purely presynaptic effect

It is generally considered that 4-AP acts presynaptically, and this view is supported by the results of experiments with *Torpedo* prisms, in which ACh release was directly measured. The ACh stores of isolated prisms were labelled using radioactive acetate as precursor, excess radioactivity was washed out, and the radioactivity appearing in the solution before and after a single stimulus was then measured (Dunant, Eder and Servetiadis-Hirt, 1980). In the presence of 4-AP, the release of radioactivity was markedly increased, in a dose-dependent manner (Fig. 1). At $10^{-4}$ M 4-AP, the amount of radioactivity released was 40 x higher than that in the absence of 4-AP.

Comparison of the potentiation of the e.p.p. area by 4-AP at different concentrations (see above) with the potentiation of ACh release (as shown in Fig. 1), gave an excellent correlation. The potentiation of synaptic transmission by 4-AP can therefore be sufficiently accounted for as due to an effect on transmitter release. The slope of the e.p.p. area/ACh release relationship, however, was found to be close to 3, and the reason for this is not yet clear. It seems unlikely that it is due to an underestimation of ACh release, since systematic errors in this measure, due to reuptake or diffusion problems, should be decreased as ACh release is increased. It may be that the 3-fold greater change in e.p.p. area over ACh release represents properties of the postsynaptic side of the nerve-electroplaque junction. That is, either there is an overloading of acetylcholinesterase during the giant e.p.p., especially at the initial peak or during the late rebound, or possibly that there is a dose-action relationship for ACh depolarisation which has a slope greater than unity.

Potentiation of ACh release starting with reduced ACh stores

It could be supposed that an increased ACh release reflects an increased ACh store of the tissue. However, measurements of the ACh stores of *Torpedo* electric tissue after a resting treatment with 4-AP showed just the opposite, i.e. a *reduction* in ACh levels. These experiments were carried out using isolated prisms and 4-AP at $10^{-4}$ M without stimulation for 60-90 min. The prisms were assayed for ACh content after being rapidly frozen in isopentane at -130°C at the end of the resting period. The total ACh content was reduced to 64 % of that of controls, and the vesicle-bound ACh by the same amount (66 %). These changes were very significant and did not appear to be due to artifacts enhanced by the presence of 4-AP, or to interference by 4-AP with the ACh assay; as shown by control experiments, and also because the use of rapid freezing before ACh extraction is expected to reduce possible changes in ACh stores occurring during manipulations of the tissue.

One reason for the decrease in resting ACh levels by 4-AP could be an increase in ACh turnover rate. In one experiment, measurement of the incorporation of radioactivity from acetate precursor into the total and bound ACh compartments showed that this may well be the explanation. As described above, the absolute amounts of ACh in each compartment were reduced compared to control prisms from the same tissue. However, after 60 min incubation with 4-AP ($10^{-4}$ M), the specific activity of ACh was significantly increased (by 52 % for total ACh, and 57 % for bound ACh) over that of controls.

Treatment with 4-AP does not appear to alter the compartmentation of ACh in *Torpedo* electric tissue, since, as described above, the bound ACh and the free ACh decreased by the same proportion after incubation with the drug. Furthermore, it was found that 4-AP treatment did not alter the identification of bound ACh with that contained in synaptic vesicles (see Marchbanks and Israël, 1971). When synaptic vesicles were isolated from prisms which had been treated with radioactive acetate and with 4-AP, they migrated as usual on sucrose gradients, and their ACh was found to have a specific activity very close to that of bound ACh from the same prisms. The extravesicular, or free ACh, most probably cytoplasmic ACh, however, had a specific activity 3 x higher.

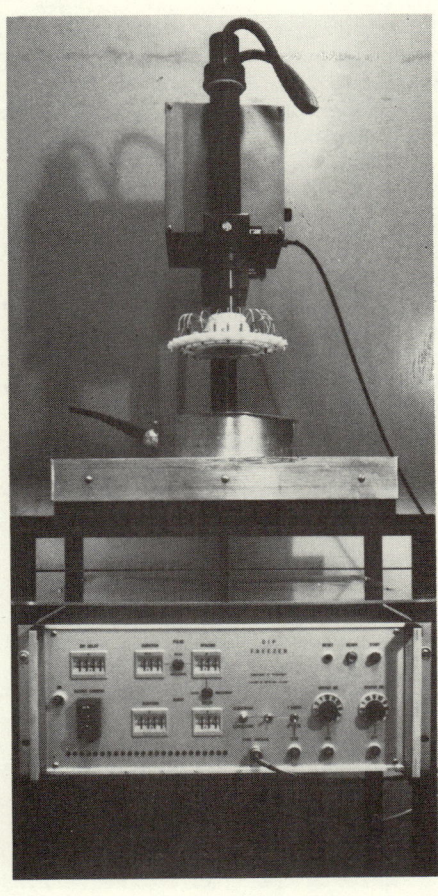

Fig. 2. Photograph of the rapid freezing-stimulator apparatus used for the experiments described in the Text. Upper : cartwheel arrangement on which up to 24 single prisms from *Torpedo* electroplaque are lightly held to small pieces of nylon cloth, by means of the Pt electrodes used for stimulating and recording. Release of a magnetic lock allows the whole arrangement to fall into a bath of isopentane maintained at $-130°C$ by liquid nitrogen. Lower : electronic apparatus which can apply various stimulation patterns to each prism with different delay intervals before release of the magnetic lock.

ACh changes in single prisms during and after a single giant e.p.p.

To analyse changes in tissue ACh at short time intervals, we used a stimulator connected to a rapid tissue freezer (Fig. 2). In each experiment with this machine, up to 24 tissue samples can be stimulated with different delays before being frozen. The results from an individual experiment can show a wide dispersion, but averaging of the results of a number of experiments enables a clear pattern of ACh changes to be obtained. Figure 3 shows the averaged results of ACh assays during a single giant e.p.p., i.e. a single impulse in the presence of 4-AP. At 100 ms time intervals, Fig. 3a, the level of total ACh was found to fall within 500 ms to between 75 and 80 % of controls without stimulus. The total ACh remained at this level for up to 1.5 s after the stimulus, and preliminary experiments have not so far indicated any restoration of the level of total ACh before 7 s. In complete contrast, no significant change was found in the level of bound ACh (Fig. 3a). Initial fluctuating changes in total ACh indicated in Fig. 3a at times less than 400 ms were analysed further in a second series of experiments using 30 ms delay intervals. The results showed a wide dispersion, even after averaging, probably because of difficulties in rigorously maintaining the same conditions for each set of prisms with these short time intervals, and also because these time intervals are approaching the limit of resolution of the rapid freezing technique (Dunant, Jones and Loctin, 1981). Nevertheless, the pooled results are encouraging, Fig. 3b, and show an initial decrease in total ACh, followed by a transient rise at 200 to 300 ms after the stimulus. The transient rise appears at the same time as the late rebound of the giant e.p.p.

The results with the rapid freezing technique are of special interest, since they may bring some light on the mechanism of transmitter release. In particular, it appears that treatment with 4-AP, because it produces an extremely large potentiation of ACh release, or in addition to this, may be in some way "coupling" the process of release to the intraterminal ACh store. The reason for thinking this is that the apparent association of a transient increase in total ACh with an increase in the postsynaptic response, the late rebound (as seen in Fig. 3b), does not occur in the absence of 4-AP. Without 4-AP, an initial fall and subsequent rise in total ACh within 200 ms has been found for stimulation at 100 Hz, but is not reflected in a change in the corresponding postsynaptic responses (Dunant, Jones and Loctin, 1981). Prolonged repetitive stimulation also produces large fluctuations in the ACh level, again without corresponding changes in the amplitude or shape of the e.p.p.s, though there is then a progressive decrease in mean ACh levels associated with a general fatigue of the response (Dunant and others, 1977).

At the present time, we have two "working hypotheses" to explain the results obtained with 4-AP. In the first, stimulation in the presence of 4-AP is assumed to produce a prolonged activation of the ACh release mechanism, such that the changes in total ACh and the postsynaptic response indicate release of a large proportion of the available ACh, followed by resynthesis and a second release of ACh. The subsequent failure is then explained as a failure of further resynthesis, possibly due to exhaustion of the metabolic supply. In the second hypothesis, a "refractoriness" of the releasing mechanism is proposed, occurring after the initial peak of the giant e.p.p., which reduces release and enables the terminals to resynthesise ACh. A subsequent relaxation from the refractory state then produces a second release of transmitter. Again, transmission may then stop because of failure of the metabolic supply. The second hypothesis is invoked to account for the observation that ACh stores do not fall to a very low level during or after the giant e.p.p. So far, however, there is no evidence for a refractoriness of the transmitter release mechanism from experiments in the absence of 4-AP (Dunant, Jones and Loctin, 1981), but it may be that this phenomenon only occurs during potent stimulation of release, as is found in the presence of 4-AP.

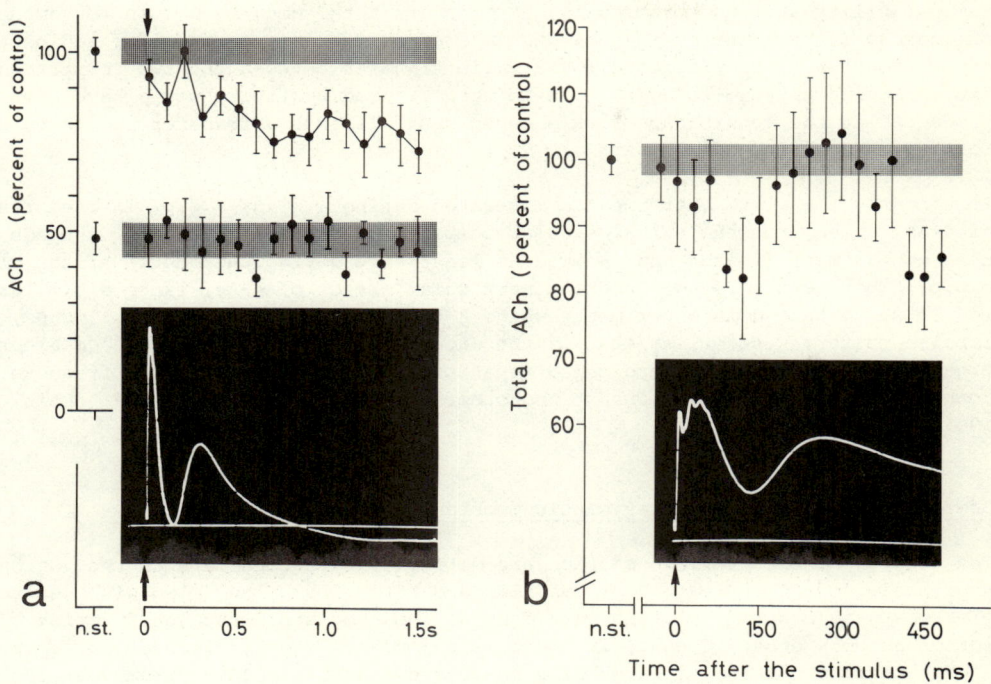

Fig. 3. Changes in total and vesicle bound ACh of prisms from *Torpedo* electroplaques during a giant e.p.p., in the presence of 4-AP ($10^{-4}$ M). a : 100 ms time intervals. Total ACh (upper points) shows an initial fluctuation, followed by a maintained decrease to 75-80 % of controls. Vesicle-bound ACh (lower points) shows no significant change. Mean values ($\pm$ s.e.m.) from 8 (upper) and 5 (lower) experiments, expressed as percent of total ACh in unstimulated controls. b : 30 ms time intervals. Total ACh shows an initial fall followed by a transient rise. The rise occurs at the same time as the rebound of the giant e.p.p. Mean values ($\pm$ s.e.m.) from 5 experiments. The electrical recordings in a and b are from one of the prisms of each of these experiments, and have been printed with the same time scales as the biochemical measurements.

## Is ACh transferred to vesicles during the giant e.p.p. ?

There is no significant change in the level of vesicle-bound ACh during or after the giant e.p.p. (Fig. 3a). To test whether this stability of vesicular ACh is due to a rapid transfer between the cytoplasmic and vesicular compartments, ACh in the terminals was labelled using radioactive acetate and changes in both radioactive and non-radioactive ACh were made at 100 ms intervals during a single giant e.p.p. The labelling was for 3 hr, and 4-AP at $10^{-4}$ M was added during washing out of the precursor. The specific radioactivity of ACh in the vesicular compartment of controls before stimulation was about one third of the specific radioactivity of the free ACh. Stimulation produced a lowering of the free ACh, as already described above, i.e. to about 80 % of controls, with a similar change in the amount of radioactivity in this compartment. The vesicular ACh showed the same stability as found previously, both in its total amount, *and* in the amount of radioactivity. There was no indication of an increase in specific radioactivity of the bount ACh, as predicted for a rapid transfer between the two compartments. (An approximately two-fold increase in specific radioactivity would have been produced, in the conditions of this experiment, if such a transfer had taken place; Corthay, Dunant and Loctin, 1981.)

It appears, therefore, that the ACh liberated during a giant e.p.p. in the presence of 4-AP, comes from the extravesicular compartment of ACh. Moreover, the ACh in this compartment is used and renewed at least once during the course of the giant e.p.p. This result is not due to a particular effect of 4-AP, since a similar result was obtained in experiments using a brief burst of impulses at 100 Hz, an impulse pattern ressembling that of the natural discharge of the *Torpedo* electric organ, or in studies with prolonged repetitive stimulation, at lower frequencies, both *in vitro* and *in vivo* (Dunant and others, 1972; Dunant, Jones and Loctin, 1981).


Changes occurring at the presynaptic membrane during the giant e.p.p.

The results of the previous section are difficult to reconcile with the vesicular hypothesis for ACh release (del Castillo and Katz, 1957), and also with the results of Heuser and others (1979) in work done on the frog neuromuscular junction. The latter authors observed that, in the presence of 4-AP, generation of an e.p.p. is accompanied by opening of large pits in active zones, resulting from vesicle-membrane interaction.

We are presently trying to solve this problem in a morphological study undertaken in collaboration with Dr. M. Garcia-Segura (Department of Morphology, Medical School, Geneva). Using our freezing machine, small pieces of electric organ were rapidly frozen at precise time intervals during transmission of a single giant e.p.p. Freezing was rapid enough at the very surface of the prisms to preserve the ultrastructure of the tissue. Thus freeze fracture could be performed after simple cryofixation, in the absence of any chemical fixative or of cryoprotectants. Two experiments were done in duplicate on two *Torpedoes*. The times chosen for freezing the tissue were (1) unstimulated controls, (2) 30 to 60 ms after the stimulus, i.e. at the peak of the large initial peak of the giant e.p.p., and (3) 570 to 600 ms after the stimulus, corresponding to the tail of the late rebound, when the potential is still at 10-15 percent of the maximum amplitude.

Large pits, probably resulting from vesicle-membrane interaction were found at a very low frequency in this tissue. They amounted to $1.25/\mu m^2$ in controls, $0.72/\mu m^2$ at the peak and $1.92/\mu m^2$ at the tail of the giant potential. Further analysis is needed to find out whether these changes are significant. In contrast, striking and reproducible changes were found in the size and distribution of intramembrane particles. At the peak of activity, small particles (< 10 nm) decreased at the P face of the presynaptic membrane and correlatively increased at the E face. Middle size and large particles ($\geq$ 10 nm) had a different behaviour, showing a large increase in both faces at the peak of activity.

All these changes of intramembranar particles recovered at the end of the giant potential. This point is important since changes in ultrastructure appearing at the end of the giant e.p.p. might well be a consequence of, rather than a morphological conterpart to, transmitter release. At these later times, the intrasynaptic pH must certainly be very low due to the large amount of ACh released and hydrolysed in the cleft.

Thus, our results on the electric organ are in discrepancy with those of Heuser and others (1979) on the frog neuromuscular junction. The discrepancy is perhaps only apparent since there was an indication that the number of large pits increases at the tail of the giant e.p.p. and, recently, Heuser and Reese (1981) showed that the occurrence of large pits at the motor nerve terminal is prominent towards the end of the e.p.p. On the other hand, Israël and others (1981) have studied the presynaptic membrane of *Torpedo* synaptosomes, when ACh release was triggered by KCl depolarization or with a toxin. They found changes in intramembrane particles very similar to those reported here.

## CONCLUSION

After treatment with 4-aminopyridine, the nerve terminals of the *Torpedo* electric organ release up to 40 times more transmitter than normal. This large release considerably depletes the transmitter store. It produces a transient increase in transmitter level, implying a rapid initiation of transmitter resynthesis. The newly synthesised transmitter is also released, producing a late rebound of the postsynaptic potential. The process of transmitter release must therefore be considered to be a highly dynamic mechanism, which acts in close cooperation with the metabolic machinery of transmitter synthesis. The changes in ACh store during release occur in the extravesicular pool of transmitter. There is no indication of a rapid transfer of ACh from cytoplasm to vesicles during release. Thus, the mechanism of ACh release must be located at the presynaptic membrane. The cytological nature of this mechanism may be revealed by study of the changes of the intramembrane particles, which occur at the same time as the transmitter is released.

## ACKNOWLEDGEMENTS

This work was supported by the "Fonds National pour la Recherche Scientifique" (grant No 3.675.0.80). We are grateful to MM. A. Masiero, J. Richez and P. Vadi for the realization of the rapid-freezing stimulator and to Mme Nicole Collet for the hard work of preparing the camera-ready manuscript.

## REFERENCES

Corthay, J., Y. Dunant, and F. Loctin (1981). Acetylcholine changes underlying transmission of a single nerve impulse in the presence of 4-aminopyridine. *J. Physiol. (Lond.)* (submitted).
Del Castillo, J., et B. Katz (1957). La base "quantale" de la transmission neuro-musculaire. In C.N.R.S. (Ed.), *Microphysiologie comparée des éléments excitables*, Colloques du C.N.R.S. No 67, pp. 245-258.

Dunant, Y., L. Eder, and L. Servetiadis-Hirt (1980). Acetylcholine release evoked by single or a few nerve impulses in the electric organ of *Torpedo*. *J. Physiol. (Lond.), 298*, 185-203.

Dunant, Y., J. Gautron, M. Israël, B. Lesbats, et R. Manaranche (1972). Les compartiments d'acétylcholine de l'organe électrique de la Torpille et leurs modifications par la stimulation. *J. Neurochem., 19*, 1987-2002.

Dunant, Y., M. Israël, B. Lesbats, and R. Manaranche (1977). Oscillation of acetylcholine during nerve activity in the *Torpedo* electric organ. *Brain Res., 125*, 123-140.

Dunant, Y., G. J. Jones, and F. Loctin (1981). Acetylcholine and ATP changes measured at short time intervals during transmission of nerve impulses in the electric organ of *Torpedo*. *J. Physiol. (Lond.)* (submitted).

Fessard, A. (1958). Les organes électriques. In P.P. Grassé (Ed.), *Traité de Zoologie*, Tome XIII. Masson, Paris. pp. 1143-1238.

Heuser, J.E., and T.S. Reese (1981). Structural changes after transmission release at the frog neuromuscular junction. *J. Cell Biol., 88*, 564-580.

Heuser, J.E., T.S. Reese, M.J. Dennis, Y. Jan, L. Jan, and L. Evans (1979). Synaptic vesicle exocytosis captured by quick freezing and correlated with quantal transmitter release. *J. Cell Biol., 81*, 275-300.

Israël, M., Y. Dunant, and R. Manaranche (1979). The present status of the vesicular hypothesis. *Prog. Neurobiol., 13*, 237-275.

Israël, M., R. Manaranche, M. Morel, J.C. Dedieu, T. Gulik-Krzywicki, and B. Lesbats (1981). Redistribution of intramembrane particles related to acetylcholine release by cholinergic synaptosomes. *J. Ultrastr. Res.* (in the press).

Marchbanks, R., and M. Israël (1971). Aspects of acetylcholine metabolism in the electric organ of *Torpedo marmorata*. *J. Neurochem., 18*, 439-448.

# Intramembrane Particles Changes: A Constant Feature of the Release Mechanism

M. Israël*, R. Manaranche*, B. Lesbats* and
T. Gulik-Krzywicki**

*Laboratoire de Neurobiologie Cellulaire, Département de
Neurochimie, C.R.N.S., Gif sur Yvette, France
**Centre de Génétique Moléculaire, Centre National de la
Recherche Scientifique, 91190 Gif sur Yvette, France

ABSTRACT

The release of acetylcholine measured with a new chemiluminescent method was triggered by KCl in presence or absence of 4 aminopyridine, and after gramicidin or calcium ionophore A 23187 actions. In all conditions studied presently and previously, cryofracture studies of the presynaptic membrane show that the release of acetylcholine is correlated to a decrease of the number of small P face intramembrane particles ($\leq 10$ nm) and to an increase of larger E face particles (8 to 16 nm). The number of synaptic vesicles remains constant and pits are not systematically found in release conditions able to deplete the cytoplasmic acetylcholine compartment.

KEYWORDS

Acetylcholine release, intramembrane particles, synaptosomes, chemiluminescent method acetylcholine, 4-aminopyridine.

INTRODUCTION

The drug 4-aminopyridine (4 AP) appears to be a useful tool to study the release of transmitter (Molgo, Lemeignan and Lechat 1975, Heuser and colleagues 1979, Dunant Eder and Servetiadis-Hirt 1980). It is probable that it enhances considerably the effect of a nerve impulse by inhibiting the repolarization of nerve terminals, leading to an increased calcium entry and to an important depletion of transmitter. Cryofracture studies of frog neuromuscular junctions electrically stimulated in presence or absence of 4 AP show that the presynaptic membrane is perforated at a sight where exocytosis is likely to take place (the active zone, identified by a double row of synaptic vesicles). In the absence of fixation, the exocytotic pits can only be seen when 4 AP is present (Heuser and colleagues 1979, Heuser and Reese 1981). This might certainly be related to the fact that acetylcholine (ACh) release has to be enhanced to increase the probability for catching a pit. Or it is possible that pits are found in presence of 4 AP because this drug changes their speed of occurrence or disappearence. It was therefore interesting to study the effect of 4 AP on pits in a situation where the drug does not increase the release of transmitter, i.e. after KCl depolarization of synaptosomes. Synaptosomes were prepared from torpedo electric organ (Israël and colleagues 1976, Morel and

colleagues 1977) and depolarized with 50 or 100 mM KCl, 4 AP did not add more to
the depolarization. The pits which were normally found after a simple KCl depolarization were much less numerous in the presence of 4 AP (Morel and colleagues 1980).

In parallel to this morphological approach a new chemiluminescent procedure for
measuring ACh and its release from tissues has been described (Israël and Lesbats
1980, 1981a, 1981b). This procedure is based on the hydrolysis of ACh by acetylcholinesterase and on the oxidation of choline to betaine and $H_2O_2$ by choline oxidase. The $H_2O_2$ generated is continuously detected by the light emission produced if
the substance luminol (5-amino-1,2,3,4 tetrahydrophtalazindion-1,4) and a catalyst
such as peroxidase are present in the incubation medium.

## PRESYNAPTIC MEMBRANE MODIFICATIONS IN THE COURSE OF ACh RELEASE

The release of ACh from torpedo electric organ synaptosomes was measured with the
chemiluminescent method after KCl depolarization in the presence or absence of 4 AP,
the Fig.1 clearly shows that 4 AP did not change the amount released. This was tested for a range of 4 AP concentrations from $10^{-5}$M to $10^{-3}$M. Analogs of 4 AP such as
3-4 diaminopyridine or 3-aminopyridine where also not efficient after KCl

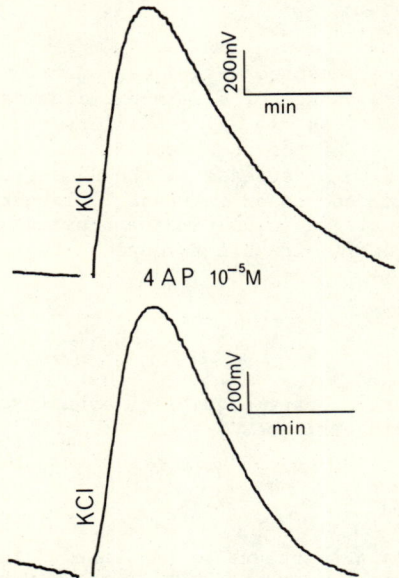

Fig. 1. Release of ACh from synaptosomes depolarized with
KCl (50 mM) in presence or absence of 4 AP $10^{-5}$M.
In this condition 4 AP does not increase ACh
release. The reaction mixture converting ACh into
a light emission consists of the physiological
solution containing choline oxidase (Sigma) horseradish peroxidase and luminol. Released ACh is
converted to choline which is oxidized, the
$H_2O_2$ generated reacts with luminol, and the light
emission is recorded. 200 mV correspond to about
40 pmol of ACh.

depolarization. This confirms a previous observation obtained with a radioactive
method for measuring ACh release from synaptosomes (Morel and colleagues 1980).

We have consequently thought that if endo-exocytotic pits (⩾20 nm) are diminished in presence of 4 AP in spite of a maintained ACh release, that it might be possible to dissociate the release of transmitter from the occurrence of pits. In a subsequent work the release of ACh from synaptosomes was triggered by two different methods either KCl depolarization or after the action of a venom extracted from the annelid <u>Glycera convoluta</u>. This venom was shown to trigger an avalanche of miniature end-plate potentials at neuro-muscular and nerve-electroplaque junctions (Manaranche, Thieffry and Israël 1980). We have found that like for KCl depolarization, Glycera venom (GV) (which releases much more ACh) did not change the number of synaptic vesicles. But in contrast to KCl depolarization, no more pits were found after GV action. This is also a marked difference with black widow spider venom which depletes the nerve terminal from its vesicles. The comparison between KCl and GV induced release showed that release of ACh could be obtained with or without the appearance of pits in the presynaptic membrane (Israël and colleagues 1980, 1981). Since a quantal release displaces a packet of some 5,000 or more ACh molecules, it appeared difficult to envisage that an avalanche of packets crossing the presynaptic membrane left no trace. Having no pits to count in the case of GV induced release, and no changes in the number of synaptic vesicles, we have tried to see if intramembrane particles were not in some way involved in the course of ACh release. The diagram fig.2 compares the intramembrane particles of P and E faces of the presynaptic membrane of synaptosomes : in different conditions 1)Synaptosomes at rest prepared in the absence of calcium) , 2) "activated" synaptosomes (in the presence of calcium) 3) after a moderated ACh release (KCl depolarization) 4) after an important ACh release (GV action). These results were established

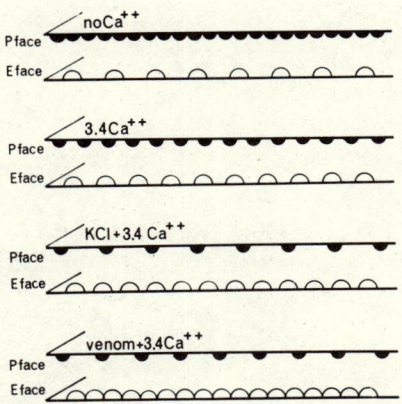

Fig. 2. Diagram representing intramembrane particle density changes in P and E faces of the presynaptic membrane. A comparison of the no calcium condition, the normal calcium control (3.4 mM) and two stimulations either KCl or venom of Glycera, show that the density of P face particles decreases, while E face particles become more numerous ●=100 P face particles ⩽ 10 nm, ⌒=50 E face particles of 8 to 16 nm. These results were described previously (Israël and colleagues 1980)

on a large statistical basis for conditions 2,3, 4 were highly significant, a description can be found in Israël and colleagues, 1980, 1981. We have in this work distinguished 3 classes of particles, in fact the absolute diameter of each class is probably within a 20 % error and it is preferable to consider the shape of histograms and distinguish small from large particles with a broader boundary. The variations of densities are rather impressive and can be summarized as follows: there is an important decrease of small P face particles ($\leqslant$10 nm) while the number of intermediate E face particles (8 to 16 nm) increases when ACh is released. In general in the course of release the synaptosomes show on the P face a decrease of the mean particle density, and on the E face an increase of the mean particle density. The partition coefficient of particles (P/E) markedly decreases in the course of release. In order to establish more firmly this correlation between intramembrane particle changes and release, we have triggered the release by two other methods : gramicidin depolarization and calcium ionophore action, and analyzed intramembrane particles modifications like for KCl and GV actions. The hypothesis is that a common ultrastructural change should be found in all these different release conditions. The particles were counted on P and E faces of cryofractured synaptosomes similar to the examples of fig.3 and 4. In parallel to the morphological analysis we have determined the content and release of ACh.

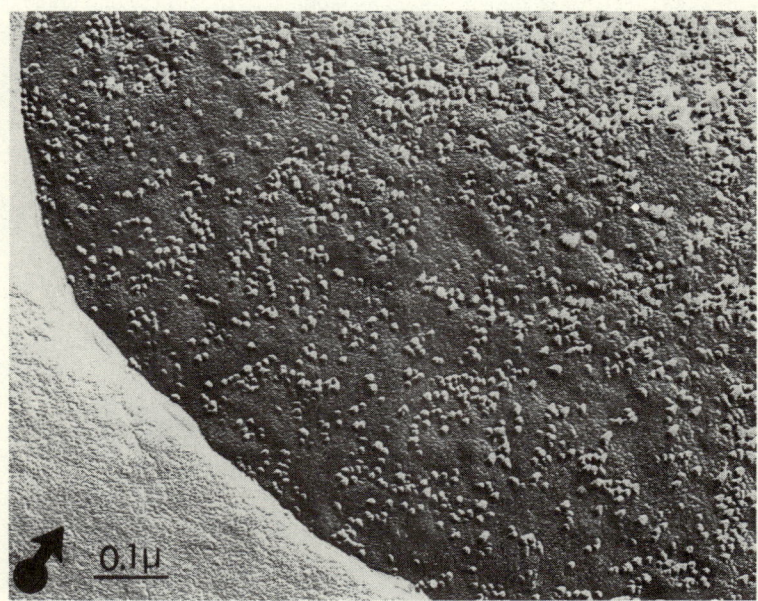

Fig. 3. Electron micrograph of a P face of a cryofractured synaptosome

SYNAPTOSOMAL ACh CONTENT AND COMPARTMENTATION

Cytoplasmic and vesicular ACh can be directly and instantly measured on synaptosomes with the chemiluminescent method. This is performed by liberating successively the two compartments in the reaction mixture which gives a light emission in proportion to the amount of ACh. The leakage of cytoplasmic ACh is first obtained by freezing

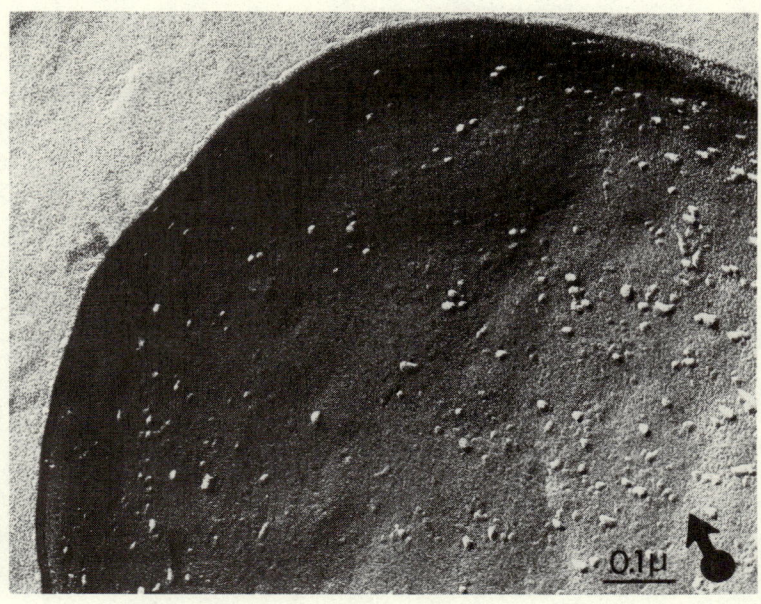

Fig. 4. Electron micrograph of an E face of a cryofractured synaptosome.

and thawing once or twice the synaptosomes. The vesicular compartment which is more resistant to freezing and thawing (vesicles are isolated from frozen tissue) is then liberated by a detergent. In both compartments the amount of choline was negligible in comparison to ACh. The Fig.5 shows the light emission induced by the leakage of ACh after the first freezing and thawing, the 2nd and 3rd trials were with little or no effect. But the detergent releases the larger ACh compartment (60 % to 75 % of the total) which has resisted to freezing and thawing. We also know from previous work that the compartment released at the first freezing has a higher specific radioactivity than the remaining ACh (Morel and colleagues 1977) this is expected since ACh is synthesized from radioactive substrates in the cytoplasm where are localized choline acetylase and a form of acetyl-CoA synthetase (Morot-Gaudry and Diebler 1979).

The cytoplasmic ACh compartment represents about 30 % of the total, several objections about its existence are ruled out presently. In contrast to intact tissue, synaptosomes can be rapidly equilibrated in different calcium containing solutions (low calcium, EGTA, or normal calcium) in all these three conditions the size of vesicular and cytoplasmic ACh compartments remained unchanged (Israël and Lesbats 1981b). This is a marked difference with intact tissue where the equilibrium between free and bound ACh is shifted towards bound ACh after relatively long incubations in low calcium media. It was also possible to rule out the objection that cytoplasmic ACh might result from the destruction of synaptic vesicles by freezing and thawing, this was done by counting the vesicles on diametral sections of cryofractured synaptosomes before or after freezing and thawing. An example of diametral section through a cryofractured synaptosome is shown Fig.6. In a normal calcium containing solution (3.4 mM) we have found, after freezing and thawing a number

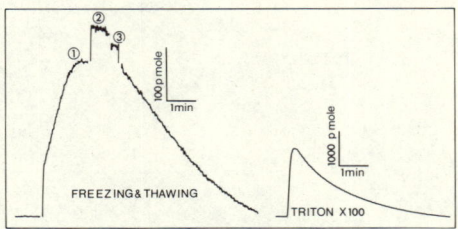

Fig. 5. Estimation of cytoplasmic and vesicular ACh with the chemiluminescent procedure. Synaptosomes are frozen and thawed in the reaction mixture, the first freezing and thawing liberates a first compartment (the ACh present in the cytoplasm) the 2nd and 3rd freezing and thawing are not efficient. But the addition of Triton X-100 liberates the vesicular compartment which is more resistant to freezing (Note the differences in scales).

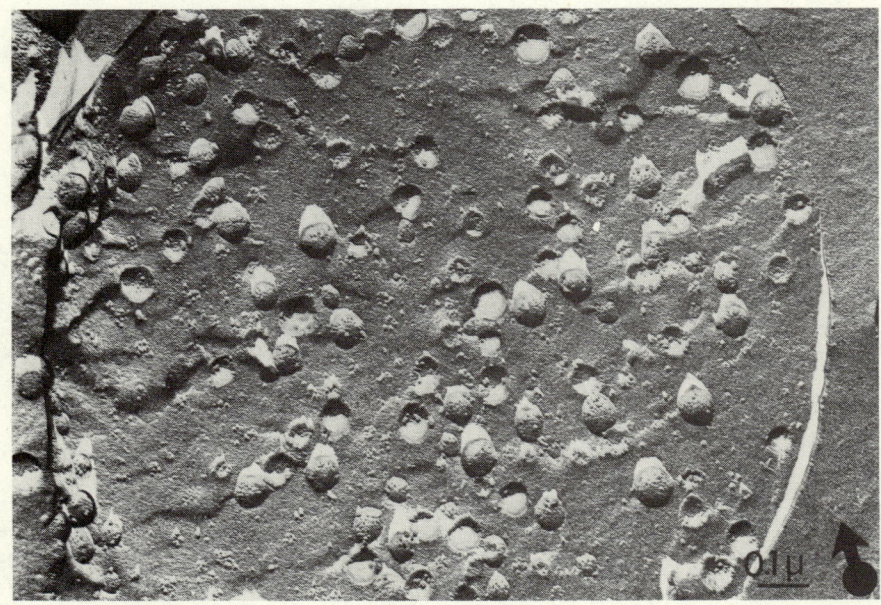

Fig. 6. Electron micrograph of a diametral section of a cryofractured synaptosome (numerous synaptic vesicles are present at 52 sec. of gramicidin action).

of synaptic vesicles equal to 118 % of control. After EGTA treatment (2 mM) frozen and thawed synaptosomes had a number of vesicles equal to 115 % of their control. The variations were not significant.

CONTINUOUS DETERMINATION OF ACh RELEASE

Examples of ACh release curves obtained with the chemiluminescent procedure are given Fig.7 synaptosomes were stimulated either with KCl or with calcium ionophore A 23 187 or with gramicidin.

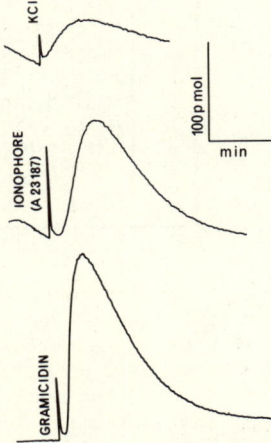

Fig. 7. Examples of ACh release curves, synaptosomes were either depolarized with KCl (115 mM) or treated with the calcium ionophore A 23187 (7 µM or gramicidin (2.4 µM). Gramicidin was more efficient than A 23187 or KCl. The chemiluminescent reaction mixture contained choline oxidase (Boehringer), luminol and horseradish peroxidase. (calcium 8 mM)

It was previously shown that the amount of ACh released is taken on the compartment characterized by freezing and thawing i.e. the cytoplasmic ACh (see Israël and Lesbats 1981). The ACh remaining in synaptosomes after triggering the release by different agents is represented in Fig. 8. It is clear that with the more powerful agents can deplete the synaptosomal ACh down to the level of the vesicular compartment. The dotted line in Fig.8 indicates in the control block the compartmentation of ACh. Such a clear depletion of synaptosomal ACh was probably obtained because ACh synthesis is not supported by a supply choline and acetate. In the long run, the vesicular stores will probably deliver ACh and ATP to the cytoplasmic pool. The accumulation of sodium, calcium or perhaps protons might signal the mobilization of the vesicular store. A parenthesis should be opened here to recall that synaptic vesicles can accumulate calcium and may well be involved in its removal from the cytoplasm (Israël and colleagues 1980). This is essential to stop the release of ACh. The ionic changes which lead to the mobilization of the vesicular store contribute to the heterogeneity of the vesicular population which might contain different concentrations of ACh, ATP and calcium at different stages of the endo-exocytotic cycle. We suspect that this cycle is related to the calcium changes in the nerve terminal, and since this cation is also the trigger for ACh

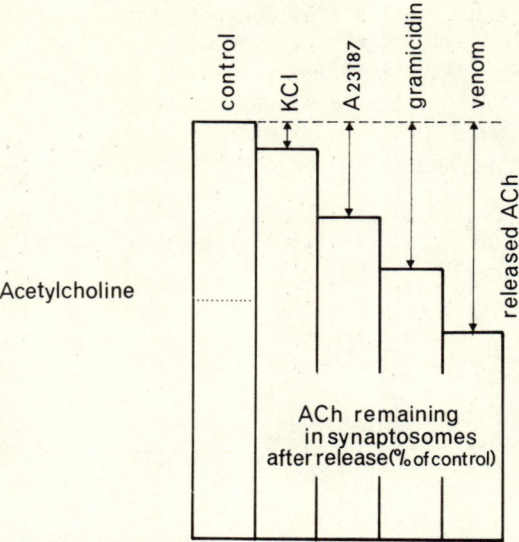

Fig. 8. ACh remaining in synaptosomes after triggering ACh release with different agents (KCl 115 mM, ionophore A 23187 7 µM, gramicidin 2.4 µM and Glycera venom 0.025 glands/ml). We have indicated in the control block by a dotted line the level of cytoplasmic (top) and vesicular (below) ACh. The most powerful agents deplete the synaptosomes until the level of vesicular ACh. The arrow is in proportion to the amount released. The remaining ACh is measured by disrupting the synaptosomes, when the release has declined, by adding Triton X 100 in the reaction mixture.

release, it is possible that in some experimental conditions it becomes possible to obtain the release of ACh, and the formation of pits within a compatible time interval. The fact that we were able to demonstrate the presence of cytoplasmic ACh and its release, without changes neither in the number of vesicles nor in the number of pits in the presynaptic membrane should question the vesicular hypothesis. The table 1 gives the number of synaptic vesicles in the course of an important ACh release triggered by gramicidin or ionophore A 23187, they were counted on diametral section of cryofractured synaptosomes. The data were not significantly different from the control.

TABLE 1  Number of synaptic vesicles after an intense ACh release triggered by gramicidin or ionophore A 23187

|  | Control | Gramicidin (5 µM) 4 min 45 sec | Ionophore A 23187 (14 µM) 4 min |
|---|---|---|---|
| Number of synaptic vesicles per µm$^2$ | 29 ± 2 (n = 17) | 31 ± 4 (n = 10) n.s. | 25 ± 4 (n = 10) n.s. |

## THE MECHANISM OF ACh RELEASE

The hypothesis we have put forward sometime ago postulates that there is in the presynaptic membrane an operative unit activated by calcium and able to release the transmitter from the cytoplasm. The important changes of intramembrane particles observed when ACh is released support this hypothesis, since they represent the only common ultrastructural change found in all the release conditions tested. There is a decrease in the number of small P face particles ($\leqslant 10$ nm) and an increase in the number of larger E face particles (8 to 16 nm). In some experimental conditions part of the larger E face particles can be pinched off with the P face masking the decrease of the small P face particles this phenomenon was not very critical in our experimental conditions. The P and E face particles undergo important changes which are more intense for conditions releasing more ACh, compare Fig. 9 and Fig. 8. The intramembrane particle density changes become more important

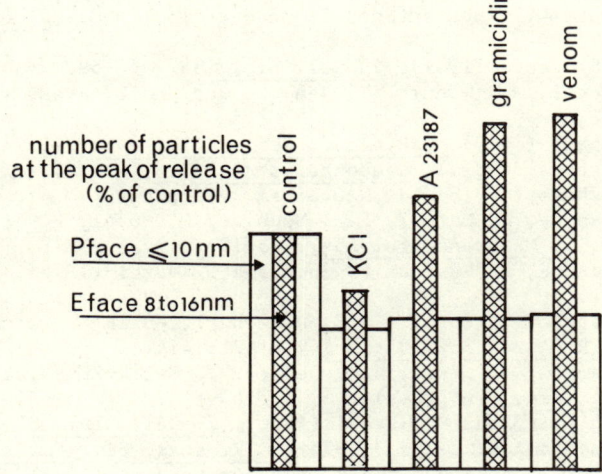

Fig. 9. Intramembrane particles of P and E faces of the presynaptic membrane at the peak of the release curve. In each block we have expressed P face small particles ($\leqslant 10$ nm) in % of control and E face particles 8 to 16 nm in % of the control For the most powerful releasing agents E face particles are more numerous while the P face becomes poor. The $\leqslant 10$ nm particles represent about 60 % of the total P face particles, while the 8 to 16 nm particles are most of the E face particles.

for the strongest release situations. The exact mechanism of these particle changes is not known, but suppose that upon calcium entry a P face particle dissociates into small units which are below the resolution of the cryofracture technique, this would lead to a decrease in the mean density of P face particles. If the reverse phenomenon association of units to form particles, occured on the E face then the mean particle density would increase. It is perhaps the momentary interaction between a P face unit and E face particle which switches on the release mechanism from a leakage regime, to a quantal or sub-quantal release. Certainly it is also possible that particle changes result from a different mechanism i.e. vertical movements of particles driven by different interactions on both sides of the membrane.

Alternatively the particle density changes might result from very rapid endo-exocytotic events which would not be caught by our methods. The collapse of the vesicle membrane in the presynaptic membrane might explain a reduction in the density of P face particles (Fesce and colleagues 1980) but it seems difficult to explain also the increased density in the E leaflet by the same mechanism.

In our final remark we would like to point out that the mechanism we propose presently explains most of the experimental observations. It is possible to imagine the release of cytosolic ACh in a quantal form, if ensured by the momentary interaction of intramembrane particles.

REFERENCES

Dunant, Y., L. Eder, and L. Servetiadis-Hirt (1980). J. Physiol. (London), 298, 185-203.
Fesce, R., F. Grohovaz, W.P. Hurlbut, and B. Ceccarelli (1980). J. Cell Biol. 85, 337-345.
Heuser, J.E., and T.S. Reese (1981). J. Cell Biol. 88, 564-580.
Heuser, J.E., T.S. Reese, M.J. Denis, Y. Jan, L. Jan, and L. Evans (1979). J. Cell Biol., 81, 275-300.
Israël, M. et B. Lesbats (1980). C.R. Acad. Sci. Paris, 291, 713-716.
Israël, M., and B. Lesbats (1981a). Neurochemistry Int.3, 81-90.
Israël, M. and B. Lesbats (1981b). J. Neurochem. (in press)
Israël, M., R. Manaranche, J. Marsal, F.M. Meunier, N. Morel, P. Frachon, and B. Lesbats (1980). J. Membrane Biol.,54, 115-126.
Israël, M., R. Manaranche, P. Mastour-Frachon, and N. Morel (1976). Biochem. J.,160 113-115.
Israël, M., R. Manaranche, N. Morel, J.C. Dedieu, T. Gulik-Krzywicki, and B. Lesbats (1980). C.R. Acad. Sci. Paris, 290, 1471-1474.
Israël, M., R. Manaranche, N. Morel, J.C. Dedieu, T. Gulik-Krzywicki, and B. Lesbats (1981). J. Ultrast. Res. (in press)
Manaranche, R., M. Thieffry, and M. Israël (1980). J. Cell Biol., 85, 446-458.
Molgo, J., M. Lemeignan and P. Lechat (1975). C.R. Acad. Sci. Paris, 281, 1637-1639.
Morel, N., M. Israël, R. Manaranche, and P. Mastour-Frachon (1977). J. Cell Biol. 75, 43-55.
Morel, N., R. Manaranche, T. Gulik-Krzywicki, and M. Israël (1980). J. Ultrast.Res 70, 347-362.
Morot-Gaudry, Y., and M.F. Diebler (1979). Biochem. J. 180, 297-301.

# Effect of Aminopyridine and Related Drugs on Catecholamine Release

S. M. Kirpekar, M. T. Schiavone and J. C. Prat

Department of Pharmacology, Downstate Medical Center,
450 Clarkson Avenue, Brooklyn, New York 11203 USA

ABSTRACT

4-aminopyridine (4-AP, 1 mM) increased noradrenaline (NA) output from the perfused cat spleen at 5 Hz by about fivefold. Enhancement of NA release by 4-AP was reversible. Output of NA induced by potassium (140 mM) was not affected. NA output was doubled at low concentrations (0.1-0.3 mM) of 4-AP, but maximal effect was obtained at 1-3 mM. At 10 mM, it induced spontaneous release of NA which was insensitive to calcium. Insignificant outputs obtained at 5 Hz in 0.1 and 0.3 mM calcium-Krebs solution were markedly enhanced by 4-AP. 4-AP enhanced release at all calcium concentrations up to 5 mM, but maximum output was obtained at 2.5 mM. 4-AP at pH 8.5 was more effective in enhancing NA release than at pH 7.4. In normal spleens the NA output per stimulus at 30 Hz was about four- and eightfold greater than at 5 and 1 Hz, respectively. Reduction of calcium concentration in the Krebs solution to 0.25 mM, while reducing outputs at all frequencies, resulted in an output at 30 Hz, which was nearly ten- and thirtyfold greater than that at 5 and 1 Hz. TEA (10 mM), which markedly enhances NA output, reversed the frequency response so that the maximum output occurred at 1 instead of at 30 Hz. Lowering the calcium concentration to 0.1 mM in the Krebs solution containing TEA, while reducing outputs at all frequencies, increased the output at 30 Hz by about fivefold over the output at 1 Hz. 4-AP, like TEA, enhanced output at lower frequencies (1 and 5 Hz) but did not appreciably affect the output at 30 Hz. The output was always greater at 5 Hz than at 1 Hz. On lowering the calcium concentration to 0.25 mM, the frequency-output relationship became steeper than the controls. 4-AP (1 mM) also enhanced the response to nicotine (50 μM) and it effectively antagonized the suppressant effects of tetrodotoxin (TTX) or calcium-free solution on release induced by nicotine. Lanthanum (1 mM) blocked the restoration of release by 4-AP in calcium-free solution. 4-AP, TEA and guanidine temporarily reversed the inhibition of NA release by guanethidine, an antihypertensive agent, during nerve stimulation or nicotine administration. Since guanethidine does not block conduction of impulses in the preterminal portion of the adrenergic neuron but blocks their propagation in the terminals, the excitation may spread to this portion of the nerve only electrotonically. Since 4-AP, TEA and guanidine are known to mobilize calcium, they may allow greater than normal amounts of calcium to enter the neuron during electrotonic depolarization to restore transmission even in the presence of guanethidine. It is suggested that 4-AP inactivates potassium current in sympathetic nerves and prolongs the duration of the action potential, thereby allowing a greater influx of calcium into the neurone to enhance release of NA. Restoration of nicotine response by 4-AP in calcium-free solution may suggest that 4-AP may mobilize a pool of tightly bound calcium presumably associated with the neuronal membrane. (Supported by USPHS Grant No. HL 22170.)

KEYWORDS

4-Aminopyridine; potassium; calcium; sympathetic nerve terminal; norepinephrine; tetraethylammonium; guanidine; guanethidine; nicotine; frequency-output relation.

INTRODUCTION

Aspects of the pharmacological actions of 4-aminopyridine (4-AP) have been known for some time, but its recent use as an anticurare agent has renewed interest in the study of 4-AP and related compounds. (For a detailed literature survey, see Bowman and Savage, 1981.)

The best-described effect of 4-AP is its ability to reduce the late potassium current in a number of excitable tissues including the voltage-clamped isolated giant axon of the cockroach (Pelhate and Pichon, 1974) and the internally perfused giant axon of the squid (Yeh, Oxford, Wu, Narahashi, 1976). Gillespie and Hutter (1975) showed that 4-AP was more effective than tetraethylammonium (TEA) in reducing the delayed potassium current in skeletal muscle fibers. At the squid giant synapse, 4-AP was shown to reduce potassium conductance in the presynaptic terminal without blocking transmission (Llinás, Walton, and Bohr, 1976). Molgó, Lemeignan, and Lechat (1977) proposed that prolongation of the presynaptic action potential at the frog neuromuscular junction by 4-AP may enhance transmitter release by increasing the calcium concentration in the nerve terminal.

The present studies examined the influence of 4-AP on NE release induced by nerve stimulation or nicotine in the cat spleen, and compared the action of 4-AP with that of TEA. The effect of 4-AP on guanethidine blockade of adrenergic transmission was also investigated. Reports on some of these findings have been previously published (Kirpekar, Kirpekar, and Prat, 1977, 1978; Kirpekar, Garcia, and Prat, 1980a,b).

METHODS

Cats weighing about 2 kg were anesthetized by ether induction, followed by chloralose (60 mg/kg). The spleens were isolated and perfused in situ with Krebs bicarbonate solution as previously described (Kirpekar and Misu, 1967). Venous samples were collected for 2 min during nerve stimulation, and control samples without nerve stimulation were taken for 2 min prior to stimulation. NE release was evoked by stimulation of the splenic nerves with supramaximal rectangular pulses of 1-msec duration at 1, 5, or 30 Hz for a total of 200 stimuli, or by rapidly injecting 0.2 ml potassium chloride solution (3.7 M) into the splenic artery. NE was assayed by a fluorometric procedure (Anton and Sayre, 1962). Alternatively, for experiments using nicotine the spleen was removed shortly after opening the abdomen, and spleen slices were prepared for in vitro studies as previously discussed (Kirpekar, Garcia, and Prat, 1980a).

RESULTS

Nerve Stimulation

<u>Graded concentrations of 4-AP and NE release</u>. In the absence of nerve stimulation, the background release of NE was usually undetectable. 4-AP (0.1-3 mM) had no

effect on the background release of NE. However, 10 mM 4-AP brought about a marked increase in the background release of NE and also in the vascular resistance. In 3 experiments, background release was increased to 54 ± 12 ng/min during perfusion with 4-AP (10 mM), and removal of calcium from the medium did not prevent release. The relationship between the concentration of 4-AP and the output of NE evoked by splenic nerve stimulation at 5 Hz is illustrated in Fig. 1. The mean control response in these trials was 0.39 ± 0.03 ng/stimulus. 4-AP enhanced the secretory response in concentrations as low as 0.1 mM, which enhanced the catecholamine output by about 60%. Maximal enhancement was observed at 1–3 mM, and the response in the presence of 10 mM 4-AP was comparable to the control output. After 20 minutes' reperfusion with normal Krebs solution following 10 mM 4-AP, the response to 5-Hz stimulation was twice as large as the initial controls. Molgó, Lemeignan, and Lechat (1977) have observed that 4-AP, at the neuromuscular junction of the frog, is effective in micromolar quantities.

<u>Effect of 4-AP on NE release induced by high potassium.</u> To compare the effect of

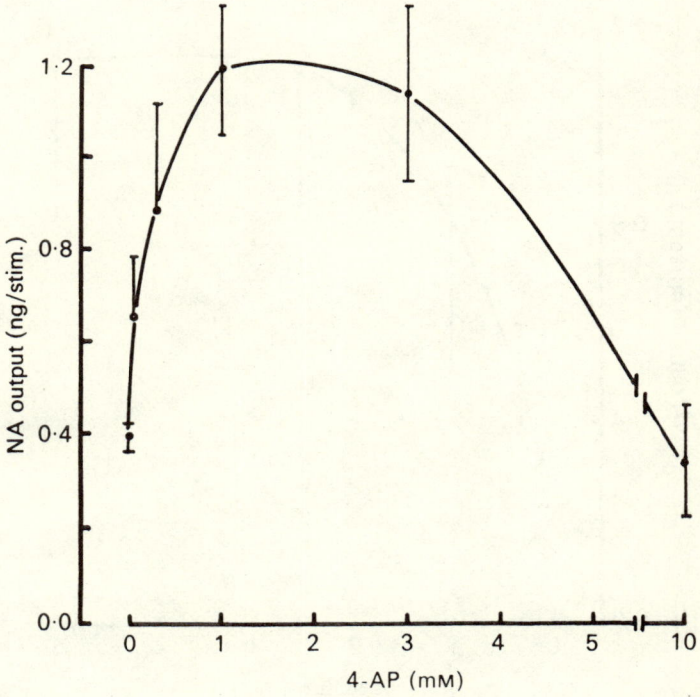

Fig. 1. Relationship between 4-AP concentration and output of NA from the perfused spleen of the cat. After obtaining the initial control output in normal Krebs solution, the spleen was consecutively perfused with Krebs solution containing 0.1, 0.3, 1, 3, and 10 mM 4-AP for 15 min each, and then again with normal Krebs solution. Splenic nerves were stimulated at 5 Hz during the last 2-min perfusion with normal Krebs solution and during perfusion with each concentration of 4-AP. Vertical lines are the S.E. of mean of 5 experiments. Release at 10 mM was obtained in 3 experiments. The sequence of doses was varied in each experiment. Curve is fitted by eye. Reproduced from Kirpekar, Kirpekar, and Prat (1977).

4-AP on NE release induced by chronic depolarization as opposed to intermittent depolarization, the perfused spleen was stimulated by injecting 0.2 ml potassium chloride solution (3.7 M) into the splenic artery. In 6 experiments, the mean control response was 68 ± 14 ng, and in the presence of 4-AP (1 mM) it was 79 ± 19.7 ng. The response in the presence of 4-AP was 120 ± 20% of the initial output, and on reperfusion with normal Krebs solution the output was 107 ± 21% of the control value. Thus, 4-AP failed to markedly enhance the secretory response to high potassium.

Effect of calcium on the enhancement of NE release by 4-AP. In low- as well as high-calcium solution, 4-AP increases the NE release evoked by splenic nerve stimulation. In the presence of 0.1-0.3 mM calcium, the NE output at 5 Hz was usually undetectable. Fig. 2 shows that, in the presence of 4-AP, secretory responses to 0.1 and 0.3 mM calcium were comparable to the control response in 2.5 mM calcium. Responses in the presence of 1 mM 4-AP were further enhanced as calcium concentration was increased up to 5 mM, but the maximal output was obtained at 2.5 mM calcium.

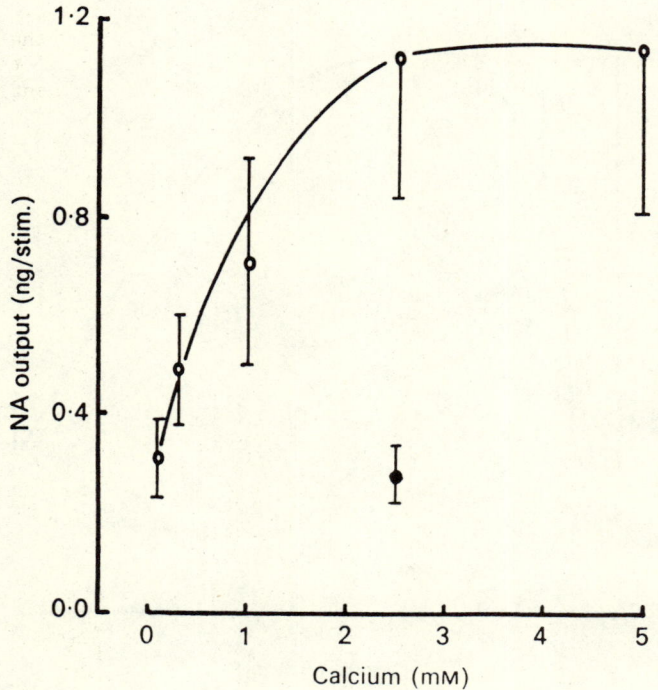

Fig. 2. Relationship between 4-AP and calcium on the output of NA from the perfused spleen of the cat. After obtaining the initial control NA output (0.28 ± 0.06 ng/stimulus, represented by ● ) in normal Krebs solution, the spleen was consecutively perfused with 4-AP (1 mM)-Krebs solution containing 0.1, 0.3, 1.0, 2.5, and 5 mM calcium for 15 min each. Splenic nerves were stimulated at 5 Hz during the last 2-min perfusion with normal Krebs solution, or during perfusion with 4-AP-Krebs solution containing different calcium concentrations. Vertical lines are the S.E. of mean of 4 experiments. Curve is fitted by eye. Reproduced from Kirpekar, Kirpekar, and Prat (1977).

Effect of pH on the enhancement of NE release by 4-AP. 4-AP exists mostly in an ionized form at physiological pH. Since studies in the internally perfused squid axon indicated that 4-AP acts equally from inside and outside the membrane (Meves and Pichon, 1975), it was of interest to determine whether 4-AP was more effective at alkaline pH, where it would exist partly as a free base. Fig. 3 shows that normal responses to splenic nerve stimulation (5 Hz) could be obtained during perfusion of the spleen with a solution at pH 8.5 (when the spleen was perfused with a solution at pH 9.0, the pH of the venous effluent was about 8.5) releasing 0.39 ± 0.08 ng NE/stimulus. At this pH, 0.1 mM 4-AP enhanced the evoked output maximally to the same extent as 1 mM at pH 7.4. At 0.3 mM, 4-AP did not further enhance release, and at 1 mM, the output was diminished. It should be noted that stimulation during perfusion with 0.3 or 1 mM 4-AP caused a marked contraction of the spleen and 50% reduction in the flow rate. Background release of NE did not increase at the lower concentrations (0.1 and 0.3 mM) of 4-AP, but at 1 mM, background release was increased to 26 ± 10 ng/min and was comparable to the release obtained with 10 mM in normal Krebs solution. Molgó, Lundh, and Thesleff (1980) reported a 3-fold enhancement in the ability of 4-AP to promote ACh release at the neuromuscular junction when the pH was increased from 7.4 to 9.0.

Effect of calcium on the frequency-output relation. Fig. 4 shows the relationship between NE output and the stimulation frequency during perfusion of the spleen with different calcium concentrations. In normal Krebs solution containing 2.5 mM

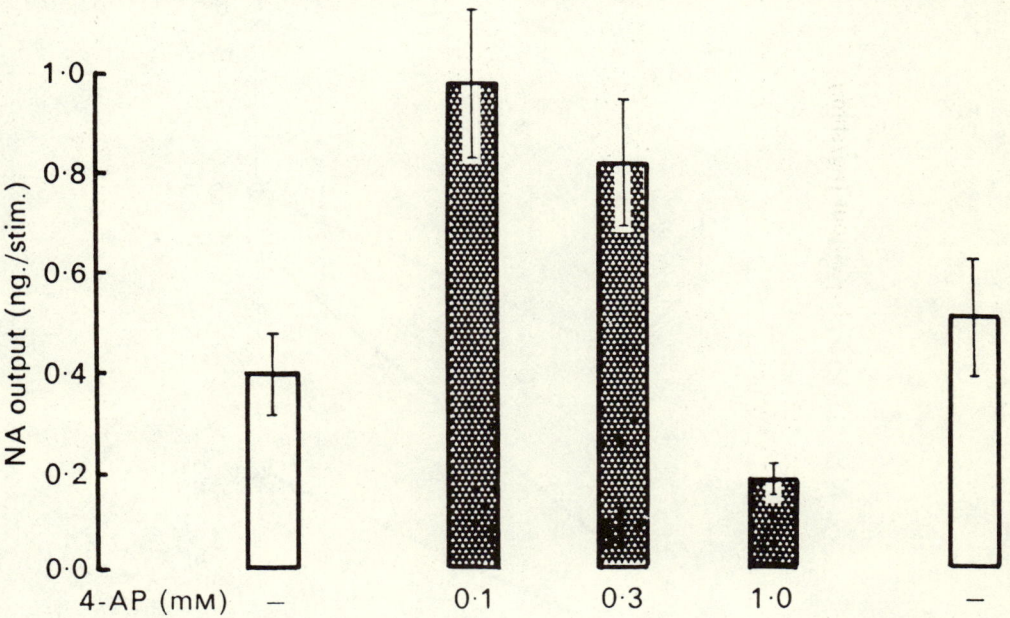

Fig. 3. Effect of 4-AP on NA output during perfusion of the spleen with a solution at pH 8.5. After obtaining the control output at pH 8.5, the spleen was consecutively perfused with this solution containing 0.1, 0.3, and 1.0 mM 4-AP, and then finally without 4-AP, for 15 min each. Splenic nerves were stimulated at 5 Hz during the last 2-min perfusion with Krebs solution (pH 8.5), or during perfusion with 4-AP solution. Vertical lines are the S.E. of mean of 7 experiments. Release at 1 mM was obtained in 3 experiments and recovery in 5 experiments. Reproduced from Kirpekar, Kirpekar, and Prat (1977).

calcium, the secretory response was doubled as the stimulation frequency was increased from 1 to 5 Hz ($P < 0.001$). The output obtained at 30 Hz was 8-fold increased over the response at 1 Hz. NE output was markedly reduced when the calcium concentration of the perfusion medium was decreased to 0.25 mM, while the frequency-output relationship was not only maintained but exaggerated. NE output was 3-fold enhanced when the stimulation frequency was increased from 1 to 5 Hz. At 30 Hz the response was 30-fold increased, as compared with the output at 1 Hz. (Relative outputs at 1, 5, and 30 Hz in the presence of low calcium were also determined on the basis of $^3$H-NE release from three spleens, and directly comparable results were obtained.) On increasing the calcium concentration to 10 mM, the outputs at 1 and 5 Hz were dramatically increased. This 4-fold increase of the calcium concentration caused little or no enhancement of the secretory response at 30 Hz. Thus, the steep frequency-output relationship observed at normal and low calcium concentrations almost disappeared, and there was no difference between responses to 1 and 5 Hz stimulation in the presence of 10 mM calcium (Fig. 4).

Effect of TEA on the frequency-output relation. TEA enhances NE output from the perfused cat spleen evoked by electrical stimulation of its sympathetic nerves (Thoenen, Haefely, and Staehelin, 1967). It was also previously shown that this enhancement is clearly demonstrated at the lower frequencies of stimulation, but is not seen at 30 Hz (Kirpekar, Wakade, and Prat, 1976). Fig. 5 shows that the

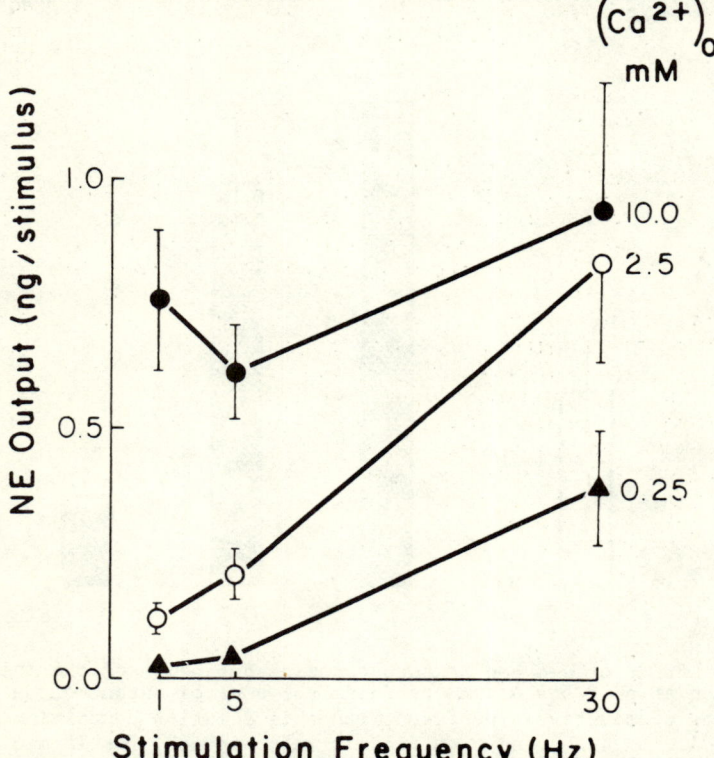

Fig. 4. Effect of calcium on the release of NE elicited by nerve stimulation in the perfused cat spleen. The splenic nerves were stimulated at 1, 5, and 30 Hz in the presence of different extracellular calcium concentrations. Data are means ± S.E. of 3 to 8 experiments. Reproduced from Kirpekar, Garcia, and Prat (1980b).

frequency-output relationship in the presence of 10 mM TEA and 2.5 mM calcium is virtually reversed from that obtained with control spleens. Thus, NE release is maximal at 1 Hz instead of at 30 Hz, and the response to 30 Hz stimulation during TEA treatment is diminished as compared to the output evoked in control spleens. At 1 and 5 Hz stimulation, 10 mM TEA enhanced NE output by 16-fold and 7-fold, respectively, while the response at 30 Hz was reduced by about 40%. When calcium was decreased to 0.1 mM in the presence of TEA, secretory responses evoked by electrical stimulation were substantially reduced, but, as seen in Fig. 5, the maximal response was once again obtained at 30 Hz, and it was nearly 5 times greater than the output at 1 Hz. Thus the effect of TEA on the frequency-output relationship was reversed by reducing the calcium concentration, although in low calcium TEA did facilitate $^3$H-NE release at all 3 stimulation frequencies. Comparable results were previously obtained in the cat spleen with 1 mM TEA (Kirpekar, Wakade, and Prat, 1976), and in the rat vas deferens using 10 mM TEA (Wakade, 1980).

<u>The frequency-output relation following reserpine</u>. The observation that TEA reduced the secretory response at 30 Hz in the presence of 2.5 mM calcium, but not when the calcium concentration was reduced, suggests that in the presence of TEA 30 Hz stimulation may lead to excessive accumulation of calcium inside the nerve terminal. Such a mechanism was previously proposed to explain PBZ's reversal of the normal frequency-response relationship (Kirpekar, Prat, and Wakade, 1975). Alternatively, reduction of the 30 Hz response in the presence of TEA may be a consequence of feedback inhibition, which becomes much less effective when NE release

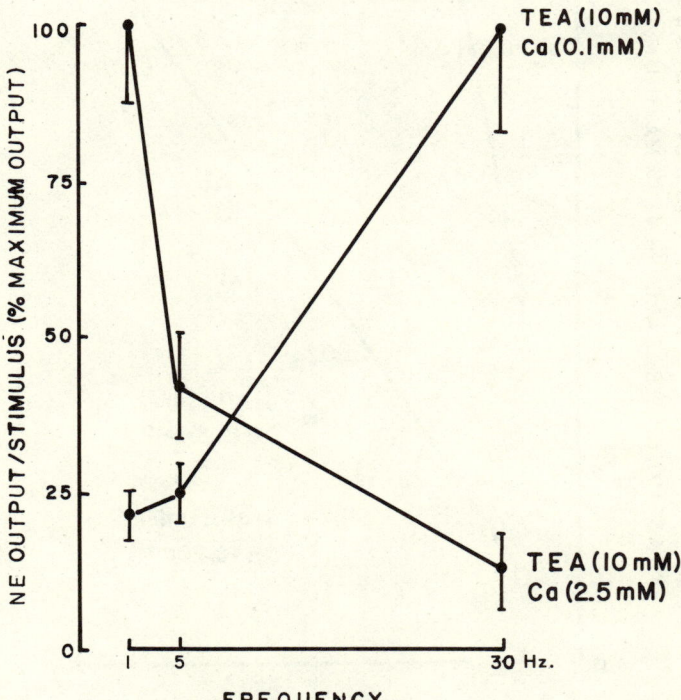

Fig. 5. Effect of TEA on the output of NE elicited by nerve stimulation in the perfused cat spleen. The splenic nerves were stimulated at 1, 5, and 30 Hz in the presence of 10 mM TEA and 0.1 or 2.5 mM calcium. Data are means ± S.E. of 4-5 experiments. Maximal outputs in 2.5 and 0.1 mM calcium + TEA were 9.28 ± 1.11 and 1.0 ± 0.18 ng/stimulus, respectively.

is reduced in 0.1 mM calcium. To rule out this possibility, experiments were conducted with in situ perfused cat spleens 2 or 3 days following reserpinization. For these trials, tissue stores were labeled with $^3$H-NE following iproniazid treatment. In these preparations endogenous stores of NE were very low, but it was possible to detect tritium release on nerve stimulation. It was found that the frequency-output relationship obtained in reserpinized spleens is comparable to that obtained in the normal spleen (Fig. 4), and that the effect of TEA is identical to that observed in the nonreserpinized cat spleens (Fig. 5).

Effect of 4-AP on the frequency-output relation. The change in the frequency-output relation in normal Krebs solution which is obtained in the presence of 4-AP is comparable to the effect of 10 mM calcium: the difference between NE outputs at low- and high-frequency stimulation are diminished, and the response to 30 Hz stimulation in the presence of 4-AP is comparable to that obtained under control conditions. However, 4-AP causes only a modest enhancement of NE release at 1 Hz (Fig. 6). The increase at 5 Hz represents a 6-fold increase in NE output, compared to the 5-Hz response in the untreated spleen. 30-Hz stimulation in the presence of 4-AP evokes a response which is not significantly greater than the 5 Hz response,

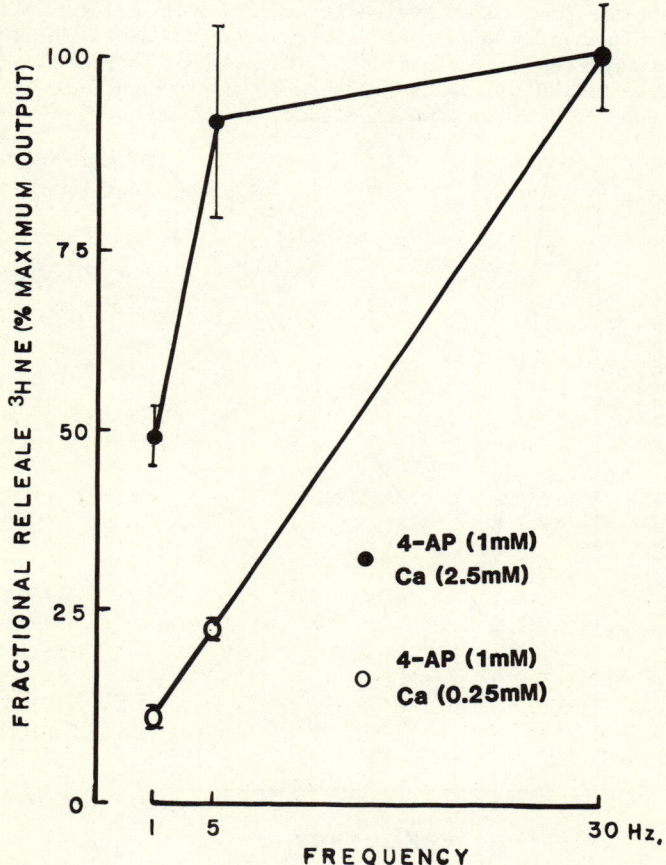

Fig. 6. Effect of 4-AP on the release of $^3$H-NE elicited by nerve stimulation in the perfused cat spleen. The splenic nerves were stimulated at 1, 5, and 30 Hz in the presence of 1 mM 4-AP. Data are means ± S.E. of 5-6 experiments. Maximal outputs at 30 Hz in 2.5 and .25 mM calcium + 4-AP were 5.68 ± 0.39 and 1.73 ± 0.13%, respectively.

and only 40% increased over the output at 30 Hz in normal Krebs solution. Thus, the potentiating effect of 4-AP was more pronounced during low-frequency stimulation (Kirpekar, Kirpekar, and Prat, 1977). The frequency-output relation obtained in the presence of 4-AP and 2.5 mM calcium is quite different from that seen for TEA in Fig. 5. On the other hand, when the calcium concentration was 10-fold reduced, 4-AP, like TEA, failed to alter the frequency- response relationship.

Additivity of TEA and 4-AP in the enhancement of electrically evoked NE release. Although both TEA and 4-AP are known to reduce potassium currents in a number of excitable cells, the differences seen in the frequency-output relationships obtained with these two agents suggest that the manner in which each agent promotes electrically evoked NE release may not be entirely the same. To further pursue this possibility, secretory responses in the perfused cat spleen were studied during electrical stimulation at 5 Hz in the presence of near-optimal doses of 4-AP (1 mM) and TEA (1 mM), administered separately and together. If TEA and 4-AP did differ in their mechanisms of enhancing NE output, then combined treatment with TEA and 4-AP would enhance the secretory response better than either treatment individually. Trials in several spleens have thus far yielded equivocal results: in some spleens, the combined treatments appear to be partially additive, while in other spleens simultaneous treatment with TEA and 4-AP failed to enhance the secretory response to 5 Hz stimulation as compared to treatments with TEA or 4-AP alone. Hirsch, Kirpekar, and Prat (1979) have reported additivity with the enhancement of electrically evoked transmitter release in the case of TEA (1 mM) and guanidine (4 mM). Guanidine appears to promote evoked NE output by increasing intracellular calcium at the nerve terminal, though it has no marked effect on the duration of the action potential. In 5 perfused spleens, guanidine caused a doubling of electrically evoked NE output, and TEA increased the response by nearly 4-fold. When guanidine and TEA were added together, the response to 5 Hz stimulation was nearly 7-fold enhanced.

## Interaction of 4-AP with Neuronal Blocking Agents

Guanethidine and 4-AP. Haeusler and co-workers (1968) have proposed that guanethidine reduces responses at the adrenergic nerve terminal by virtue of its local anesthetic action. Alternatively, guanethidine may depress NE release by limiting the access of calcium to sites in the postganglionic sympathetic nerve endings with which calcium interacts to promote NE release (Kirpekar, Kirpekar, and Prat, 1978). Since 4-AP appears to both prolong depolarization and enhance the calcium entry evoked by electrical stimulation, the present experiments sought to determine if 4-AP could reverse guanethidine's blockade of NE release evoked by nerve stimulation. In control trials, following 15-min treatment with 0.3 µg/ml guanethidine, the response to splenic nerve stimulation (10 Hz) remained depressed during subsequent perfusion with guanethidine-free Krebs solution; after 90 min, the evoked release remained at only 15% of the control value. The reduced NE release after guanethidine was restored to the initial value during perfusion with 1 mM 4-AP for 15 min. During subsequent stimulations at 15-min intervals, the response to nerve stimulation increased gradually on subsequent stimulation, and after 60 min of 4-AP treatment the response was nearly twice the control output. Responses of the perfusion pressure to stimulation were also suppressed by guanethidine, and greatly enhanced during 4-AP perfusion. Following removal of 4-AP the secretory response declined, after 15 min, to 60% of the control response. When evoked NE output declined to 30% of the control output, 4-AP was reintroduced and the NE release was again enhanced to approximately twice the control output. Thus, 4-AP temporarily reverses the guanethidine blockade of NE release. Similar results have been obtained with TEA (Kirpekar, Kirpekar, and Prat, 1977).

Adrenergic blocking properties of a new guanidine derivative. Misu and co-workers (1976) have reported that the guanidine derivative 4,7-exo-methylene-hexahydroisoindoline-ethyl-guanidine-hemisulfate (No. 865-123) is comparable to guanethidine in its ability to block responses to postganglionic nerve stimulation in isolated rabbit atria although, unlike guanethidine, it showed no local anesthetic properties. This laboratory has recently examined the effects of No. 865-123 on NE secretion in the perfused cat spleen as evoked by electrical stimulation of the splenic nerve. Preliminary trials indicated that blockade by No. 865-123 (10 μM) was slower in onset than the sympathetic blockade imposed by guanethidine, but at the end of 30-min treatment with No. 865-123 the response to 5 Hz stimulation was completely blocked. During subsequent perfusion with normal Krebs solution this blockade was maintained for several hours. 4-AP not only reversed the blockade by No. 865-123, but also nearly doubled the secretory response to 5 Hz stimulation for at least 50 min following perfusion of 4-AP. TEA and guanidine also reversed the inhibitory effects of No. 865-123, although the inhibitory effect of this agent partially reappeared upon washout of TEA or guanidine. These observations suggest that a neuronal blocking agent need not have local anesthetic activity to produce blockade of adrenergic transmission.

Nicotine at the Sympathetic Nerve Terminal

Effect of TTX on release of $^3$H-NE by nicotine. Secretory responses to nicotine at the sympathetic nerve terminal were studied in preparations of cat spleen slices previously labeled with $^3$H-NE. During a 5-min incubation period, 50 μM nicotine released 0.8 ± .08% of the tissue $^3$H-NE stores. On increasing the nicotine concen-

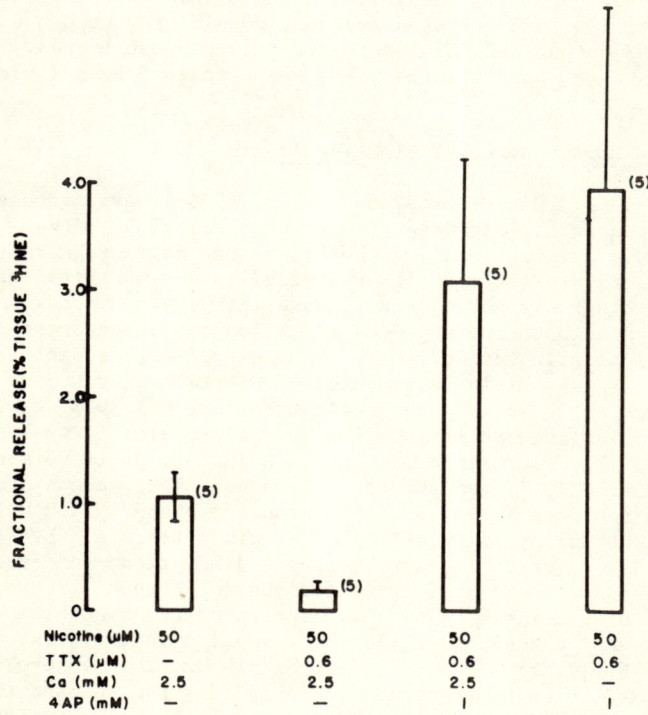

Fig. 7. Effect of 4-AP on the inhibitory effect of TTX on NE release by nicotine. 4-AP reverses the TTX blockade both in calcium-containing and calcium-free solutions. Reproduced from Kirpekar, Garcia, and Prat (1980a).

tration to 2 mM, release was further increased to 2.73 ± 0.39% (P < .001). Similar results were obtained from iproniazid-treated slices. In the presence of TTX (0.6 μM), the response to 50 μM nicotine was substantially reduced, and the low dose of nicotine released only 0.15 ± 0.04% of tissue radioactivity (P < .001). Out of 26 trials, release was blocked by 50% or less in only 3 preparations. TTX had no effect, however, on the response to 2 μM nicotine (Kirpekar, Garcia, and Prat, 1980a).

Effect of 4-AP on TTX blockade of NE release. Since 4-AP antagonized the blockade of NE release by neuronal-blocking agents, it was of interest to determine the effect of 4-AP on TTX blockade of $^3$H-NE release. In the spleen slice preparation, 4-AP (1 mM) caused a 4-fold enhancement of spontaneous release from both control and TTX-treated slices. This effect was observed in the presence and in the absence of calcium, as well as after 40-min exposure to EGTA. When the effects of 4-AP on nicotine-evoked release were tested, this basal release was always subtracted from stimulated samples. Fig. 7 shows that 4-AP dramatically reversed the inhibitory effect of TTX on NE release by nicotine. In the presence of 4-AP (1 mM) and TTX, nicotine evoked a secretory response which was almost 3 times greater than the control output. Since 4-AP appears to potentiate NE release by facilitating calcium entry (Kirpekar, Kirpekar, and Prat, 1977), it seemed possible that 4-AP might reverse the TTX-blockade by virtue of the enhanced calcium influx. Experiments were thus conducted to determine whether the TTX-reversal by 4-AP would be abolished in calcium-free medium. Fig. 7 shows that removal of calcium

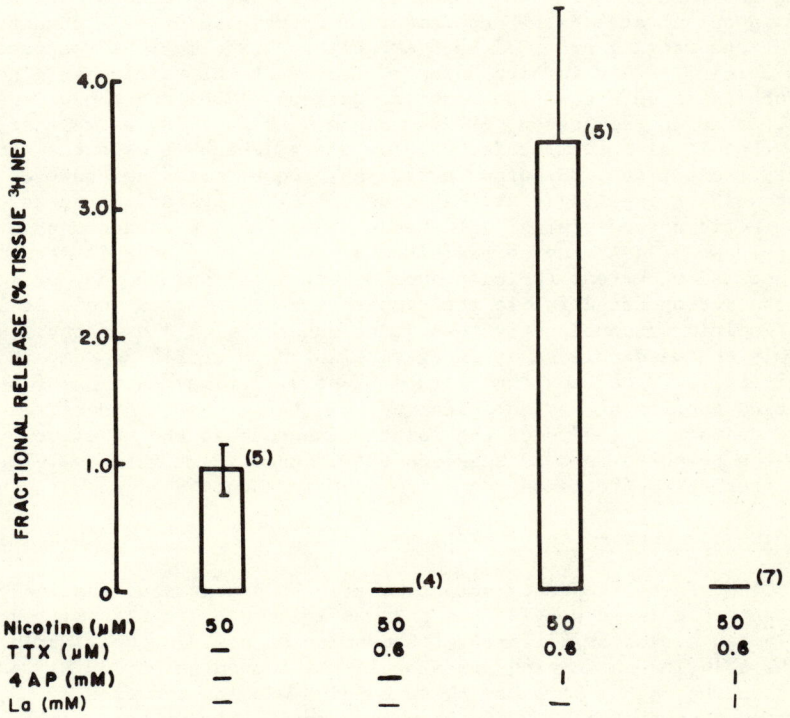

Fig. 8. Effect of lanthanum (La) on restoration of TTX blockade of nicotine-induced release of NE by 4-AP. Note that 4-AP restored TTX blockade of nicotine-induced release of NE, and that La blocked this response. Reproduced from Kirpekar, Garcia, and Prat (1980a).

did not block the nicotine response in the presence of 4-AP and TTX. Thus, during treatment with 4-AP and TTX, nicotine released 3.09 ± 1.16 and 3.9 ± 1.71% of tissue $^3$H-NE in normal and calcium-free Krebs solution, respectively. In the absence of TTX, 4-AP similarly enhanced the response to nicotine in calcium-free Krebs. However, these responses were almost completely abolished when the tissues were previously incubated for 40 min in calcium-free EGTA (1 mM) solution.

Effect of lanthanum on $^3$H-NE release. Since 4-AP failed to enhance nicotine-evoked $^3$H-NE output following treatment with EGTA, it seemed that the response evoked by nicotine and 4-AP in calcium-free Krebs solution may have been due to incomplete washout of minute amounts of calcium remaining in the tissue extracellular space. To evaluate this possibility, trials were carried out in the presence of lanthanum, an ion which selectively blocks calcium transport in a variety of tissues (Van Breeman, Aaronson, and Loutzenhiser, 1978). Fig. 8 shows that nicotine, in the presence of lanthanum (1 mM) did not release $^3$H-NE from spleen slices exposed to TTX and 4-AP ($P < .001$). This inhibitory effect was seen in the presence of normal calcium and in calcium-free solution. Nearly complete blockade of release by lanthanum would suggest that the restoration of nicotine response in calcium-free solution containing TTX and 4-AP was due to mobilization of extracellular calcium.

DISCUSSION

4-AP enhanced the amount of NE which appeared in the venous effluent during stimulation of the splenic nerves at 5 Hz. It was found that 4-AP blocked NE reuptake somewhat, but this property alone was not sufficient to account for a nearly 5-fold increase in output at 5 Hz. Enhancement of NE release by 4-AP occurred in calcium concentrations ranging from 0.1 to 5 mM, although the maximal response was obtained in 2.5 mM calcium. 4-AP is also known to facilitate NE release from nerve endings of the rabbit vas deferens (Johns and co-workers, 1976) and the rat portal vein (Leander, Arner and Johansson, 1977). Since 4-AP facilitates release, it is possible that it also facilitates calcium entry, which is essential for evoked transmitter secretion. NE output evoked by excess potassium, however, is not enhanced by 4-AP, suggesting that 4-AP does not directly facilitate calcium entry at the sympathetic nerve terminal. Instead, the selective enhancement of nerve-induced release by 4-AP may be explained by the ability of this agent to block the delayed potassium current (Pelhate and Pichon, 1974) and thereby prolong the duration of the action potential in the sympathetic nerve; this would prolong the period of calcium channel activation, thus enhancing calcium entry. 4-AP more effectively enhanced release at an extracellular pH of 8.5 as compared to 7.4. This may simply reflect the fact that with a pK of 9.17, less than 2% of 4-AP is present as uncharged species at physiological pH, and the drug would more readily penetrate the nerve endings as the pH of the solution approaches the pK value. The influence of pH on the response to 4-AP suggests that 4-AP may act intracellularly to produce its characteristic effects on potassium inactivation.

4-AP and the Frequency-Output Relationship

Early studies of the frequency-output relationship suggested that calcium may play an important role in modulating the changes in adrenergic transmitter release from the cat spleen evoked by different frequencies of stimulation. During perfusion with Krebs solution containing 2.5 mM calcium, the output at 30 Hz was 8-fold greater than the output at 1 Hz. When calcium was lowered to 0.25 mM, the difference between responses at low and high frequencies became more marked, and the output at 30 Hz became nearly 30- to 40-fold greater than the output at 1 Hz. On the other hand, increasing the calcium concentration diminished the difference between responses to low- and high-frequency stimulation, so that secretory responses at 1 and 5 Hz were almost comparable to the output obtained at 30 Hz. This change in the relationship largely reflected a preferential enhancement of the outputs at 1 and 5 Hz. In fact, the output at 30 Hz in high-calcium solution was not significantly different from the output in normal Krebs solution at this frequency. These results, then, suggest that the increase in NE release associated with the increase in stimulation frequency may reflect the greater availability of calcium to the sympathetic nerve terminals as the stimulation frequency is increased.

The frequency-output relationship observed in the presence of TEA suggests that sufficiently high concentrations of calcium may actually reduce NE output. Kirpekar, Wakade, and Prat (1976) previously reported that, in the presence of 1 mM TEA, the response to 30-Hz stimulation is 60% of the response to 5-Hz stimulation in the cat spleen during perfusion with 2.5 mM calcium-Krebs solution. Feedback inhibition is not likely to play a role in the relationship, since the present results indicate that TEA has a similar effect in the reserpinized spleen. On the other hand, during perfusion with Krebs solution containing 0.1 mM calcium, TEA did enhance NE output at all three frequencies, but the maximal secretory response was obtained at 30 Hz. Since NE output in both normal and reserpinized spleens is markedly reduced at 30 Hz as compared to 1 Hz, and low calcium reverses this relationship, it appears that the reduced release at 30 Hz is not due to failure of conduction of impulses, but instead may have something to do with the intraneuronal calcium concentration. It is possible, then, that at 30 Hz excessive calcium accumulates within the nerve terminal and this may, in turn, desensitize the release process. Because 4-AP and TEA both block the late potassium current associated with action potentials at nerve terminals, it is generally presumed that both agents enhance NE output in response to nerve stimulation by increasing calcium entry secondary to prolongation of the action potential. This is supported by the observation that TEA and 4-AP are not additive in their ability to enhance NE release evoked by splenic nerve stimulation.

In this context, the finding that TEA and 4-AP modify the frequency-output relationship in different ways is a puzzling observation. TEA completely reverses the relationship, so that secretory responses decline as the stimulation frequency is increased from 1 to 30 Hz. Although 4-AP, on the other hand, fails to reverse the frequency-output relationship, the response to 30-Hz stimulation in the presence of 4-AP is not significantly different from the response to 5 Hz stimulation. This observation may be related in some way to the proportion of time the nerve membrane remains depolarized. As the stimulation frequency increases, the proportion of time the membrane is depolarized also increases; thus, at higher frequencies of electrical stimulation, TEA or 4-AP will tend to lose their ability to increase the proportion of time during which the nerve terminal is depolarized. This explanation is supported by the finding that TEA is more effective in enhancing responses of the anococcygeus muscle to field stimulation of the motor adrenergic nerves at low than at high frequencies of stimulation (Gillespie and Tilmisany, 1976). Another explanation previously considered in the context of the TEA response is the possibility that responses at high frequencies and in the presence of an agent such as TEA or 4-AP may be limited by excessive accumulation of calcium at the nerve terminal. This explanation is supported by the observation that 4-AP, like TEA, fails to modify the frequency-output relation when the calcium concentration is reduced. Two obvious differences, however, remain unexplained. First, 4-AP, unlike TEA, fails to substantially increase the secretory response to 1 Hz stimulation. Secondly, while the response to 30-Hz stimulation during 4-AP treatment is not significantly different from the NE release evoked at 5 Hz, TEA reduced the 30-Hz response with respect to the output at 5 Hz as well as in comparison with the control output at 30 Hz. Nonetheless, the effects of 4-AP and TEA on secretory responses evoked by postganglionic nerve stimulation are roughly comparable.

## 4-AP and Guanethidine

The inhibitory effect of guanethidine on NE release from the cat spleen by nerve stimulation was dramatically reversed by 4-AP and TEA. Guanethidine blockade was similarly reversed by treatment with guanidine (Hirsch, Kirpekar, and Prat, 1979). In addition, the sympathetic blockade imposed by the guanidine derivative No. 865-123, which is devoid of local anesthetic activity (Misu and co-workers, 1976), is also reversed by 4-AP, TEA and guanidine. All three agents are known to enhance calcium concentration in the nerve terminals (Lundh, Leander and Thesleff, 1977). TEA and 4-AP are presumed to enhance NE release by blocking the potassium current and thus prolonging the duration of the action potential; as a result, calcium channels remain open longer, and more calcium is allowed to enter. However, guanidine does not affect inactivation of the potassium current; it mobilizes calcium in nerve terminals by enhancing its influx, and possibly by interfering with intracellular binding (Hirsch, Kirpekar, and Prat, 1979; Lundh, Leander, and Thesleff, 1977; Matthews and Wickelgren, 1977). Thus, although guanidine, like 4-AP or TEA, mobilizes intracellular calcium at the adrenergic nerve terminal, a different mechanism appears to be involved; yet all three agents antagonize the inhibitory effects of guanethidine or No. 865-123 on adrenergic transmission. It is possible, then, that TEA, 4-AP and guanidine allow greater than normal amounts of calcium to accumulate inside the nerve terminals during an action potential to reverse the blockade of NE release by guanethidine and related agents. The adrenergic blockade produced by guanethidine could have its origin in the local anesthetic properties of the agent. However, the fact that a guanidine derivative with no local anesthetic action effectively blocks adrenergic transmission, and that its blockade is reversed by calcium-mobilizing agents, strongly suggests that guanethidine and its congeners may reduce neurotransmitter release by some mechanism other than, or in addition to, local anesthetic action.

## 4-AP and Nicotine

In the incubated spleen slice preparation of the cat, TTX blocked the secretory response evoked by a low dose of nicotine, while 4-AP markedly enhanced the response. TTX had no effect, however, on the nicotine response in the presence of 4-AP. The TTX blockade of transmitter release probably means that the low dose of nicotine used in this study activated presynaptic nicotine receptors and caused sufficient localized depolarization of the sympathetic nerve terminals to generate propagated activity which is directly responsible for NE release. TTX, by blocking this regenerative activity, markedly reduces NE release. At a 40-fold higher concentration, nicotine would cause a massive depolarization by increasing the cation permeability independent of any effect on the voltage-sensitive sodium channel. This membrane activation would promote calcium influx into the nerve terminals, and thus trigger NE release. It was surprising, however, that comparable enhancement of the nicotine response by 4-AP was observed in the presence of TTX, even when no calcium was added to the incubation medium. Since lanthanum blocked the secretory response of nicotine in TTX and 4-AP solution, it would appear that the influx of residual calcium remaining in the intracellular space, or more probably from an extracellular pool of tightly bound calcium, was partly responsible for release. The 4-AP response to nicotine was also blocked by prolonged incubation in a calcium-free solution containing EGTA. Kirpekar and Prat (1978) have demonstrated that NE release may be evoked from TTX- and TEA- treated cat spleen slices in response to electrotonic depolarization of sympathetic nerve terminals, and they attributed the release to a regenerative calcium entry into the adrenergic nerve terminal. It is therefore possible that a prolonged entry of residual calcium in the present trials may have occurred as a result of potassium conductance blockade by 4-AP to restore the nicotine response in the presence of TTX.

It seems unlikely, however, that restoration of NE release in the presence of 4-AP could be explained solely on the basis of calcium influx. Kirpekar, Kirpekar, and Prat (1977) previously reported that supraoptimal doses of 4-AP enhance spontaneous release of NE. It is therefore conceivable that 4-AP may enhance calcium influx not only by blocking potassium conductance, but also by mobilizing a pool of calcium presumably associated with the neuronal membrane. The EGTA experiments suggest that calcium bound to high-affinity sites may play a role in this response.

Conclusions

4-AP enhances NE release mainly as a consequence of its ability to block the potassium channel and prolong the duration of the action potential, thereby promoting a greater influx of calcium ions into the nerve terminal. Additionally, 4-AP may enhance calcium influx not only by blocking potassium conductance, but also by mobilizing a pool of calcium which may be bound to high-affinity sites on the neuronal membrane.

REFERENCES

Anton, A.H., and D.F. Sayre (1962). A study of the factors affecting the aluminum oxide trihydroxyindole procedure for the analysis of catecholamines. J. Pharmac. exp. Ther., 138, 360-375.

Bowman, W.C., and A.O. Savage (1981). Pharmacological actions of aminopyridines and related compounds. Reviews in Pure and Applied Pharmacological Sciences (in press).

Gillespie, J.I., and O.F. Hutter (1975). The action of 4-aminopyridine on the delayed potassium current in skeletal muscle fibers. J. Physiol., 252, 70-71 P.

Gillespie, J.S., and A.K. Tilmisany (1976). The action of tetraethylammonium chloride on the response of the rat anococcygeus muscle to motor and inhibitory nerve stimulation and to some drugs. Br. J. Pharmac., 58, 47-55.

Haeusler, G., H. Thoenen, W. Haefely, and A. Mürlimann (1968). Durch Acetylcholin hervorgerufene antidrome Aktivität im kardialen Sympathicus und Noradrenalin friesetzung unter Guanethidin. Helv. Physiol. Pharmac. Acta, 26, CR352-CR354.

Hirsch, J., S.M. Kirpekar, and J.C. Prat (1979), Effect of guanidine on release of noradrenaline from the perfused spleen of the cat. Br. J. Pharmac., 66, 537-546.

Johns, A., D.S. Golko, P.A. Lauzon, and D.M. Paton (1976). The potentiating effects of 4-aminopyridine on adrenergic transmission in the rabbit vas deferens. Europ. J. Pharmacol., 38, 71-78.

Kirpekar, M., S.M. Kirpekar, and J.C. Prat (1977). Effect of 4-aminopyridine on release of noradrenaline from the perfused cat spleen by nerve stimulation. J. Physiol., 272, 517-528.

Kirpekar, M., S.M. Kirpekar, and J.C. Prat (1978). Reversal of guanethidine blockade of sympathetic nerve terminals by tetraethylammonium and 4-aminopyridine. Br. J. Pharmacol., 62, 75-78.

Kirpekar, S.M., A.G. Garcia, and J.C. Prat (1980a). Action of nicotine on sympathetic nerve terminals. J. Pharmac. exp. Ther., 213, 133-138.

Kirpekar, S.M., A.G. Garcia, and J.C. Prat (1980b). Calcium and frequency-dependent release of norepinephrine. Biochem. Pharmacol., 29, 3029-3031.

Kirpekar, S.M., and Y. Misu (1967). Release of noradrenaline by splenic nerve stimulation and its dependence on calcium. J. Physiol., 188, 219-234.

Kirpekar, S.M., and J.C. Prat (1978). Effect of tetraethylammonium on noradrenaline release from cat spleen treated with tetrodotoxin. Nature (Lond.) 276, 623-624.

Kirpekar, S.M., J.C. Prat, and A.R. Wakade (1975). Effect of calcium on the relationship between frequency of stimulation and release of noradrenaline from the perfused spleen of the cat. Naunyn-Schmiedeberg's Arch. Pharmacol., 287, 205-212.

Kirpekar, S.M., A.R. Wakade and J.C. Prat (1976). Effect of tetraethylammonium and barium on the release of noradrenaline from the perfused cat spleen by nerve stimulation and potassium. Naunyn-Schmiedeberg's Arch. Pharmacol., 294, 23-29.

Leander, S., A. Arner, and B. Johansson (1977). Effects of 4-aminopyridine on mechanical activity and noradrenaline release in the rat portal vein in vitro. Europ. J. Pharmacol., 46, 351-361.

Llinás, R., K. Walton, and V. Bohr (1976). Synaptic transmission in squid giant synapse after potassium conductance blockage with external 3- and 4-aminopyridine. Biophys. J., 16, 83-86.

Lundh, H., S. Leander, and S. Thesleff (1977). Antagonism of the paralysis produced by botulinum toxin in the rat. J. Neurol. Sci., 32, 29-43.

Matthews, G., and W.O. Wickelgren (1977). Effects of guanidine on transmitter release and neuronal excitability. J. Physiol., 266, 69-89.

Meves, M., and Y. Pichon (1975). Effects of 4-aminopyridine on the potassium current in internally perfused giant axons of the squid. J. Physiol., 251, 60-62P.

Misu, Y., H. Nishio, T. Hosotani, and S. Hamano (1976). A new guanidine derivative: Dissociation of the adrenergic neuron blocking activity from local anesthetic activity. Japan. J. Pharmacol., 26 , 367-375.

Molgó, J., M. Lemeignan, and P. Lechat (1977). Effects of 4-aminopyridine at the frog neuromuscular junction. J. Pharmac. exp. Ther., 203, 653-663.

Molgó, J., H. Lundh, and S. Thesleff (1980). Potency of 3,4-aminopyridine on mammalian neuromuscular transmission and the effect of pH changes. Europ. J. Pharmacol., 61, 25-34.

Pelhate, M., and Y. Pichon (1974). Selective inhibition of potassium current in the giant axon of the cockroach. J. Physiol., 242, 90-91P.

Thoenen, H., W. Haefely, and H. Staehelin (1967). Potentiation by tetraethylammonium of the response of the cat spleen to postganglionic sympathetic nerve stimulation. J. Pharmac. exp. Ther., 157, 532-540.

Van Breemen, C., P. Aaronson, and R. Loutzenhiser (1978). Sodium-calcium interactions in mammalian smooth muscle. Pharmacol. Rev., 30, 167-208.

Wakade, A.R. (1980). A maximum contraction and substantial quantities of tritium can be obtained from tetraethylammonium-treated $^3$H-noradrenaline preloaded, rat vas deferens in response to a single electrical shock. Br. J. Pharmac., 68, 425-436.

Yeh, J.Z., A.S. Oxford, C.H. Wu, and T. Narahashi (1976). Interactions of aminopyridines with potassium channels of squid axon membranes. Biophys. J., 16, 77-81.

# Some Differences in the Blockade of Potassium Permeabilities by Apamin and the Aminopyridines

D. H. Jenkinson

Department of Pharmacology, University College London,
Gower Street, London WC1E 6BT, UK

ABSTRACT

Apamin, a polypeptide from bee venom, has been found to block receptor-initiated increases in the potassium permeability of smooth muscle and liver cells. Its actions differ from those of the aminopyridines in that only calcium-dependent potassium permeabilities are affected, and that very low concentrations are needed.

KEYWORDS

Apamin; aminopyridines; calcium-activated potassium permeability; liver cells; smooth muscle; potassium channels.

INTRODUCTION

Other chapters in this volume illustrate the progress that can result from the discovery of agents which selectively block specific processes in synaptic transmission. A recent addition to the armamentarium is the polypeptide apamin which was considered to merit some mention in a Symposium primarily devoted to the aminopyridines because of the common feature that both substances block potassium permeabilities, albeit of a different kind.

Apamin is found in bee venom, and it was first described by Habermann & Reiz in 1965. The sequence of its 18 amino-acids is known from the work of Shipolini, Bradbury, Callewaert & Vernon (1967) and of Haux, Sawerthal & Habermann (1967), and is illustrated in Fig. 1. (For studies of the three dimensional structure, see Bystrov and co-workers, 1980).

Habermann and his colleagues found apamin to be a centrally acting neurotoxin: parenteral administration of a lethal dose causes motor hyperactivity in mammals, leading to generalised convulsions and death. Though the cellular mechanism of the action on the CNS is not yet known, a good deal has been done to characterise it, and the interested reader is referred to the excellent reviews of Habermann

(1972; 1982) and of Granier & van Rietschoten (1980); for an account of apamin in relation to other arthropod toxins, see O'Connor & Peck (1978).

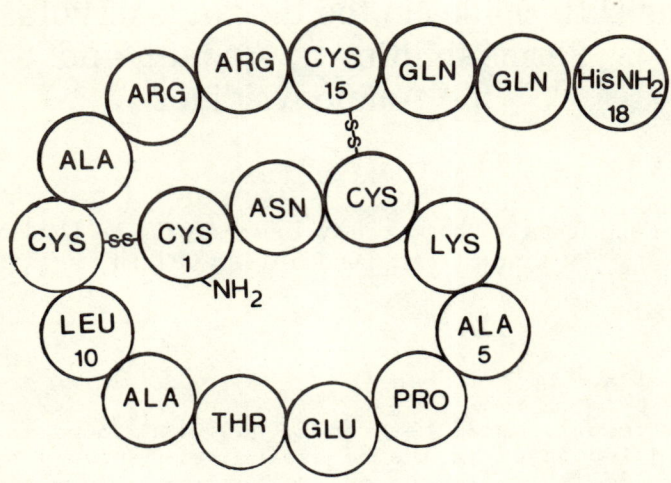

FIG. 1. Structure of apamin.

PERIPHERAL ACTIONS OF APAMIN

The pioneering work of M. F. Shuba, I. Vladimirova and their colleagues in Kiev has shown that apamin also has specific peripheral actions, and these are the main subject of the present article. The Kiev group (Baidan, Vladimirova, Miroshnikov & Taran, 1978; Vladimirova & Shuba, 1978) discovered that apamin was remarkably effective in blocking the response to stimulation of the nonadrenergic, noncholinergic (NANC) inhibitory nerve supply to guinea-pig stomach and intestinal smooth muscle. Moreover, the same low concentrations of apamin blocked the response to applied ATP, a candidate for the neurotransmitter mediating NANC inhibition. It has since been found, however, that apamin is not a specific ATP antagonist; it also blocks the inhibitory actions of other agents, including bradykinin (Ferrero, Cocks & Burnstock, 1980) and catecholamines (Banks and co-workers, 1979; Maas & den Hertog, 1979; Muller & Baer, 1980; Vladimirova & Shuba, 1980) on the same smooth muscles. Pharmacological analysis has shown that it is the response to $\alpha$- rather than to $\beta$-adrenoreceptors that is antagonised (see Fig. 2). Similarly, apamin affects only the inhibitory response to the type of purinergic receptor described as $P_2$ on the classification introduced by Burnstock (1978): the $P_1$ receptors remain functional (Brown & Burnstock, 1981). Since the inhibitory influence of $\alpha$-adrenoreceptors, as well as of ATP acting through $P_2$ receptors, on intestinal smooth muscle is known to be largely attributable to a rise in the potassium permeability of the cell membrane, Banks and co-workers suggested that apamin acted by blocking this permeability increase.

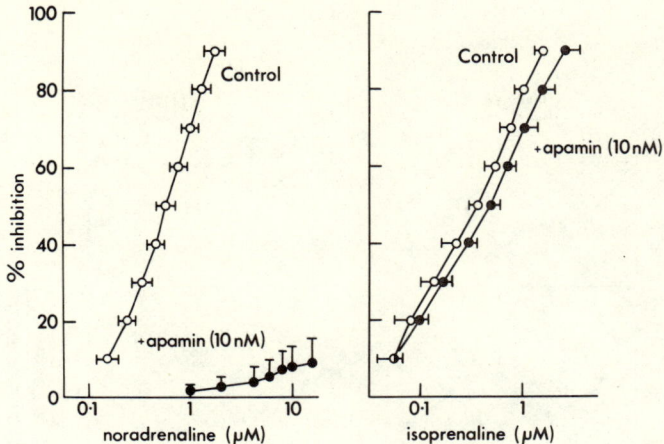

Fig. 2. Apamin (10 nM) blocks the inhibitory effect of α- but not β-adrenoreceptor activation on the spontaneous contractile activity of isolated intestinal smooth muscle (guinea-pig taenia caeci). From Jenkinson (1981).

Support for this has come from experiments with two quite different tissues. den Hertog and his co-workers at Groningen have applied electrophysiological and radioisotopic methods to the study of the action of apamin on receptor-induced changes in the potassium permeability of the taenia of the guinea-pig caecum. One of their findings is illustrated in Fig. 3, which shows that apamin at 100 nM reduces the increase in $^{42}K$ efflux caused by both adrenaline and ATP, and attributable to a rise in $P_K$. Using electrophysiological methods, it was demonstrated that apamin converts the hyperpolarization initiated by α-adrenoreceptors to a depolarization. The abolition of the hyperpolarization, and the reduction in the concomitant fall in membrane resistance, can be explained as a consequence of blockade of the increase in $P_K$, though the nature of the ionic currents which underlie the depolarization thereby unmasked is as yet not completely certain; calcium ions may well be involved (Maas and co-workers, 1980; den Hertog, 1981).

Additional evidence for the blocking actions of apamin on potassium permeabilities has been obtained with a quite different tissue, guinea-pig liver. Perhaps surprisingly, the liver cells of most species possess receptors which initiate an increase in the potassium permeability of their membranes. Most work has been done with guinea-pig liver which has been found to respond in this way to noradrenaline, ATP and angiotensin II. The response is blocked by low concentrations of apamin, just as in intestinal smooth muscle (Banks and co-workers, 1979; Burgess, Claret & Jenkinson, 1981). Moreover, apamin converts the hyperpolarization which α-adrenoreceptors initiate in liver cells to a small depolarization (D. G. Haylett, personal communication), again paralleling the findings with smooth muscle.

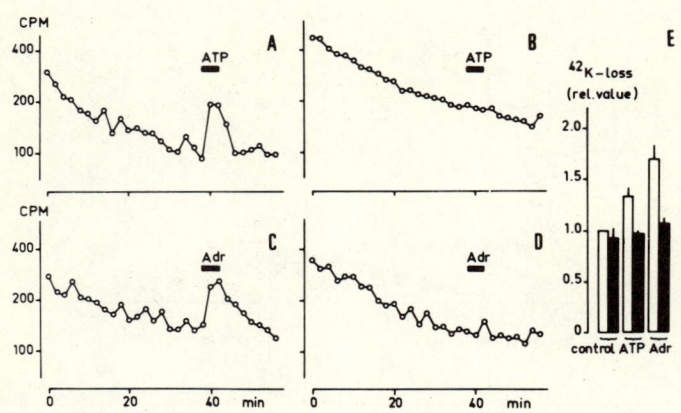

Fig. 3. Apamin (100 nM, present in B and D) blocks the increases in $^{42}$K efflux which follow the application of either ATP (400 μM, A and B) or adrenaline (3 μM, C and D) to strips of guinea-pig taenia caeci. The histograms (E) show the mean increases in $^{42}$K; the black bars indicate the values observed in the presence of apamin. From Maas and co-workers (1980), with permission.

There is reason to think that both in intestinal smooth muscle (Bülbring & Tomita, 1977, den Hertog, 1981) and in liver cells (Haylett, 1976; Weiss & Putney, 1978; Burgess, Claret & Jenkinson, 1979,1981) the increase in $P_K$ which follows receptor activation is triggered by a rise in cytosolic calcium. In guinea-pig liver, the increase in $[Ca^{++}]_i$ is reflected by an increase in $^{45}$Ca efflux, and is likely to underlie the increase in glucose release that follows α-adrenoreceptor activation (Haylett & Jenkinson, 1972; Haylett, 1976; Osborn, 1978). As Fig. 4 shows, apamin does not affect the latter responses when applied at a concentration (10 nM) sufficient to block the increase in $P_K$ (as assessed by changes in the efflux of $^{42}$K). This provides further evidence that apamin is not a receptor antagonist: it seems to interfere either directly with the potassium channels which open in response to receptor activation, or with the mechanism linking the rise in $[Ca^{++}]_i$ to channel opening.

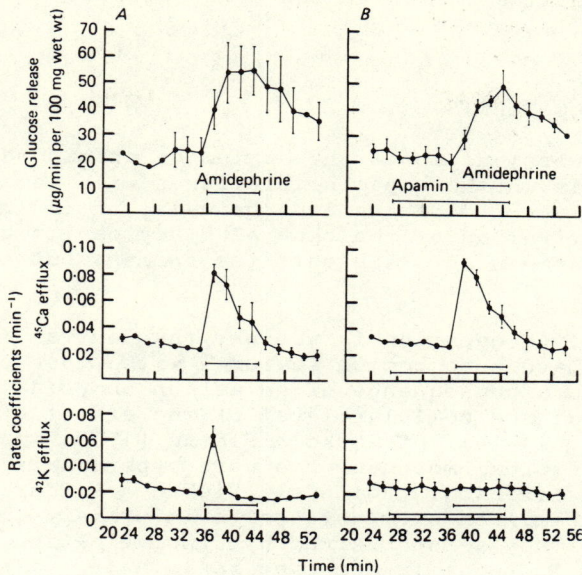

Fig. 4. Left. The α-adrenoreceptor agonist (-)-amidephrine (10 μM) increases the release of glucose (top), $^{45}$Ca (middle) and $^{42}$K (bottom) from rabbit liver slices.

Right. Apamin (10 nM) selectively inhibits the increase in $^{42}$K efflux. From Burgess, Claret & Jenkinson (1981), with permission.

## APAMIN IN RELATION TO THE AMINOPYRIDINES

Though the aminopyridines and apamin both block potassium permeabilities, several features distinguish them. Apamin is effective at much lower concentrations, 5-10 nM being enough for near maximal inhibition. Also, apamin can act within seconds (Burgess, Claret & Jenkinson, 1981) whereas block by aminopyridines is generally much slower, as discussed in other chapters in this volume. Perhaps the most striking difference is that apamin, unlike the aminopyridines, appears (on present evidence) to influence only calcium-activated potassium permeabilities, and not all of these. Thus, the well characterized 'Gardos effect' in red cells is quite unaffected (Burgess, Claret & Jenkinson, 1981). Apamin's lack of action on other ion permeabilities is well illustrated by the experiments of Baidan and co-workers (1979) who have shown that there is no effect on the end-plate potential or the miniature end-plate potentials in frog skeletal muscle. This implies that it blocks neither the presynaptic potassium channels that are so sensitive to aminopyridines in this preparation (Molgo, Lemeignan & Lechat, 1977), nor the postsynaptic channels which are opened by the action of nerve-released acetylcholine. The same workers have also shown that apamin has little effect on inhibitory postsynaptic potentials recorded from snail parietal ganglia. Nor is the hyperpolarizing action of either acetylcholine or ATP on the sinus venosus of the frog heart inhibited (Vladimirova & Shuba, 1980).

FINAL COMMENTS

Several major questions about the action of apamin have still to be settled. One is whether apamin interferes with potassium permeabilities directly, by blocking ion channels, or indirectly, by inhibiting the activation of the channel by cytosolic calcium. The speed at which apamin acts suggests the former, but the evidence is not decisive.

A second unresolved question is whether the central 'neurotoxic' effects (which have some common features with those of the aminopyridines) are also a consequence of an action on potassium permeability. The only study at the cellular level of the effect of apamin on CNS neurones in situ is that of Görke & Pierau (1979) working on pigeons. They found that spinal motoneurones were hyperpolarized, though the IPSP was little affected. Dimpfel, Pierau & Haider (1979) examined the action of apamin on excitable cells in primary cultures derived from rat CNS. They also observed hyperpolarization which was accompanied by an increase in membrane resistance. In discussing their findings, they inclined to the view that either sodium or chloride permeability became reduced.

Finally, we may note that methods for the labelling of apamin have been described (for references see Cavey, Vincent & Lazdunski, 1979 and Habermann, 1982), as has the production of antibodies against it (Komissarenko and co-workers, 1981). These advances will help greatly in the study of the action of apamin, and could lead to the isolation of the target ion channels, or the structure that controls them.

REFERENCES

Baidan, L. V., I. A. Vladimirova, A. I. Miroshnikov and G. A. Taran (1978). Deistuie apamina na sinapticheskviv peredachu v razlichnykh tipakh sinapsov. Dokl.Akad.Nauk SSSR, 241, 1224-1227. (Available in translation: Doklady Natural Sciences, (1979) 241 373-376.
Banks, B. E. C., C. Brown, G. M. Burgess, G. Burnstock, M. Claret, T. M. Cocks and D. H. Jenkinson (1979). Apamin blocks certain neurotransmitter-induced increases in potassium permeability. Nature, 282, 415-417.
Brown, C. M. and G. Burnstock (1981). Evidence in support of the $P_1/P_2$ purinoceptor hypothesis in the guinea-pig taenia coli. Br. J.Pharmac., 73, 617-624.
Bülbring, E. and T. Tonita (1977). Calcium requirement for the $\alpha$-action of catecholamines on guinea-pig taenia coli. Proc.R.Soc.B, 197, 271-284.
Burgess, G. M., M. Claret and D. H. Jenkinson (1979). Effects of catecholamines, ATP and ionophore A23187 on potassium and calcium movements in isolated hepatocytes. Nature, 279, 544-546.
Burgess, G. M., M. Claret and D. H. Jenkinson (1981). Effects of quinine and apamin on the calcium-dependent potassium permeability of mammalian hepatocytes and red cells. J.Physiol.,Lond.,317,67-90.

Burnstock, G. (1978). A basis for distinguishing two types of purinergic receptor. In R. W. Straub and L. Bolis (Eds.), Cell Membrane Receptors for Drugs and Hormones. Raven Press, New York. pp. 107-118.

Bystrov, V. F., V. V. Okhanov, A. I. Miroshnikov and Y. A. Ouchinnikov (1980). Solution spatial structure of apamin as derived from NMR study. FEBS Letters, 119, 113-117.

Cavey, D., J-P. Vincent and M. Lazdunski (1979). A search for the apamin receptor in the central nervous system. Toxicon, 17, 176-179.

den Hertog, A. (1981). Calcium and the α-action of catecholamines on guinea-pig taenia coli. J.Physiol.Lond., 316, 109-125.

Dimpfel, W., F-K. Pierau and S. G. Haider (1979). Electrophysiological studies on the effects of the neurotoxin apamin on cultured neurones. In B. Ceccarelli and F. Clementi (Eds.) Advances in Cytopharmacology, Vol. 3. Raven Press, New York, pp. 395-399.

Ferrero, J. D., T. Cocks and G. Burnstock (1980). A comparison between ATP and bradykinin as possible mediators of the responses of smooth muscle to non-adrenergic non-cholinergic nerves. Eur.J. Pharmac. 63, 295-302.

Görke, K. and F. K. Pierau (1979). Response of spinal sensory neurones and motoneurones of pigeons to the neuropeptide apamin. Pflügers Arch.Physiol., 382, R 39.

Granier, C. and J. van Rietschoten (1980). Chemical structure, biological and pharmacological activities of apamin, and their relations. In D. Eaker and T. Wadström (Ed.), Natural Toxins. Pergamon Press, Oxford. pp. 481-486.

Habermann, E. (1972). Bee and wasp venoms. Science, N.Y. 177, 314-322.

Habermann, E. (1982). Apamin. Pharmacol. and Therap. In the press.

Habermann, E. and K. G. Reiz (1965). Ein neues Verfahren zur Gewinnüng der Komponenten von Bienengift, insbesondere des zentralwirksamen Peptids Apamin. Biochem.Z., 341, 451-466.

Haux, P., H. Sawerthal and E. Habermann (1967). Sequenzanalyse des Bienengift-Neurotoxins (Apamin) aus seinen tryptischen und chymotryptischen Spaltstücken. Hoppe-Seylers Z.Phys.Chem., 348, 737-738.

Haylett, G. G. (1976). The effects of sympathomimetic amines on $^{45}Ca$ efflux from liver slices. Br.J.Pharmac., 57, 158-160.

Haylett, D. G. and D. H. Jenkinson (1972). The receptors concerned in the actions of catecholamines on glucose release, membrane potential and ion movements in guinea-pig liver. J.Physiol.,Lond., 225, 751-772.

Jenkinson, D. H. (1981). Peripheral actions of apamin. Trends in Pharmacological Sciences. In the press.

Komissarenko, S. V., S. V. Vasilenko, E. G. Elyakova, E. A. Surina and A. I. Miroshnikov (1979). Immunochemistry of apamin - bee venom neurotoxin - I. Radioimmunoassay with apamin and its derivatives. Molec.Immunol., 18, 533-536.

Maas, A. J. J. and A. den Hertog (1979). The effect of apamin on the smooth muscle cells of the guinea-pig taenia coli. Eur.J. Pharmac., 58, 151-156.

Maas, A. J. J., A. den Hertog, R. Ras and J. van den Akker (1980). The action of apamin on guinea-pig taenia caeci. Eur.J.Pharmac. 67, 265-274.

Molgo, J., M. Lemeignan and P. Lechat (1977). Effects of 4-aminopyridine at the frog neuromuscular junction. J.Pharmac.exp.Ther. 203, 653-663.

Muller, M. J. and H. P. Baer (1980). Apamin, a non-specific antagonist of smooth muscle relaxants. Naunyn-Schmiedebergs Arch.exp. Path.Pharmak., 311, 105-107.

O'Connor, R. and M. L. Peck (1978). Venoms of Apidae. In S. Bettini (Ed.), Arthropod Venoms. Heffter's Handbuch der exp. Pharmakol., 48, 613-659.

Osborn, D. (1978). The alpha adrenergic receptor mediated increase in guinea-pig liver glycogenolysis. Biochem.Pharmac. 27, 1315-1320.

Shipolini, R., A. F. Bradbury, G. L. Callewaert and C. A. Vernon (1967). The structure of apamin. Chemical.Comm., 679-680.

Vladimirova, A. I. and M. F. Shuba (1978). Strychnine, hydrastine and apamin effect on synaptic transmission in smooth muscle cells. Neurofiziologija, 10, 295-299.

Vladimirova, I. A. and M. F. Shuba (1980). Effect of apamin on norepinephrine inhibitory action in smooth muscles. Physiological Journal (Kiev), 26, 547-552.

Weiss, S. J. and J. W. Putney (1978). Does calcium mediate the increase in potassium permeability due to phenylephrine or angiotensin II in the liver? J.Pharmac.exp.Ther., 207, 669-676.

## DISCUSSION OF THE THIRD SESSION

Dr. Fastier: Dr. Marshall, as I shall be mentioning later, methyl-thiouronium has considerable $K^+$-channel blocking activity. Although much less potent than 4-aminopyridine it nevertheless might prove useful for some therapeutic purposes because of its relative inability to excite the central nervous system. About 30 years ago I suggested that methyl-thiouronium should be tried as an alternative to guanidine in the treatment of myasthenia gravis. Potency ratios might well differ from one tissue to another, depending on the importance of penetrability.

Dr. Marshall: I am aware of the $K^+$-channel blocking activity of methyl-thiouronium but as I understand it the potency of the compound is considerably less than that of 4-aminopyridine. However, obviously the development of compounds related to methyl-thiouronium could be of interest.

Dr. Thesleff: Phencyclidine is a potent $K^+$-channel blocker (100 µM) indicating that there may be a number of chemically different blockers of that ionic channel.

Dr. Marshall: I am aware of the $K^+$-channel blocking activity of phencyclidine. It also blocks endplate channels at the neuromuscular junction. The central effects of phencyclidine are not reversed by 4-aminopyridine, as has been shown by Agoston and co-workers, whereas they showed that ketamine can be antagonized by 4-aminopyridine. Presumably phencyclidine blocks most of the $K^+$-channels and hence 4-aminopyridine cannot work.

Dr. Polak: Dr. Dunant, how do you know that you do not loose an important part of your vesicles from the "bound" store during homogenization? That is, how sure are you that your "bound" ACh represents the complete vesicular store?

Dr. Dunant: We demonstrated in our series of experiments that bound ACh is qualitatively identical to vesicular ACh also after rapid-freezing and 4-aminopyridine treatment. Free ACh contains the most recently synthesized transmitter and behaves as a distinct compartment. The recent work of M. Israel and co-workers (see this Symposium) on Torpedo synaptosomes is a good demonstration that all the free ACh is almost certainly cytoplasmic and all the bound ACh is vesicular.

Dr. Thesleff: If I understood you correctly you first freeze the tissue and then thaw it to determine the ACh content in vesicles respectively cytoplasm. Could not such procedures interfere with the distribution of ACh between the two compartments?

Dr. Dunant: The frozen pieces of tissue were broken into two fragments. The first one was used to measure the total ACh content, which was carefully extracted to prevent any hydrolysis during thawing. All the significant changes were seen in this total ACh. The second fragment was pulverized and then homogenized at 10°C in iso-osmotic medium. Synaptic vesicles are resistant to this treatment and keep their ACh and ATP content. We have verified this by isolating vesicles also under other conditions of rapid-freezing and 4-aminopyridine. The conclusion is that all the bound ACh is probably vesicular. The question of whether a small fraction of free ACh is, or is not, associated with special vesicles is more difficult to answer but there seems to be little evidence for it, see the report by Dr. Israel at this Symposium. Thus, we think that our condition of freezing minimizes the risk of ACh redistribution during extraction and assay.

Dr. Bergman: Dr. Israel, something is not clear to me in your experiments on synaptosome depolarization. Assuming that 4-aminopyridine selectively blocks the $K^+$-channels, would you expect the same $K^+$-induced depolarization in the presence and in the absence of 4-aminopyridine?

Dr. Israel: Yes if $K^+$-depolarization also involves a potassium permeability through channels other than those blocked by 4-aminopyridine.

Dr. Bergmann: Did you find the same relation between free ACh and bound ACh in the tissue without freezing? Does the ratio change after several hundred electric stimuli? Does it suggest that vesicular ACh is not serving as a precursor of free ACh? Can ACh be synthesized by the cytosol after separation from the vesicles?

Dr. Israel: Free ACh has also been measured indirectly by the difference between total and vesicular or bound ACh. In that case the tissue is not frozen and thowed as for the direct measurements obtained on synaptosomes. After several hundred electrical stimuli free ACh decreases and there is no change in vesicular ACh and the number of synaptic vesicles remains constant. ACh is synthesized in the cytosol since the enzyme cholineacetylase is a cytoplasmic enzyme.

Dr. Yanagisawa: Dr. Schiavone, have you tried the effect of TTX on the spontaneous release of catecholamines by high concentrations of 4-aminopyridine? I have some data which suggest that TTX reduces the spontaneous release of neurotransmitters from the autonomic nervous system.

Dr. Schiavone: We have not examined this question.

Dr. Löffelholz: You have shown that 4-aminopyridine increased the TTX sensitive release of NA caused by nicotine in low concentrations. I wonder if you have studied the effect of 4-aminopyridine on the transmitter release caused by high concentrations of nicotine, which is TTX-insensitive and due to sustained depolarization. I assume that 4-aminopyridine has no effect under the latter condition, unless desensitization of the nicotine receptor was affected.

Dr. Schiavone: We did look at the response to 2mM nicotine in the presence of 4-aminopyridine. 4-aminopyridine does not change the response.

Dr. Bergmann: Dr. Jenkinson, does apamin injected peripherally penetrate into the CNS? This would be quite surprising.

Dr. Jenkinson: There is a good deal of evidence both from physiological experiments and from the use of radiolabelled derivatives to show that apamin enters the CNS (see Habermann, E. and E. Hovarth, Toxicon, 18, 549-560, 1980, and Vincent, J.P., H. Schweitz and M. Lazdunski, Biochemistry, 14, 2521-2525, 1975). It is indeed surprising!

Dr. Bowman: Are there transmitter-activated, calcium-activated, potassium channels that are not blocked by apamin?

Dr. Jenkinson: The action of apamin has so far been examined in detail in only a few tissues (intestinal smooth muscle, red blood cells, hepatocytes). It does not seem to block the calcium-activated increase in potassium permeability which occurs when noradrenaline is applied to rat salivary glands *in vitro* (K. Koller, unpublished observations).

# Miscellaneous Actions of Aminopyridines and Related Compounds: Poster Communications

*Chairmen:* W. C. Bowman, S. Thesleff and P. Lechat

# The Action of Morphine Dependence on the Convulsive Effect of 4-Aminopyridine and Other Drugs

V. Aleman Aleman and D. Martinez De Munoz

Departamento de Neurociencias, Centro de Investigación y de
Estudios Avanzados del I.P.N., Apartado Postal 14-740,
14, D. F., México

In recent years, it has been shown that either single intraventricular or thalamic dorsomedialis nucleus injections of morphine or enkephalin, were able to produce convulsive effects. These convulsions were blocked by naloxone. In 1975 Mannino and Wolf found that single morphine injections lowers the pentylenetetrazol (PTZ) threshold in mice, but did not in morphine dependent mice. Similarly we wanted to test the effect of 4-aminopyridine (4-AP) and other convulsive drugs in morphine dependent rats but in the absence of a challenge dose of morphine.

Thirty days old rats were made morphine dependent by a six days schedule of twice a day injections of increasing doses of morphine. Thirty minutes after the last injection, the convulsive drugs were tested in control and morphine dependent rats. The drugs used were 4-AP, PTZ, bicuculline, strychnine and mercaptopropionic acid.

The drugs that exhibited greater change on their convulsive effects were 4-AP and PTZ. The percentage of rats treated with 4-AP that had convulsions increased from 8.0 % for the control group to 44 % for the morphine dependent rats and in the PTZ treated rats increased from 83 % to 100 % respectively. With 4-AP the seizure lasting time increased from 20 seconds in the control rats to 36 seconds in the morphine dependent group. In the case of PTZ this increase was from 16.8 to 27.5 seconds respectively. The seizure latency in the 4-AP treated rats increase from 740 seconds for the control group to 1736 seconds for the morphine dependent rats, and in the case of PTZ treated rats it decreased from 106 to 78 seconds respectively. The percentage of deaths produced by the convulsive effect in the case of 4-AP treated rats increased from 8.3 % for the control group to 31 % for the morphine dependent rats, in the PTZ treated rats this increase was from 25 to 40% respectively. These results indicate that in morphine dependent rats, 4-AP and PTZ have stronger convulsive effects as compare with rats that have not been treated with morphine.

On the other hand, strychnine and mercaptopropionic acid seemed to have some apperent opposite effects, thus the percentage of rats that were treated with strychnine and had convulsions decreased from 58 % for the control group to 17 % for the morphine treated rats and in the case of mercaptopropionic acid treated rats decreased from 100 % to 75 % respectively. The above results seemed to indicate that the morphine dependent group of rats decreased the convulsive effects of both strychnine and mercaptopropionic acid.

# Antagonism to Dopaminergic Stereotypy, and Convulsant and Hypertensive Effects by 2-Amino-4-Methylpyridine

F. Bergmann

Department of Pharmacology, The Hebrew University-Hadassah
Medical School, Jerusalem 91 000, Israel

2-Amino-4-methylpyridine (2-AMP) resembles morphine in some pharmacological properties, but differs from the opiate in others. Thus implantation of morphine into the lateral thalamus of rats causes stereotyped behavior (1), but deposition of 2-AMP into this region is ineffective. Thalamic application of apomorphine also evokes stereotypy. Thus this effect is due to direct or indirect activation of dopamine receptors; on this mechanism 2-AMP has no influence. On the other hand, systemic morphine suppresses stereotyped behavior, caused by injection of apomorphine or by thalamic implantation of morphine, and a similar inhibition is produced by systemic 2-AMP. The antagonistic effect of either morphine or 2-AMP against stereotypy is abolished by pretreatment of the rats with p-chlorophenylalanine and may therefore be ascribed to activation of an inhibitory serotonergic mechanism.

Large i.v. doses of 2-AMP produce convulsions in wake rabbits, but are rather ineffective in cats under pentobarbitone anesthesia or in spinal or pithed cats. Whenever seizures appear, they are accompanied by a sharp and prolonged rise of blood pressure, in marked contrast to the morphine-induced hypotension. The question arises whether the hypertension evoked by 2-AMP in wake rabbits, is a secondary phenomenon, induced by the seizures, or represents a primary, independent action. In anesthetised or spinalised cats, low doses of 2-AMP cause hypertensive responses in the absence of epileptic fits. Furthermore, if the seizures of wake rabbits are suppressed by valium or by small, subnarcotic doses of pentobarbitone, 2-AMP still causes pressure rises, although at a somewhat reduced scale. Regitine has no effect on the hypertensive responses to 2-AMP.

---

(1) Bergmann, F., M. Chaimovitz, V. Pasternak (Na'or) and A. Ramu (1974). Brit. J. Pharmacol., 51, 197 - 205.

# 4-Aminopyridine (4AP) Enhances Acetylcholine Output from the Rat Cerebral Cortex in vivo

R. Corradetti*, P. Mantovani*, K. Löffelholz**
and G. Pepeu*

*Department of Pharmacology, University of Florence, Italy
**Pharmakologisches Institut der Universitat, Mainz,
Federal Republic of Germany

The effect of 4AP administration on cortical acetylcholine (ACh) output was investigated in adult male Wistar rats under urethane (1.2 g/Kg i.p.) or pentobarbital (45 mg/Kg i.p.) anaesthesia.
A small Perspex cylinder filled with eserinized Ringer solution was applied on the exposed cerebral cortex. The composition of the Ringer solution was the following: NaCl(mM) 150, KCl 5.6, $CaCl_2$ 1.6, $NaHCO_3$ 5.9, glucose 5.5 and eserine sulphate 0.15. The solution in the collecting cylinder was removed every 10 min and its ACh content was determined by bioassay on the dorsal muscle of the leech.
In urethane anaesthetized rats the control ACh output was $0.98 \pm 0.16$ ng/min/$cm^2$ and the administration of 4AP (3 mg/Kg i.p.) was followed by a rapid increase in ACh output lasting at least 40 min. The increase in ACh output was paralleled by a decrease in the depth of anaesthesia and at the peak was $244 \pm 35$ % larger than the basal output.
In pentobarbital anaesthetized rats, in which ACh basal release was $1.52 \pm 0.24$ ng/min/$cm^2$, 4AP elicited a slow increase in ACh output which 60 min after administration was 3 fold larger than prior administration. However pentobarbital sleeping time was not modified by 4-aminopyridine.
These findings provide a direct evidence that 4-aminopyridine is a potent ACh releasing agent also in mammalian CNS and may explain some of the central effects of 4-aminopyridine.

This investigation was supported by the grant n° 79.01950 from CNR.

# 4-Aminopyridine as a Tool to Elucidate Different Actions of Botulinum A and Tetanus Toxin at the Mouse Neuromuscular Junction

F. Dreyer and A. Schmitt

Rudolf Buchheim-Institut für Pharmakologie, Frankfurter Straße 107, D-6300 Giessen, Federal Republic of Germany

Tetanus toxin (TeTx) produces a block of neuromuscular transmission in the isolated mouse diaphragm, similar to the action of botulinum A toxin (BoTx) (Habermann et al., Naunyn-Schmiedeberg's Arch. Pharmacol. 311: 33, 1980). After the development of a complete paralysis using equipotent toxin concentrations, 4-aminopyridine (4-AP) failed to restore the muscle twitch tension. On the other hand it is reported that in muscles of BoTx poisoned animals the nerve evoked transmitter release is restored by 4-AP (Lundh et al., J. Neurol. Sci. 32: 39, 1977). To elucidate these differences TeTx (1 µg/ml) as well as BoTx (5 ng/ml) paralyzed diaphragms were studied with intracellular recording techniques. When the nerve was stimulated with 50 Hz, about 1 % of the nerve impulses caused transmitter release at poisoned endplates. However in the presence of 4-AP (100 µmol/l) considerable differences in the nerve induced transmitter release were observed comparing both toxins. In the BoTx poisoned muscles endplate potentials ($epp_N$) made up of several quanta could be recorded immediately with the first nerve stimulus of a 50 Hz train. The $epp_N$ were strongly correlated to the action potential with similar synaptic delays compared to unpoisoned preparations. However, in the TeTx poisoned muscles not only the nerve had to be stimulated for 2 - 3 sec with 50 Hz to observe any transmitter release, but also surprisingly instead of recording $epp_N$, only a marked increase of post-stimulus miniature endplate potential (mepp) frequency was recorded. The latencies of these responses following the action potentials varied between 1 msec and seconds with a maximum frequency around 5 msec. Such an effect on mepp-frequency could not be observed in BoTx poisoned muscles. Increasing both toxin concentrations ten times shortened considerably the time courses of muscle paralysis development, but did not change the electrophysiological findings indicating that the differences are not due to different toxin concentrations. The data on the TeTx poisoned motor nerve endings demonstrate a distortion of the phasic secretion of quanta in response to nerve action potentials. From these findings it could be postulated that TeTx and BoTx act at different sites of the depolarization-transmitter releasing process.

# Antagonism of the Myoneural Activity of Antibiotics, Local Anesthetics and General Anesthetics By 4-APYR

F. F. Foldes*, D. B. S. Rao*, K. Thomas**, I. Leung**, G. Bikhazi** and H. Nagashima*

*Department of Anesthesiology, Montefiore Hospital and Medical Center and Albert Einstein College of Medicine, Bronx, N.Y. 10467, USA
**Department of Anesthesiology, University of Miami School of Medicine, Miami, Florida 33101, USA

The neuromuscular (NM) block induced by competitive inhibitors of acetylcholine (ACh) can be reversed by anticholinesterases. The myoneural block caused by many other compounds, however, cannot be antagonized by cholinesterase inhibitors. In the present study the effects of 4-aminopyridine (4-APYR) on the inhibition of the isometric twitch tension (P) by the latter type compounds (e.g., antibiotics, local anesthetics, halogenated inhalation anesthetics, dantrolene, verapamil) have been investigated. The experiments were carried out on the rat phrenic nerve hemidiaphragm preparation, suspended in mammalian Krebs' solution at 37°C aerated with 95% $O_2$ - 5% $CO_2$ and stimulated at 0.1 Hz directly or indirectly by supramaximal impulses of 2 and 0.2 msec respectively. NM transmission was blocked by d-tubocurarine in the experiments with direct stimulation. The inhibitory effect of antibiotics and local anesthetics on P was greater during indirect than during direct stimulation ($p < 0.001$ for the differences of ED50 with direct and indirect stimulation). In contrast halogenated inhalation anesthetics, halothane, enflurane and isoflurane and dantrolene and verapamil were equally potent inhibitors of P during direct and indirect stimulation. During indirect stimulation the myoneural effects of the aminoglycoside type antibiotics, neomycin, streptomycin, gentamycin, kanamycin and except for tetracaine, those of the ester type local anesthetics, cocaine, procaine and 2-chloroprocaine as well as those of the halogenated inhalation anesthetics were completely antagonized by $5 \times 10^{-6}$M 4-APYR. The same concentration of 4-APYR, however, only partially antagonized the myoneural effects of polymyxin B, colistin and dantrolene and it had little or no effect on those of the antibiotics, lincoin or cleocin or the amide type local anesthetics lidocaine, mepivacaine, etidocaine and bupivacaine or that of verapamil. During direct stimulation only the myoneural effects of the inhalation anesthetics and dantrolene were antagonized by 4-APYR. On the basis of the generally accepted mode of action of 4-APYR and the differences observed in the potency and reversibility by 4-APYR of their myoneural effect during direct and indirect stimulation the probable site(s) and mechanism(s) of action of the various compounds may be inferred. It appears that the myoneural effect of the aminoglycoside type antibiotics is due to inhibition of presynaptic ACh release. The site and mechanism of action of the polypeptide and other type antibiotics may be different. Except for tetracaine, the myoneural effect of the ester type local anesthetics may be due to the blockage of the $Na^+$ and those of amide type agents to that of the $K^+$ channels of the postjunctional membrane. The site of action of inhalation anesthetics, dantrolene and verapamil is probably the muscle fiber.

# Increased Tetanic Fade Produced by 3,4-Diaminopyridine in the Presence of Neuromuscular Blocking Agents

A. J. Gibb, I. G. Marshall and W. C. Bowman

Department of Physiology and Pharmacology, University of Strathclyde, Glasgow G1 1XW, UK

In the presence of tubocurarine, aminopyridine enhances the rundown of trains of endplate potentials (Lundh, 1978; Illes & Thesleff, 1978; Molgó et al,1979). It is possible that this effect may reflect a prejunctional action of tubocurarine, acting to reduce transmitter mobilisation. We have now studied the ability of 3,4-diaminopyridine (DAP) to enhance the fade of tetanic tension (50 Hz for 1.9 sec) produced by a range of non-depolarizing neuromuscular blocking agents in the isolated rat phrenic nerve-hemidiaphragm preparation. DAP alone (50 µM) increased twitch and tetanic tension by 256 ± 17% and 21 ± 7% respectively, and caused only 2.5 ± 0.9% tetanic fade. Concentrations of neuromuscular blockers that produced 26 ± 8.6% tetanic fade under equilibrium conditions were chosen and DAP (50 µM) was added. Tetanic fade significantly increased from 36 ± 8% to 47 ± 7% (difference = 11 ± 2%) in Org NC 45 (1.5 µM), from 23 ± 8% to 49 ± 8% (difference = 26 ± 7%) in tubocurarine (0.25 µM) and from 25 ± 9% to 62 ± 6% (difference = 39 ± 7%) in hexamethonium. With atracurium, breakdown occurs in the tissue bath and hence fade in the presence of DAP was compared with fade occurring at the same time in separate preparations exposed to atracurium (4.26 µM) alone. Fade increased from 20 ± 5% to 53 ± 4% (difference = 33 ± 9%). The postjunctionally active snake toxin erabutoxin b (0.325 µg/ml) produced no tetanic fade and in DAP only 15 ± 5% fade could be measured. The increase in fade produced by DAP was significantly greater in hexamethonium than in Org NC 45. There was no significant difference between Org NC 45 and tubocurarine or between hexamethonium and tubocurarine. The fade produced by combinations of neuromuscular blockers and DAP was partially reversed by neostigmine (0.25 µM).

Assuming that maintainance of tetanic tension is at least partially a reflection of transmitter mobilisation (Bowman, 1980) we postulate that the different increases in tetanic fade reflect the abilities of different neuromuscular blocking drugs to block a prejunctional cholinoceptor involved in a positive feedback control of mobilisation. The results suggest that the order of affinities for those cholinoceptors is hexamethonium > atracurium > tubocurarine > Org NC 45 >> erabutoxin b.

References

Bowman, W.C. Anesth. Analg. (Cleve.)., 59, 935 (1980).
Illes, P. & Thesleff, S. Br. J. Pharmac., 64, 623 (1978).
Lundh, H. Brain Res., 153, 307 (1978).
Molgó, J., Lemeignan, M. & Lechat, P. Eur. J. Pharmac., 53, 307 (1979).

Acknowledgements. AJG is an S.R.C. CASE award scholar. Org NC 45 and atracurium were gifts from Organon Scientific Development Group and the Wellcome Research Laboratories respectively. Erabutoxin b was supplied by Dr. A.L. Harvey.

# Effect of 4-Aminopyridine on the Electrical Activity of the Hippocampus and the Cerebellum

G. Gogolák, K. Czech and Ch. Stumpf

Institute of Neuropharmacology, University of Vienna and Department of Neuropharmacology, Brain Research Institute, Austrian Academy of Sciences, Währingerstr. 13a, 1090 Vienna, Austria

4-Aminopyridine (4-AP) has been shown to elicit hippocampal theta rhythm followed by seizure like activity (SLA) in the hippocampus (HC) and subsequently in the neocortex (Co) (Wi.kli.Wschr.92, 734, 1980). This effect was prevented or attenuated by anticholinergic agents (Naunyn-Schmiedeberg's Arch.Pharmacol.Suppl.to 313, 124,1980), and therefore investigations were aimed at revealing whether the cholinergic innervation of the HC from the septum contributes to the SLA induced by 4-AP.

In six male rats electrolytic lesion of the medial septum was carried out under anesthesia (pentobarbital). Six to ten weeks after surgery the rats were immobilized (alcuronium; intubation under propanidid anesthesia), and the EEG was monitored from the HC and the Co. In addition, two or a maximum of four mg/kg 4-AP elicited SLA in the HC and Co, whereas HC theta rhythm was only present in the control rats. These findings indicate that 4-AP-induced seizures in the HC are not mediated by cholinergic septo-hippocampal projection.

The observation that in non-immobilized rabbits bursts of intensive tremor preceed the beginning of generalized seizures promted us to investigate the action of 4-AP on the cerebellum (Cb). These experiments were carried out on immobilized (alcuronium) rabbits. Recordings were taken from the HC, and Co (both by macroelectrodes) as well as from the Cb (macro- or microelectrodes). Under the influence of 4-AP (2-4 mg/kg) a 15-17 Hz rhythm repeatedly appeared in the cerebellogram. In addition, Purkinje cells (medial vermis) discharged with increased frequency and/or with rhythmic burst pattern. These effects preceeded and accompanied the SLA in the HC.

The present pilot study shows that 4-AP has various effects on the central nervous system; the mechanism of these actions as well as the relationship between changes in the Cb activity and the tremor, both induced by 4-AP, will be the object of further experiments.

# Cardiac Effects of 4-Aminoquinoline on Mammalian and Amphibian Isolated Preparations
# An Electrophysiological Study

S. Guerrero, L. Novakovic, J. Campos and M. Penna

Department of Pharmacology, Faculty of Medicine, University of Chile
P.O. Box 16387, Santiago 9, Chile

4-Aminopyridine stimulates the release of transmitters at cardiac level, causes positive inotropism (Thesleff,1980), depresses sinus node activity and prolongs action potential repolarization (Guerrero and Novakovič,1980). The present study concerns the effects of an aminopyridine related compound 4-aminoquinoline (4-AQ) on automatism, contractility and refractory period of isolated cat and frog myocardial preparations. In addition, 4-AQ effects on impulse conduction of frog desheathed sciatic nerves and on membrane potentials of frog atrial fibres were studied. Conventional electrophysiological techniques were used for both intra and extracellular recordings. 4-AQ dose-dependently (60-480 $\mu$M) depressed heart rate of the cat right auricle with a simultaneous enhancement of isometric tension (n=12). In the frog atria 4-AQ (80-1280 $\mu$M) also caused bradychardia. The drug (320 $\mu$M) significantly prolonged the effective refractory period (ERP) of trabecular muscles from the frog left auricle. In untreated papillary muscles of the cat 4-AQ (60-480 $\mu$M) produced positive inotropism accompanied by increase of the mean rate of force development ($p<0.001$; n=12). Both effects were absent in preparations previously exposed to 30 nM pindolol, or in muscles obtained from reserpine treated animals. ERP of untreated as well as treated (pindolol or reserpine) papillary muscles was dose-dependently prolonged by 4-AQ ($p<0.01$). This effect was reversible after washing. 4-AQ (1.5-15 mM) reversibly decreased compound action potential amplitude, slowed conduction speed and prolonged the relative refractory period of frog desheathed nerves in a concentration-related manner. Activity ratio relative to procaine was 0.42. In untreated or atropine-treated frog sinus venosus, intracellular recording revealed that 4-AQ slowed spontaneous firing rate (n=30). At the same time a depression of the maximum diastolic potential amplitude, decline of phase 4 and prolongation of the action potential duration was observed. In contractile cells of the frog atrium 4-AQ (0.15-1.5 mM) also prolonged action potential duration, while 0.5-1.5 mM depressed upstroke velocity ($p<0.05$). All these effects were reversible. No changes of the membrane resting potential were recorded. 4-AQ inotropic effect seems to be mediated by the release of catecholamines. It is known that this drug stimulates the release of acetylcholine at the neuromuscular junction and induces the appearance of "giant" miniature end-plate potentials (Molgô and co-workers,1980). The effects on myocardium or nerve refractoriness could be explained by inhibition of gNa, gK or both. Prolongation of cardiac action potentials is probably related to gK blockade.

Thesleff,S. (1980) Neuroscience, 5, 1413-1419.
Guerrero,S., Novakovič,L., (1980) Eur. J. Pharmacol., 62. 335-340.
Molgô,J., Lemeignan,M., Lechat,P.and Thesleff,S.(1980).Neurosci.Lett.Suppl.5, S 367.
(Supported by Grants B.181-804 and B.1355-811-4, University of Chile).

# Facilitatory Effects of Aminopyridines on Synaptic Transmission in the Sixth Abdominal Ganglion of the Cockroach

B. Hue*, M. Pelhate*, J. J. Callec** and J. Chanelet*

*Laboratoire de Physiologie, U.E.R. Médecine, 49045 Angers, France
**Laboratoire de Physiologie Animale, Université Rennes I, 35042 Rennes, France

Aminopyridines (AP) are known to facilitate synaptic transmission at central synapses (1,2) as well as at peripheral synapses (3,4). The effects of AP were studied by electrophysiological methods at cercal-nerve, giant-interneurone synapses of the cockroach sixth abdominal ganglion where acetylcholine is the main excitatory neurotransmitter (5,6).

At low concentrations ($10^{-6}$ to $10^{-5}$M), AP and particularly 4-aminopyridine (4-AP) -the most potent isomer- increased the postsynaptic background activity, namely the frequency and amplitude of unitary EPSPs and IPSPs. Moreover both evoked EPSPs and IPSPs were greatly enhanced in amplitude. At the presynaptic level, 4-AP triggered action potentials in the cercal nerves XI (recorded with external electrodes). These "antidromic" action potentials appeared singly or repetitively especially after subthreshold electrical stimulation of cercal nerves XI. Monosynaptic correlation with unitary EPSPs was observed. Synaptic depressant effect of $Mg^{2+}$ was antagonized by 4-AP. All these effects were observed without changes in the resting potential, the postsynaptic membrane resistance, the sensitivity of the postsynaptic cholinoceptors, and the equilibrium potentials of ions involved in postsynaptic events. It is suggested that AP facilitate central synaptic transmission by an increase in transmitter release.

Higher concentrations of AP ($10^{-4}$ to $10^{-2}$M) always induced depolarizations of postsynaptic membranes even after blockade of muscarinic and nicotinic receptors by atropine and d-tubocurarine. 2-AP and 3-AP were approximately 10 times more potent and produced a more reversible depolarization than 4-AP. These postsynaptic depolarizing effects of AP were not induced by activation of postsynaptic cholinoceptors.

References : (1) HUE B, PELHATE M, CALLEC JJ & CHANELET J (1975), C.R.Soc.Biol. 169, 876-882. (2) JANKOWSKA E, LUNDBERG A, RUDOMIN P & SYKOVA E (1977), Brain Res. 136, 387-392. (3) SCHAUF CL, COLTON CA, COLTON JS & DAVIS FA (1976), J.Pharmac.exp.Ther. 197, 414-425. (4) MOLGO J, LEMEIGNAN M & LECHAT P (1977), J.Pharmac.exp.Ther. 203, 653-663. (5) CALLEC JJ (1974), In "Insect Neurobiology",ed.JE Treherne, 119-178, North-Holland American Elsevier. (6) SATTELLE DB (1980), Adv. Insect Physiol. 15, 215-315.

# The Effect of 3-,4-AP and 3,4-DAP on the Evoked Activity of the Pyramidal Cell Layer (CA 1,2) of the Hippocampus An *in vitro* Study

U. Kuhnt and M. Szente

Department of Comp. Physics, University of Szeged, Szeged, Hungary

Aminopyridines (AP) are used as experimental epileptogenic agents. However, the used form of application does not allow definite conclusions about the concentrations of the drugs on the place of action. We therefore choose a superfusion slice preparation, where the drugs were mixed to the medium immediately before the tissue chamber. We compared the effects of 3-,4-AP and 3.4-DAP on the fieldpotential of the hippocampal pyramidal cell- (CA 1,2) and dendritic layer of the guinea pig. 3 M NaCl filled pipettes (resistance below 4 MOhm) served as recording ,tungsten in glass as stimulation electrodes. Double stimuli,150 ms separated,were repeated all 3s throughout the experiments. Drugs were applied for 10 min and at least 75 min recovery time elapsed before another drug/concentration was applied. For each response 20 stimuli were averaged. 3-,4-AP and 3.4-DAP lead with the concentrations used (2mM, 50 µM, 25/50 µM) regularly to a facilitation of the first response. The increase of the population spike (PS) might comprise several 100 %. The facilitation of the first response might be preceeded by a short lasting depression. This depression, however, was never observed during the application of 3-AP. Under certain stimulus conditions a second PS might develop in response to the first stimulus, which vanishes during the recovery time. After the application of 4-AP and 3.4-DAP an over 200 ms long afterpotential might develop, which appears regularly later than the primary facilitation and disappears earlier. The recovery after a ten min application depends as well on the concentration of the drug as on the stimulus strength and on the condition of the slice. However in most cases the recovery took at least 1.5 h. The changes of the different APs on the second response are more dramatical and the pattern of facilitation and depression are more complicated. Regularly an early facilitation is seen often followed by a depression. The first response increases more than the second.
In controles the first response is usually smaller than the second response. In the dendritic area the responses behave similar, however the afterpotential is never observed. Furthermore the time course of the recovery is faster. The extracellular equivalent of the evoked EPSP behaves basically similar as the PS. The antidromic evoked response shows only after 3.4-DAP a clear increase, which however is weaker than the orthodromic facilitation.
We can conclude that 3.4-DAP is the most potent facilitatory AP of the three different APs studied. Maximal effects are reached with concentrations of 25-100 µM. Besides the facilitation a late hyperpolarization can develop. All three APs block the potentiation of the second response, which is regular seen in controles. Experiments to elucidate the action of APs on the single cell level are in progress.

# Fast and Slow Automatic Activity of Squid Giant Axons Induced by 4-Aminopyridine

E. Lammel and K. Mandrek

Physiologisches Institut der Philipps-Universität, Deutschhausstr. 2,
D-3550 Marburg/Lahn, Federal Republic of Germany

4-Aminopyridine (4-AP, 1 mmol/l) induces automatic activity in giant axons of Loligo forbesi. A rapid spike process (frequency 100 - 150 Hz) can be distinguished from slow oscillations of the membrane potential in the range of 1 - 5 Hz (K.Golenhofen and K.Mandrek, J.Physiol.284,69-70P,1978). In order to analyze the underlying mechanism the inhibitory effect of 4-AP on the kinetics of the potassium current was investigated in voltage-clamp experiments. 4-AP decreased both the rate of rise (turning on) and the height of the potassium conductance $g_K$ on depolarizing clamp pulses as described by Meves and Pichon (J.Physiol.267,511-532,1977). The effect of 4-AP on the time course of decay of $g_K$ on repolarization (turning-off) was investigated with short test pulses of different amplitudes $U_T$, thereby eliminating the effect of the unknown shift in K-reversal potential due to K-accumulation in the periaxonal space during current flow ($g_K = \Delta I_m/\Delta U_m$; $\Delta I_m$: difference in current related to difference in $U_m$, at given times in consecutive runs). In contrast to the turning-on, the turning-off kinetics was found to be unaffected by 4-AP. The results were interpreted under the assumption that 4-AP combines only with closed K-channels and that the reaction obeys first-order kinetics (cf. Meves and Pichon). A differential equation: $db/dt = \alpha \cdot [4-AP] \cdot (1-n^4) \cdot (1-b) - \beta \cdot b$, with b being the fraction of K-channels occupied by 4-AP was incorporated into the set of Hodgkin-Huxley (HH) equations. The voltage dependent rate constants $\alpha$ and $\beta$ were determined from the experimental data. Numerical solutions of the equations agreed with the experimental findings in resembling all features of the rapid spiking process. (1) Automatic spike generation was associated with a small depolarization. (2) The spike frequency f could be modulated by current application (de-and hyperpolarizing currents de-and increasing f). (3) Simulation of treatment with reduced 4-AP concentrations led to rapid subthreshold oscillations. The computational results indicate that the rapid spiking process is related to an almost steady blockade of a major fraction of K channels (showing little time variation within a spiking period). The slow oscillation process could not be simulated, even when K-accumulation in the periaxonal space was taken into account. Possible reasons are discussed.

Supported by the Deutsche Forschungsgemeinschaft (Ma722/2,3)

# The Ability of 4-Aminopyridine and 3,4-Diaminopyridine to Cross the Blood-Brain Barrier can Account for Their Difference in Toxicity

M. Lemeignan, H. Millart, N. Letteron, D. Lamiable,
J. Josso, H. Choisy and P. Lechat

Laboratoire Associé du C.N.R.S. n°206, Paris, France and
Laboratoire de Pharmacologie, Centre Hospitalier
Régional, Reims, France

As far as we know, only 4-aminopyridine (4-AP) has been used in clinical practice for treatment of human neuromuscular diseases, but its usefulness has been limited by its central nervous system (CNS) stimulant effect.

3,4-diaminopyridine (3,4-DAP) has been shown to be 6 to 10 times more potent than 4-AP in increasing evoked transmitter release at the neuromuscular junction *in vitro* and 2 times less convulsant and toxic than 4-AP after acute i.v. injection in mice.

The present study was undertaken in order to further compare the toxicity, the CNS stimulant action and the ability of 4-AP and 3,4-DAP to cross the blood-brain barrier (Bbb).

The results obtained were as follows: a) 3,4-DAP was less toxic than 4-AP in rats and mice after acute administration (table 1). b) When chronically administered to young rats, 3,4-DAP (8 mg/kg p.o. twice a day during 7 weeks) did not modify the rate of growth of the animals when compared to controls, whereas 4-AP (4 mg/kg p.o. twice a day, 7 weeks) significantly slowed it. c) In anesthetized rats (urethane 1.3g/kg i.p.) slow venous infusion of the drugs induced the appearance of a progressively developping convulsive state, the doses triggering clonic convulsions were respectively 75.9 ± 3.7 and 17.1 ± 0.4 mg/kg for 3,4-DAP and 4-AP. Moreover tonic extension was not observed in rats treated with 3,4-DAP. d) The concentrations of the drugs were measured by a HPLC method in the cerebrospinal fluid (CSF) and in the serum of anesthetized rats (urethane) 5 min after i.v. injection of 4-AP (7 mg/kg) or 3,4-DAP (16 mg/kg). The concentration of 3,4-DAP in the CSF was lower than that of 4-AP. The ratios of the concentrations found in the CSF to those found in the serum were significantly higher with 4-AP than with 3,4-DAP (Fig. 1).

In conclusion, 3,4-DAP does not cross the Bbb as easily as 4-AP and this can account for its lower than 4-AP CNS stimulant action and toxicity *in vivo*.

|  | $LD_{50}$ mg/kg | | |
|---|---|---|---|
|  | i.v. mouse | i.v. rat | p.o. rat |
| 4-AP | 7.5 | 6.3 | 31 |
| 3,4-DAP | 16 | 19.5 | 60 |

Table 1

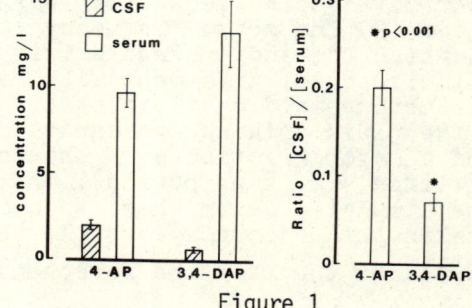

Figure 1

# Action of 4AP and TEA on Presynaptic Currents in Mammalian Motor Endings

A. Mallart and J. L. Brigant

Unité de Physiologie Neuromusculaire, Laboratoire de
Neurobiologie Cellulaire, C.N.R.S., Gif sur Yvette, France

We have investigated the mechanism by which the K channel blockers 4AP and TEA enhance evoked transmitter release.

Since the nodes of Ranvier of mammalian nerves lack K channels, we first looked for their possible presence at the motor endings. Then we investigated how the delayed K current can affect the inward Ca current.

To this purpose we recorded extrinsic currents at motor endings from the triangularis sterni muscle of the mouse by focal electrodes. We observed that, under normal conditions, inward current is recorded only at the transition between myelinated and non myelinated portions of the axon while outward current is found everywhere else. A late component of the outward current can be suppressed by 4AP or, better, by TEA , indicating that it corresponds to delayed IK. The suppression of IK unmask an inward current which correspond to ICa since it can be blocked by cobalt ions or be enhance by Ca rich solutions.

Our results show that :i) the action potential does not invade actively the terminal arborization but depolarizes it by electrotonic propagation, and ii) IK brings back rapidely the membrane potential to its resting level, thus impairing the development of ICa.

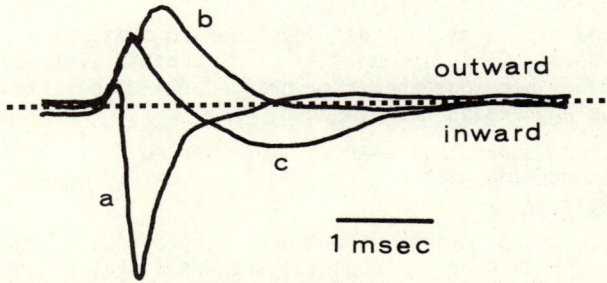

Fig. 1. Superimposed recordings showing I Na at the initial portion of the endings (a), I K preceded by passive current at the main portion of the endings (b) and I Ca after blocking I K by TEA (c). Each record is the average of 20 sweeps.

# Protein Synthesis in Brain Subcellular Fractions Effect of 4-Amino-Pyridine

D. Martinez de Munoz

Departamento de Neurociencias, Centro de Investigación y de Estudios Avanzados del I.P.N., Apartado Postal 14-740, 14, D. F., México

4-amino pyridine (4-AP) is a potent stimulating drug that at high doses produces convulsions. We have shown that $\gamma$-hydroxi, $\gamma$-phenyl caproamide (YPCA) is a protecting agent against convulsions induced by: pentylenetetrazol, thiosemicarbazide, electroshock, kindling and others.

The involvement of protein synthesis as a regulation process of the functional state of the nervous system is widely recognized. Therefore the brain functional state should be specially sensitive to agents which modify this process. Inhibition of brain protein synthesis has been observed by several convulsant drugs such as: 3-mercaptopropionic acid, 2-amine-4-pentenoic acid (allylglicine) pentylenetetrazol and others. Some anticonvulsant drugs, such as diphenylhydantoine (DPH) produce inhibition of protein synthesis but the molecular bases of their action are unknown.

The purpose of the present study was to study the effects of 4-AP on the protein synthesis *in vivo* in subcellular fractions and to evaluate the protective effect of YPCA in convulsions induced by 4-AP.

YPCA, 60 mg Kg$^{-1}$ intraperitoneally, produced a powerful protection against tonic-clonic convulsions and/or death elicited by 4-AP 10 mg Kg$^{-1}$, in mice. When YPCA was compared with some of the most used anticonvulsant drugs, it was shown that diazepam and YPCA are more potent than nembutal and DPH against convulsions induced by 4-AP.

Rats were injected with a mixture of radiolabelled aminoacids and then with 4-AP at subconvulsant doses (0.5 - 4.0 mg Kg$^{-1}$), for protein synthesis determination. Subcellular fractions were obtained from brain cortex and radioactivity incorporated in acid insoluble proteins was measured.

The results obtained shown that 4-AP at 1.0 - 1.5 mg Kg$^{-1}$ increases protein synthesis in synaptosomes and mitochondria and at 2.0 - 4.0 mg Kg$^{-1}$ it remains as the control.

In conclusion YPCA is an anticonvulsant drug very effective against seizures induced by 4-AP and this drug at subconvulsant doses does not inhibit protein synthesis in brain subcellular cortex otherwise it is considerably increased.

# Effects of 4-Hydroxypyridine on Transmitter Release at the Neuromuscular Junction

G. Montoya*, J. Molgo, M. Lemeignan and P. Lechat

Institut de Pharmacologie, Laboratoire Associé du C.N.R.S. n° 206,
15, rue de l'Ecole de Médecine, 75006 Paris, France

Aminopyridines are drugs known to block $K^+$ channels in excitable membranes, to have pronounced convulsant effects on the central nervous system and to increase evoked transmitter release at the neuromuscular junction. Other group of drugs which share some common properties with the aminopyridines concerning its effects on $K^+$ currents in nerve membranes and in the central nervous system are the hydroxypyridines (Kirch and Narahashi, 1978; Lemeignan, Molgo and Letteron, unpublished). The fact that 4-hydroxypyridine (4-HP) was found to be less toxic than 4-aminopyridine (4-AP) in its effects on the central nervous system prompted us to study the effects of 4-HP at the frog neuromuscular junction by using conventional electrophysiological techniques.

The results obtained show that 4-HP (1-10mM) greatly increased stimulus evoked transmitter release in junctions in which the normal release of transmitter was reduced by increasing extracellular $Mg^{++}$ and reducing $Ca^{++}$. Similarly 4-HP dose dependently was able to restore from complete blockade neuromuscular transmission in curarized preparations when stimulated at low frequency. However, during tetanic stimulation only the 1st response in the train was facilitated while the successive responses were depressed in comparison to the controls.

4-HP had no effect on the time course of the synaptic potentials and there was no evidence that the drug in the concentrations used had any postsynaptic effect.

Focal extracellular recordings revealed that 4-HP increased the latency of the evoked responses and that this effect was mainly due to a prolongation of the synaptic delay. Spontaneous quantal release was unaffected by 4-HP in resting junctions or in junctions depolarized by increasing the external $K^+$ concentration.

Furthermore, the drug markedly increased the frequency of miniature end-plate potentials appearing after repetitive stimulation (0.5-100 Hz). The drug also increased the duration of indirectly elicited muscle action potentials in preparations in which excitation-contraction was uncoupled. From the analysis of dose-response curves it appears that 4-HP is considerably less active than 4-AP concerning its effects on evoked transmitter release. Moreover, 4-HP effects on evoked transmitter release are more readily reversible than the effects of 4-AP. The difference in activity observed between 4-HP and 4-AP do not seem to be related to their degree of ionization at physiological pH. In conclusion, although 4-HP is less toxic and less active than 4-AP, its effects at the neuromuscular junction are very similar to those of 4-AP and probably related to its ability to block $K^+$ channels in the nerve terminal.

Kirsch, G.E. and Narahashi, T. (1978) <u>Biophys. J.</u> 22, 507

*Supported by DGRST. Present address: Universidad de Concepcion, Concepcion, Chile.

# 4-Aminopyridine Analogs of Novel Chemical Structure

Y. Ohta, I. Chaudhry, I. Lalezari and F. F. Foldes

Departments of Anesthesiology, Montefiore Hospital and Medical Center and Albert Einstein College of Medicine, Bronx, New York 10467, USA

In various <u>in vitro</u> and <u>in vivo</u> animal preparations 4-aminopyridine (4-APYR) not only antagonizes the neuromuscular (NM) blocking effect of competitive (nondepolarizing) muscle relaxants (MR), but also those of other compounds (e.g., certain antibiotics and local anesthetics, botulinum A toxin) that cannot be reversed by anti-ChE. 4-APYR was also found to be effective in the treatment of carcinomatous neuropathy (Eaton-Lambert syndrome). Unfortunately, the clinical usefulness of 4-APYR is limited by its unwanted CNS and cardiovascular effects. In attempting to eliminate these side effects several analogs of 4-APYR were synthetized and tested in the rat <u>in vitro</u> phrenic nerve - diaphragm and the <u>in vivo</u> sciatic - tibialis anterior preparation. The ability of the compounds to influence the course of pentobarbital anesthesia in rats was also investigated. Of the compounds synthetized so far 4, p-acetyl-aminobenzenesulfonyl-4-aminopyridine (LF-1), 4-pyridylcarbonic acid ethyl ester (LF-5), 1-(4-pyridyl)-2, 2-diethylurea (LF-10), and 1(4-pyridyl)-2, 2-diethylurea (LF-11) had similar antagonistic effect as 4-APYR on the pancuronium (see table) and d-tubocurarine (d-Tc) induced NM block <u>in vitro</u> and <u>in vivo</u>. <u>In vitro</u> except for LF-5 the new analogs were more potent ($p < 0.05$ to 0.01; Student's $t$ test) antagonists of NM block than 4-APYR. <u>In vivo</u> LF-1 and LF-5 were less potent ($p < 0.001$ and 0.02) and LF-10 and LF-11 were about as potent as 4-APYR. In contrast to 4-APYR none of the new compounds increased the intra-arterial blood pressure in anesthetized rats. However, LF-1 and LF-10 similarly to 4-APYR delayed the onset ($p < 0.01$ to 0.001) and prolonged the duration of pentobarbital anesthesia in rats. The investigation of the influence of LF-5 and LF-11 on pentobarbital anesthesia and the pharmacological screening of other 4-APYR analogs is in progress.

Antagonism of the Pancuronium Induced NM Block by 4-APYR Analogs

| Compound | M.W. | In Vitro | | In Vivo | |
|---|---|---|---|---|---|
| | | ED50* | ED90† | ED50* | ED90† |
| 4-APYR | 94.11 | 2.55±0.33‡ | 10.96±1.45 | 0.29±0.04 | 1.18±0.36 |
| LF-1 | 291.32 | 1.79±0.03 | 5.41±0.31 | 1.04±0.07 | 3.82±0.14 |
| LF-5 | 167.11 | 2.49±0.23 | 8.26±0.94 | 1.55±0.22 | 4.29±0.85 |
| LF-10 | 165.19 | 0.87±0.06 | 3.17±0.43 | 0.13±0.01 | 0.43±0.06 |
| LF-11 | 193.25 | 0.85±0.07 | 2.43±0.16 | 0.20±0.01 | 0.59±0.03 |

* and † Indicate concentrations ($10^{-6}$M) <u>in vitro</u> and doses (mg.kg$^{-1}$) <u>in vivo</u> which increase twitch tension from < 10% to 50 and 90% of control respectively.
‡Mean±SEM of 4 experiments.

# Excitatory Action of Imidazole on Evoked Transmitter Release from the Phrenic Nerve and on Potassium-stimulated $^{45}$Ca Uptake by Synaptosomes in the Rat

J. A. Ribeiro, M. L. Dominguez and A. M. Sá-Almeida

Centro de Biologia, Instituto Gulbenkian de Ciência, 2781 Oeiras, Portugal

Imidazole stimulates several excitable tissues, but its effect on neuromuscular transmission is as yet unclear, it can facilitate (e.g. Ribeiro et al., 1979 - Arch. int. Pharmacodyn., 238, 206) or depress (Standaert et al., 1976 - J. Pharmacol. exp. Ther., 199, 553) neuromuscular transmission. So the present work was undertaken to study further the effects of imidazole on transmitter release from the phrenic nerve endings of the rat. We also tested imidazole on the compound action potential of the frog-sciatic nerve, and as calcium is considered a primum mobile on transmitter release we investigated the effect of imidazole on the uptake of $^{45}$Ca by a rat-brain synaptosome rich-preparation.

End-plate potentials were recorded in the conventional way. Imidazole (0.5 - 5 mM) reversibly increased the quantum content of the evoked end-plate potentials and the mean amplitude of the miniature end-plate potentials in preparations in which transmission was partially blocked with high magnesium and/or low calcium concentrations. In solutions with low calcium concentrations imidazole caused a smaller effect on the mean quantal content of the evoked end-plate potentials. Imidazole also reversibly increased the amplitude of the evoked end-plate potentials in preparations in which transmission was blocked with tubocurarine ($2 \times 10^{-6}$ M). In unstimulated preparations imidazole (5 mM) decreased the frequency of miniature end-plate potentials.

Imidazole (5 - 10 mM) was devoid of effect on the compound action potential of the frog-sciatic nerve.

In the synaptosome rich-preparation $^{45}$Ca uptake was measured in control media, and in depolarizing media containing 71 mM potassium. Imidazole (0.5 - 4 mM) enhanced the potassium stimulated uptake of $^{45}$Ca but had little or no effect on unstimulated synaptosomes.

It is concluded that the excitatory effect of imidazole on the evoked release of the transmitter can be interpreted in terms of the increased calcium influx which it produced. The depressing effect on the frequency of miniature endplate potentials might result from changes in the mechanisms that regulate intracellular free calcium.

# Aminopyridine Effects on Molecular Models in Myopathic States

## G. K. Roussev, D. Paskov and T. Jirkolova

Laboratory of Biological and Organic Chemistry, 2, Buket St.,
1618 Sofia, Bulgaria and Research Laboratory of Pharmachim,
16, Iliensko Shaussee St., 1220 Sofia, Bulgaria

Since 1968 the effect of 4-aminopyridine.HCl (Pymadin) has been studied in various myopathic states of rats and mice: post immobilization atrophy, E-avitaminosis muscular dystrophia, hereditary muscular dystrophia of $dy^{2J}$ line; intoxication adynamia after physical effects, severe fatigue. In all cases, the drug had a therapeutic effect, determined by Ingle and swimming tests. The search of pharmacomolecular mechanisms was carried out on models of myofibril proteins: contraction of isolated myofibrils, ATP-ase activity of A myosin, superprecipitation of native actomyosin in the presence of $Ca^{2+}$ or EGTA, dimerization of G-actin, aggregation of tropomyosin from troponin, formation of synthetic and native actomyosin. The reactions among the myofibril proteins, isolated from myopathic animals, proved to be inhibited as compared with the proteins of healthy animals, each myopathy being characterized by a definitive type of molecular damages. 4-aminopyridine, as well as some of its derivatives, added to the reaction mixtures in a concentration of 1 μM, normalize the reactions, the effect being best in case of muscular dystrophia. The reactions of native actomyosin formation proved to be best restored among the models studied by us.

Two possibilities of aminopyridine favourable molecular effect are discussed: 1. Mobilization of Ca ions retained in the isolated myofibril proteins; 2. Effect on redox processes accompanying the intermolecular reactions.

# Effects of Pyridine on the Frog Rectus Abdominis Muscle

## M. J. Rowan and P. L. Chambers

Department of Pharmacology, University of Dublin,
Trinity College, Dublin 2, Ireland

The pyridine ring is usually considered to exert a powerful depressant effect on transmission at the skeletal neuromuscular junction (Bochefontaine, M., C.R. Séances Soc. Biol., 1883, VII (IV), 5). Somewhat surprisingly, pyridine has also been shown (Valenzuela, F. and Huidobros, F., J. Pharmacol. exp. Ther., 1948, 92, 1) to augment stimulation of the quadriceps femoris and soleus muscles of the cat in vivo induced by various methods. In the present study a somewhat similar augmentation of response by pyridine has been observed and studied on the frog isolated rectus abdominis muscle.

Although pyridine (0.5-12.0 mM) only slightly increased the amplitude of indirectly stimulated contractions, the dose-response curve for acetylcholine evoked contractures was clearly shifted to the left and is considered to be an augmentation of the response. The dose response curve for this effect was of the inverted U type, the optimal concentration being approximately 3 mM. The effect was readily reversible. The amplitude of maximal contractures was not affected. Neither increasing the pyridine pretreatment period from 2 minutes to 8 minutes nor raising the pH of the frog-Ringer solution from 7.4 to 9.0 altered the augmentation of acetylcholine evoked contractures. Contractures of the rectus abdominis muscle which were evoked by carbachol were also increased in the presence of pyridine although to a lesser extent. However, those evoked by tetramethylammonium were not significantly changed. Although pretreatment of the tissues with eserine ($3 \times 10^{-5}$M) did not appear to significantly affect the degree of augmentation produced by pyridine on either acetylcholine or carbachol evoked contractures, a larger concentration of eserine ($1.5 \times 10^{-4}$M) antagonized these effects of pyridine. The contractures elicited by either carbachol or tetramethylammonium however were antagonized by the larger concentration of eserine.

High concentrations of pyridine ($\geqslant$ 15 mM) produced reversible contractures of the rectus abdominis. The effect was dose-dependent. Mild tachyphylaxis was observed especially in the case of high concentrations of pyridine. The dose-response curve for these contractures was shifted to the right by d-tubocurarine. A similar shift of the dose-response curve was also produced by eserine ($1.5 \times 10^{-4}$M).

One of the authors, M.J.R., was in receipt of financial support from the Department of Education of the Government of the Republic of Ireland while these experiments were being performed.

# 4-Aminopyridine and Pre-synaptic Modulation of Transmitter Release in *Aplysia*

T. Shimahara

Laboratoire de Neurobiologie Cellulaire du C.N.R.S.,
91190 Gif sur Yvette, France


In an identified synapse of Aplysia, the synaptic output is sensitive to presynaptic soma potential; a presynaptic hyperpolarization induces a decrease of the postsynaptic potential (P.S.P.) evoked by the presynaptic spike. Since a reduction of this presynaptic spike amplitude is observed at the same time, it appears that the reduction of P.S.P. amplitude is due to a decrease of presynaptic spike amplitude.

In the present experiment the effect of presynaptic membrane potential on the postsynaptic potential was studied in an identified synapse of Aplysia (Aplysia californica). In order to examine the ionic mechanism involved in the presynaptic spike potential, the voltage clamp technique was used. As in many excitable cells, the inward current is reduced when the test pulse is preceeded by a depolarizing conditioning pulse. On the other hand, it also decreases if the conditioning pulse is hyperpolarizing. This phenomenon could be due to the superimposition on the early inward current of 4-aminopyridine (4-AP) sensitive early outward potassium current. Such a depression could result in the observed decrease of the presynaptic spike. To test this hypothesis, I have applied 10 mM 4-AP on the preparation and studied the effects of prepulses on the inward current. After treatment with 4-AP the inward current is less affected by hyperpolarizing conditioning pulses. Under current clamp condition, external application of 4-AP abolishes the anomalous reduction of the action potential by hyperpolarizing pulses, and the P.S.P. amplitude becomes quite independent of the presynaptic soma potential.

These results suggest that a 4-AP sensitive early outward potassium current modulates transmitter release in Aplysia neurones.

# Naloxone, 4-Aminopyridine and Physostigmine as Antagonists of Morphine in Rabbits

R. L. Sia, P. Westra and H. Wesseling

Institutes of Anaesthesiology and Clinical Pharmacology,
University Hospital Groningen, Oostersingel 59,
9713 EZ Groningen, The Netherlands

A comparative study of naloxone, 4-aminopyridine and physostigmine on the respiratory depressant and analgesic effects of morphine was done in conscious rabbits. Arterial blood gases ($Po_2$ and $Pco_2$), end-tidal $Pco_2$, respiratory frequency and analgesia (stimulation threshold; ear flick method) were measured. Morphine 2.5 mg kg$^{-1}$ decreased respiratory frequency on average by 63% and $Pao_2$ on average by 20% and increased $Paco_2$ on average by 23% and $Petco_2$ and stimulation threshold resp. 2.3 and 2.8-fold compared with the control values. Naloxone 0.05 mg kg$^{-1}$ and 4-aminopyridine 1.25 mg kg$^{-1}$ restored respiratory frequency, $Pao_2$, $Paco_2$, $Petco_2$ and stimulation threshold to control levels after resp. 2 and 5-10 min. Physostigmine 0.2 mg kg$^{-1}$ restored respiratory frequency to a mean of 52% of control and $Paco_2$ to near control values, but this action was of short duration compared with naloxone and 4-aminopyridine. The influence of physostigmine on morfine-induced analgesia was not statistically significant (fig. 1). The mode of action of 4-aminopyridine is probably dual; the morphine-induced respiratory depression is antagonized by increasing Ach and the analgesic effect of morphine is reversed by another mechanism as pointed out by the action of physostigmine.

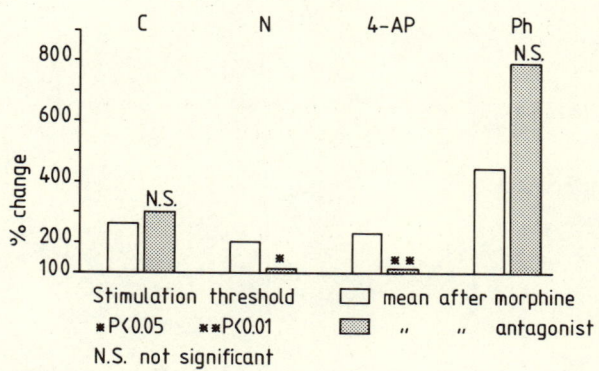

# Anti-Curare Action of 4-Aminopyridine and 4-Aminopyridine-like Substances

V. Sobek

Laboratory for the Research of Infectious Diseases, Faculty of Paediatrics, Charles University, 180 81 Prague 8—Bulovka, Czechoslovakia

We have been compared and analysed the action of following substances: 4-aminopyridine, pyrocatechin, tetraethylammonium and caffeine on the arrest of respiration and cardiac depression induced by aminoglycosidic antibiotics. Out of these four substances, caffeine was ineffective, tetraethylammonium had only cardiostimulating activity. Pyrocatechin did not affect the reduced contractility of the cardiac muscle, so that the only suitable substance was 4-aminopyridine. The latter had a similar effect as calcium, i. e. it increased blood pressure and restored respiration. It acted even in the case when other therapeutic agents were ineffective, i. e. in cases of calcium resistance and potentiated the effect of calcium and neostigmine.

# 4-Aminopyridine Reversal of Morphine Analgesia

A. S. Tung, and B. W. Brandom

University of Pittsburgh School of Medicine, Department of Anesthesiology, Pittsburgh, PA 15261, USA

4-Aminopyridine (4AP) reversal of morphine analgesia was assessed because while morphine sulfate (MS) inhibits the release of neurotransmitters involved with pain transmission,[1] 4AP enhances calcium-dependent neurotransmitter release.[2] 4AP has been used clinically to reverse non-depolarizing muscle relaxants[3] and ketamine-diazepam anesthesia. The usefulness of 4AP in these circumstances may be due to an ability to block potassium conductance, create a regenerative calcium current and thus enhance neurotransmitter release.[2] These events may also diminish morphine induced analgesia.

Analgesia was measured by tail flick and hot plate tests. The response latencies in these tests were converted to maximal possible effect (%MPE) .MPE=(Postinjection latency - baseline)/(cutoff time - baseline). All drugs were given i.p.

| $\bar{X} \pm$ SEM | MS-10 | 4AP-2 | MS&saline | MS&4AP-0.5 | MS&4AP-1.0 | MS&4AP-2.0 |
|---|---|---|---|---|---|---|
| %MPE TFL | 88±10 | 3±6 | 65±12 | 48±32 | 10±8 | 22±16 |
| %MPE HPL | 36±17 | 59±14 | 34±18 | 48±21 | 55±21 | 100±0 |

Statistically significant ($P<0.5$) results are as follows. MS 10 mg/kg elevated both the tail flick (TFL) and hot plate (HPL) latencies. 4AP alone did not affect the TFL but increased the HPL. In addition, all three doses of 4AP caused a significant reduction of the MS induced increase in TFL. On the other hand, 4AP at 2mg/kg resulted in a potentiation of the MS effect on the HPL.

As indicated by the results of the TFL (a monosynaptic spinal reflex) 4AP did reverse MS analgesia. Analgesia reversal was not demonstrated by the HPL because the end point of the hot plate test was indicated by the animal's ability to lick or tap its hind paw. This behavior would require multisynaptic supraspinal function which was affected by the central excitatory action of 4AP. A clinical implication of these results is that while attempting to antagonize muscle relaxant or anesthetic effects in postoperative patients with 4AP, incidental reversal of much needed narcotic analgesia may occur.

1. Mudge AW, Leeman SE and Fischback GD: Enkephalin inhibits release of substance P from sensory neurons in culture and decreases action potential duration. Proc Natl Acad Sci USA 76:526-530, 1979.
2. Lundh H: Effects of 4-aminopyridine on neuromuscular transmission Brain Res 153:307-318, 1978.
3. Miller RD, Booij LHD, Agoston S, et al: Potentiation of neostigmine and pyridostigmine by 4-aminopyridine in man. Anesthesiology 50:416-420, 1979.

# 4-Aminopyridine as Antagonist of the Cardiovascular and Neuromuscular Depressant Effects of Kanamycin in Rats

T. Uchiyama, M. Lemeignan and P. Lechat

Institut de Pharmacologie, Laboratoire Associé du C.N.R.S.
n° 206, 15, rue de l'Ecole de Médecine, 75006 Paris, France

4-Aminopyridine (4-AP) has been shown to antagonize the neuromuscular blockade produced by some aminoglycoside antibiotics in vivo and in vitro (1). This work was undertaken to study if 4-AP could antagonize both the cardiovascular and neuromuscular depressant effects of kanamycin (KM) in anesthetized and conscious rats.

For this purpose, in anesthetized rats (urethane, 1.3 g/kg i.p.), directly and indirectly elicited maximal twitch tensions of the tibialis anterior muscle in situ were recorded together with the mean arterial blood pressure (AP) and heart rate (HR). Kanamycin infusion (70 mg/ml, 0.2 ml/min i.v.) induced progressively a decrease in twitch tension and in HR and AP. 4-AP (2.8 mg/kg s.c.) raised significantly the KM doses inducing cardiovascular or neuromuscular depressions. KM infusion to chronically catheterized conscious rats induced a spontaneous head drop that was taken as a sign of the neuromuscular block and a decrease in HR and AP. 4-AP (2.8 mg/kg s.c.) also antagonized these effects of KM but was less active than in anesthetized rats.

4-AP enhances the evoked neurotransmitter release at various types of synapses probably by increasing the influx of calcium in nerve terminals (2). Furthermore the depressant effects of KM in conscious rats were potentiated by a decrease in serum total calcium level (3). Therefore it was of interest to study the effect that hypocalcemia has on the actions of 4-AP in vivo and whether it modifies the antagonism of 4-AP toward KM depressant actions. Hypocalcemic states were obtained by s.c. injection of synthetic salmon calcitonin (CT: 1,000 mU/kg; mean serum total calcium obtained: $7.2 \pm 0.2$ mM/l). 4-AP dose-dependently increased both indirectly and directly elicited muscle twitches being more efficient on indirectly elicited ones. Hypocalcemia potentiated this action and increased the efficacy of 4-AP to reduce the effects of KM infusion in conscious rats.

The results show that 4-AP antagonizes both the cardiovascular and neuromuscular KM-depressant effects and that hypocalcemia potentiates the effects of 4-AP. This may be explained if it is assumed that hypocalcemia, which by itself, can induce repetitive firing in nerve and muscle fibres, potentiates the ability of 4-AP to induce repetitive discharges in motor and ganglionic nerve terminals.

(1) Y.N. SINGH, A.L. HARVEY and J.G. MARSHALL (1978) Br. J. Anaesth., 50, 109-117.
(2) S. THESLEFF (1980) Neuroscience, 5, 1413-1419
(3) T. UCHIYAMA, M. LEMEIGNAN, J. MOLGO and P. LECHAT (1981) Arch. int. Pharmacodyn. 249, 275-288.

# Further Actions of Aminopyridines on Muscle and Nerve: Short Communications

*Chairman:* P. Lechat

# Effects of 4-Aminopyridine on Mammalian Peripheral and Central Neurones

M. Galvan, P. Grafe and G. ten Bruggencate

Department of Physiology, University of Munich, Pettenkoferstr. 12, 8000 Munich 2, Federal Republic of Germany

We have studied the effects of 4-aminopyridine (4AP) on neurones in the rat isolated superior cervical ganglion and the guinea-pig isolated olfactory cortex slice. All experiments were performed at 30°C in Krebs' solution; neurones were impaled with $K^+$-acetate filled microelectrodes. Bath application of 0.1-1.0 mM 4AP to ganglia frequently resulted in the appearance of spontaneous EPSPs and/or spikes, without a detectable change in membrane potential or resistance. These potentials were completely blocked by hexamethonium or tetrodotoxin and thus most probably arise as a result of a release of acetyl-choline from presynaptic structures. Somatic action potential duration was only marginally affected by 1 mM 4AP, prolongations of upto 60% were observed. Vagus nerve B- and C-fibre potentials were prolonged by 100 µM 4AP, but A-fibre potentials were unaffected.

In the brain slice, application of 3-10 µM 4AP led to very powerful seizure discharges. These were preceeded by a massive increase in the frequency and amplitude of spontaneous postsynaptic potentials. In addition, we recorded marked oscillations of membrane potential and extracellular $K^+$ and $Ca^{++}$ concentrations. EPSPs elicited by orthodromic stimulation tended to be reduced in amplitude but were followed by several membrane potential "after oscillations". A late hyperpolarizing potential (possibly an IPSP) was abolished in the seconds before seizure onset. During the seizures, cells discharged repetitively and extracellular $K^+$ rose to over 10 mM. These dramatic abnormal neuronal discharges were observed in cells which exhibited no change in resting membrane potential, input resistance, or soma action potential duration. The fibre spike recorded from the lateral olfactory tract was prolonged by about 100% in 10 µM 4AP.

Our results suggest that 4AP has actions on mammalian neurones and synapses, which cannot be simply explained by its well described blockade of axonal delayed rectifier currents.

Supported by the Deutsche Forschungsgemeinschaft.

# Interactions of Aminopyridines and Related Compounds with Ionic Channels in the Isolated Cockroach Axon

M. Pelhate*, B. Hue*, Y. Pichon** and J. Chanelet*

*U.E.R. Médecine, Lab. Physiologie, 49045 Angers, France
**Lab. Neurobiologie Cellulaire du C.N.R.S.,
91190 Gif sur Yvette, France

We have shown previously (1) that, in insect axons, 4-aminopyridine (4-AP) modify excitability and increase the duration of the action potential through a selective inhibition of the potassium conductance. The present experiments have been performed to compare, on this same preparation, the isolated giant axon of Periplaneta americana, the effects of 4-AP with those of its isomers : 2 and 3-aminopyridines (2 and 3-AP) and some of its derivatives : 3,4-diaminopyridine (3,4-DAP), 4-aminoquinoline (4-AQ) and 9-aminoacridine (9-AA). Ionic currents corresponding to various depolarizations have been recorded using the voltage-clamp technique.

The results can be summarized as follows : (a) Whereas the pyridine nucleus alone has very little effect even at high concentrations (about 10% inhibition for 10 mM) 4-AP and its isomers and derivatives all depress the potassium conductance at micromolar concentrations ; (b) The slope of the dose-response curve as well as the apparent dissociation constant (Kd) change with the membrane voltage and the nature of the molecule. For a 100 mV depolarization, the efficacy decreased according to the following sequence : 3,4-DAP (Kd: $1.8 \times 10^{-5}$M) > 4-AP (Kd: $3 \times 10^{-5}$M) > 3-AP (Kd: $5 \times 10^{-5}$M) > 2-AP (Kd: $2 \times 10^{-4}$M) > 9-AA (Kd: $2.7 \times 10^{-4}$M) > 4-AQ (Kd: $3.7 \times 10^{-4}$M) ; (c) Apart from 9-AA which induces inactivation after an apparently normal opening of the potassium channels in very much the same way as internally applied tetraethylammonium (2), all the other compounds block the potassium channels at rest. This blocking decrease during the course of the depolarizations (voltage dependent 'clearing' of Meves and Pichon (3) ; (d) 4-AQ and 9-AA modify both sodium and potassium conductances whereas the other molecules only affect the latter.

These data indicate that at least three molecular factors are involved in channel blockage : lipid solubility, presence of a quaternary ammonium and size.

References : (1) PELHATE M, HUE B, PICHON Y and CHANELET J (1974),C. R.Acad.Sci., Paris, 278, p.2807. (2) ARMSTRONG CM & HILLE B (1972), J.Gen.Physiol. 59, p.388. (3) MEVES H & PICHON Y (1975), J. Physiol. London, 251, 60P.

# 4-Aminopyridine-induced Alteration in the Receptive Field of Cuneate and Gracile Neurones

N. E. Saadé*, N. R. Banna*, A. J. Khoury*, S. J. Jabbur**
and P. D. Wall***

*Faculty of Sciences, Lebanese University, Hadeth-Beirut, Lebanon
**Faculty of Medicine, American University of Beirut, Lebanon
***Department of Anatomy, University College, London, UK


As no true regeneration of neurones occurs in the mammalian central nervous system (CNS) once development and differentiation are complete, plasticity in the adult CNS needs to be based on other processes. Two mechanisms could produce a new response in a neurone following the loss of its normal input: sprouting of intact axons to occupy the area left by the degenerating input, or the opening up of polysynaptic pathways which had previously been inhibited by the normal input. The unmasking of ineffective synapses in the adult animal could offer an alternative to the above suggestions as a mechanism of plasticity of CNS connections. The following experiments were designed to test this last mechanism by the local application of 4-aminopyridine (4-AP) to cuneate and gracile neurones to determine if any expansion or reduction in their receptive fields (RF) could be detected.

Adult male cats were anesthetized with Nembutal (35 mg/kg i.p.) and the head placed in a stereotaxic instrument. Holes were drilled in the parietal bone to allow the placement of coaxial electrodes in the two medial lemnisci (coordinates A5, L4.5, V1.8). They were subsequently paralyzed with Flaxedil, artificially respired and subjected to bilateral pneumothorax. Body temperature, end tidal $CO_2$ and blood pressure were monitored and maintained within the normal physiological range. The dorsal column nuclei were exposed and single units recorded with double-barrelled glass electrodes.

Forty one single unit responses of both relay and nonrelay cuneate and gracile neurones were studied in response to natural stimulation. The nature and extent of the peripheral field were determined first in stable units, then 4-AP was released locally using one of three techniques: microiontophoresis, baroejection (WPI nanoliter pump) or localized surface application. The units studied were distributed as follows: 15 responded to hair movement, 16 to touch, 2 to light pressure, and 8 to hair and touch. In 32 units, the receptive field was increased in area after the local application of 4-AP. The onset of this expansion in receptive field was rapid (within one minute). It persisted for 10-20 min and was frequently reversible. In 4 units, a reduction in receptive field area was observed after 4-AP application. No change in the extent of the receptive field could be noted in 5 cells. Since 4-AP increases nerve impulse-evoked transmitter release nonspecifically, it is likely that its application in the vicinity of neurones causes the activation of otherwise ineffective synapses on the dendrites of these neurones.

# Effect of 4-Aminopyridine on the Desensitisation of the Rat Diaphragm Caused by Carbachol

O. Vital Brazil and M. D. Fontana

Department of Pharmacology, Faculty of Medical Sciences, State
University of Campinas, Campinas, São Paulo, Brazil

4-Aminopyridine reverses the inhibitory effect produced by crotoxin on the depolarisation induced by carbachol (Vital Brazil et al., 1979). Crotoxin, without binding to the acetylcholine receptor sites, stabilizes the receptor protein in a conformation which exhibits a high affinity for agonists, that is, in a state similar to the desensitized state (Bon et al., 1979). There is, therefore, strong evidence that 4-aminopyridine is able to stabilize the cholinergic receptor in its low affinity resting conformation. In the present research, the effect of 4-aminopyridine on the desensitization produced by prolonged interaction of an agonist with the receptor was investigated.

The experiments were carried out in the isolated rat diaphragm. Measurement of transmembrane potential was done with glass microelectrodes filled with 3 M KCl using standard techniques. Desensitisation was induced by adding carbachol to the Tyrode solution bathing the preparation (temperature of bath $37^{\circ}C$). 4-Aminopyridine was added either before carbachol or after it when the end-plates repolarized in spite of the presence of carbachol in the bath.

In the experiments in which 4-aminopyridine was added before carbachol the agonist produced permanent depolarization, that is, 4-aminopyridine prevented desensitization of the receptors. When it was added after repolarization, the end-plates depolarized to the same extent as before desensitization. It concluded that 4-aminopyridine has the unique property of stabilizing the receptors of end-plate in the undesensitized state, reversing them to this state when they are already desensitized.

Bon, C., Changeux, J.O., Jeng, T.W. and Fraenkel-Conrat, H. - Postsynaptic effects of crotoxin and its isolated subunits. Eu. J. Biochem., $99$: 471, 1979.

Vital Brazil, O., Fontana, M.D. and Heluany, N.F. - Effect of 4-aminopyridine on neuromuscular blockade produced by crotoxin. Toxicon, $17$ (Suppl. $N^{\circ}$. 1): 16, 1979.

# The Effects of 4-Aminopyridine on Neuromuscular Block Produced by Succinyldicholine

### N. N. Durant, C. Lee and R. L. Katz

Department of Anesthesiology, UCLA Medical Center,
Los Angeles, California 90024, USA

The failure of 4-aminopyridine (4-AP) to reverse neuromuscular block produced by succinyldicholine (SDCh) has been shown on the isolated rat diaphragm and also in the anaesthetized cat. This raises the possibility that SDCh may inhibit the prejunctional action of 4-AP or alternatively that the increased release of acetylcholine produced by 4-AP does not overcome the postjunctional block produced by SDCh. The present electrophysiological study was undertaken to investigate the effect of 4-AP on SDCh block at the frog neuromuscular junction using conventional voltage clamp techniques to eliminate depolarization. The muscle was exposed to 30 µM SDCh for 45 min before 4-AP was added to the organ bath.

| Min | 15 | 30 | 45 | 75 | 105 | 135 |
|---|---|---|---|---|---|---|
| [4-AP] µM | - | - | - | 30 | 100 | 300 |
| Amp (nA) | 180±66 | 50±10 | 26±4 | 55±6 | 88±13 | 49±4 |
| τ (msec) | 2.1±0.3 | 1.9±0.2 | 2.1±0.2 | 1.8±0.2 | 1.9±0.3 | - |
| 5/1 at 5Hz | 158±23% | 105±8% | 102±7% | 69±2% | 45±5% | 44±3% |

Table 1. The effects of SDCh and 4-AP on endplate currents recorded at a holding potential of -90 mV. The trains of 5 stimuli at 5 Hz (5/1 at 5 Hz) were carried out as separate experiments (N=5).

Table 1 shows that 4-AP (30 to 300 µM) did increase the amplitude of endplate currents (EPCs) depressed by SDCh but not sufficiently to overcome the neuromuscular block. No significant effect of either drug on the single exponential decay constant (τ) was observed. At some endplates repetitive EPCs were observed in response to single nerve stimuli in the presence of all of the concentrations of 4-AP studied. The decline of EPC amplitude during a train of 5 nerve stimuli at a frequency of 5 Hz, which is characteristic of 4-AP (Illes & Thesleff, Br.J.Pharmacol., 64: 623, 1978), was observed with 4-AP in the presence of SDCh (5/1 at 5 Hz). These two observations suggest the prejunctional effects of 4-AP are not abolished by SDCh.

It is concluded that SDCh does not prevent the action of 4-AP on the nerve terminal and that the increased release of acetylcholine due to 4-AP does not overcome the postjunctional block due to SDCh because of desensitization.

# Chemical Modulators: Their Molecular Characteristics and Kinetics of Actions

T. Maeno

Department of Physiology, Shimane Medical University,
Izumo 693, Japan

The kinetics of competitive interaction of aminopyridines and aminoglycoside antibiotics on the release mechanism of the available acetylcholine quanta were studied by calculating the fractional release ($P$) from the tetanic rundown during short train stimulations of the endplate potentials recorded on the curarized frog muscle with conventional microelectrode techniques. To explain the marked facilitatory effect of 4-aminopyridine (4AP) on $P$ and the antagonistic effect of neomycin and streptomycin thereupon, I would like to propose the following simplified schemes.

1) It is well established that the flow of Ca ions into the nerve terminal is essential for depolarization-secretion coupling. I assume that four Ca ions combine with the specific release process X to trigger a complicated chain of events of the transmitter release and that $P$ is related normally to the amount of $Ca_4X$ complex.

2) The chemicals which modify the transmitter output by acting on the Ca-dependent release process X may be defined the chemical modulators. The chemical modulators can be divided further into two classes; $i.e.$ accelerators and depressors. A drug which has the facilitatory action fundamentally identical to that of 4AP is termed accelerator (A). The combination of A with $Ca_4X$ presumably modifies allosterically the action of the $Ca_4X$ complex to augment profoundly the evoked release. Thus, $P$ in the presence of an accelerator may be considered to be related to the sum of the above two forms of release. Depressor (D) such as neomycin also reacts with the Ca-bound release process X, but inhibits the transmitter release; $i.e.$

$$4Ca + X \xrightleftharpoons{K_{Ca}} Ca_4X \xrightarrow{P_{Ca}} \text{normal evoked release}$$

$$A + Ca_4X \xrightleftharpoons{K_A} A\text{-}Ca_4X \xrightarrow{P_A} \text{accelerated evoked release}$$

$$D + Ca_4X \xrightleftharpoons{K_D} D\text{-}Ca_4X \longrightarrow \text{depressed release}$$

Consequently, the accelerator and depressor compete for occupancy of the Ca-bound X site. $P$ in the presence of both A and D was calculated to be

$$P = (P_{Ca} + P_A[A]/K_A)/\{(1 + K_{Ca}/[Ca])^4 + [A]/K_A + [D]/K_D\}$$

which agreed well with the obtained data. Common feature of the chemical modulators is characterized by a hexagonal skeleton with at least two nitrogen atoms attached at or within the hexagonal ring. Several aromatic and heterocyclic diamines act as accelerators, and derivatives of alicyclic diamine show depressor activity.

# DISCUSSION OF THE FIFTH SESSION

Dr. Ulbricht: Dr. Galvan, what is the 4-aminopyridine concentration to block 50% of your "A" current?

Dr. Galvan: The A-type current recorded from rat sympathetic neurons was blocked about 50% by 1 mM 4-aminopyridine. It would be interesting to know if such a current exists in cortical neurons and can be blocked by lower concentrations.

Dr. Glover: My colleague Peter Gage, working in collaboration with J.W. Moore, has recently shown that 4-methyl-2-aminopyridine which has a similar but weaker convulsant action in intact animals has little effect on $K^+$ conductance in the giant axon of the squid. This is in keeping with the suggestion that the convulsant action of 4-aminopyridine is not due to a blockade of $K^+$ channels of the type found in peripheral nerves.

Dr. Galvan: This is an interesting observation which obviously needs further investigation.

Dr. Jankowska: Could not the depression of IPSPs that you found in your preparation be due to activation of some neurons? Parallel to the development of the convulsant discharges, such neurons might interfere with the activity of those interneurons which are responsible for the IPSPs depressed by 4-aminopyridine.

Dr. Galvan: In fact the pattern of inhibition we recorded was phasic. The IPSPs disappeared just before onset of seizure activity and then reappeared in the interseizure period. We think that this may be in some way related to the massive increase in spontaneous activity occurring before seizures. Spontaneous potentials are transiently abolished after seizures due to a fall in the electric resistance of the cell and in this phase the IPSPs reappear.

Dr. Ulbricht: Dr. Pelhate, which is the 9-aminoacridine concentration needed to block 50% of the $Na^+$ current?

Dr. Pelhate: About $10^{-4}$ M blocks 50% after 10 minutes. $2 \times 10^{-4}$ to $5 \times 10^{-4}$ M blocks completely the sodium current in the cockroach axon within 15 minutes.

Dr. Pichon: In squid axon 9-AA blocks both channels when injected in the axon. The 50% block of the $K^+$ current is obtained for about 10 times smaller concentrations (about 50 uM) than for sodium channels (500 uM). The block of $Na^+$ channel is frequency dependent indicating that channels should be open before the block can occur. There is no effect of 9-AA if applied from the outside. We have no indication that these results can be extended to coackroach axon.

Dr. Sellin: Was there a difference between the concentration of 4-aminoquinoline required to block the $K^+$ channel compared to the $Na^+$ channel?

Dr. Pelhate: 4-aminoquinoline is in the range of one order of magnitude less potent as a $Na^+$-channel blocker.

Dr. Bergmann: Did you test the effect of 4-aminopyridine separately on excitatory and inhibitory fibres of the cockroach?

Dr. Pelhate: All the experiments have been done with "artificial nodes" 100 μm long of giant axons 40 μm in diameter. The giant axon dissected was from a giant interneuron of the ventral nerve group. These giant interneurons are considered to be excitatory neurons.

Dr. Jankowska: Dr. Saadé, would you mind commenting on some points related to the interpretation of your very clearcut results? One of them concerns the existence of experimental evidence for silent synapses; silent in the sense that they do not give rise to any PSPs. Would it not be better to stick to the term "ineffective" throughout? In view of other data on the action of 4-aminopyridine your observations should be fully compatible with an increase in amplitude of EPSPs evoked by stimuli applied at the outskirts of the receptive fields of your cells. EPSPs evoked by such stimuli might be too small to discharge the cells before the injection of 4-aminopyridine and their effects would remain undetectable with extracellular recording, but they could be sufficiently large to be recorded after 4-aminopyridine.

Dr. Saadé: Our previous work concerns only ineffective synapses, which cannot normally evoke the firing of the cell. By intracellular recording we can only detect PSPs. Application of 4-aminopyridine can enhance the efficacy of these synapses. In silent synapses, according to one theory of plasticity, more branches of an axon are produced during embryonic development than are required for normal functioning of the final working circuit. These branches of the terminal arborisation may not be normally functional, but small variations in the structure or in the impinging controls, as may be brought about by injury, could conceivably switch these axons from a blocked, inactive state, to a conducting one (Wall, 1976). "Silent synapses" cannot be detected by the mean of electrophysiological recording. Histological studies of neurons after degeneration can give indirect evidence for their existence.


Dr. Schiavone: Dr. Vital-Brazil, does 4-aminopyridine reverse the carbachol induced desensitization by an interaction with the receptor or with some mechanism beyond the receptor-activation step?

Dr. Vital-Brazil: I really do not know the mechanism by which 4-aminopyridine is able to stabilize the receptor in its resting non-desensitized conformation.

Dr. Schiavone: What was the $Ca^{2+}$ concentration in the preparation before $Ca^{2+}$ was added to antagonize the 4-aminopyridine induced restoration of the carbachol response? Did you measure changes in the contractile response in the course of your experiments?

Dr. Vital-Brazil: The $Ca^{2+}$ concentration was 1.8 mM, the usual concentration in Tyrode's solution. We have not yet studied contractile responses but intend to study the effects of 4-aminopyridine on phase I and phase II type of neuromuscular block by recording the tension of indirectly evoked twitches.

Dr. McArdle: J.-P. Changeux and his colleagues have shown that when the ACh receptor is solubilized in a detergent it is stabilized in a high affinity state for the agonist. This form of the receptor Changeux refers to as desensitized. If the receptor is isolated in the presence of lipid it does not appear in the high affinity state. Therefore, I wonder if 4-aminopyridine can overcome desensitization through an action on membrane lipids surrounding the receptor proteins and not on the protein itself?

Dr. Vital-Brazil: I do not know, but it is possible. I believe that 4-aminopyridine overcomes desensitization by acting on the lipids of the receptor rather than on the protein itself.


Dr. Galvan: Dr. Durant, you showed that 300 µM 4-aminopyridine restored EPC amplitude to approximately control values. Why do you conclude that it cannot reverse suxamethonium block?

Dr. Durant: Since we did not measure EPCs in the absence of suxamethonium, which would be the true control EPCs, it cannot be said that 300 µM 4-aminopyridine restored EPC amplitude to control values. In other experiments we have measured EPC amplitude in transected frog muscle fibres and these amplitudes were at least 2 times larger than any of the EPCs measured in the presence of suxamethonium + 4-aminopyridine. Furthermore, we found no evidence that 4-aminopyridine produced any restoration of twitch responses to indirect stimulation. Thus, we conclude that although

4-aminopyridine increased EPC amplitude it did not completely reverse the effects of suxamethonium.

Dr. Bergmann: Did you try to apply eserine or neostigmine to your preparation treated with suxamethonium and 4-aminopyridine?

Dr. Durant: No, we did not apply eserine or neostigmine to our preparation. We did some twitch experiment with our preparation (frog cutaneous pectoris muscle) in response to nerve stimulation. In these experiments neostigmine did not restore the twitch response abolished by suxamethonium.

Dr. Foldes: We have observed that the suxamethonium induced neuromuscular block of the rat hemi-diaphragm preparation cannot be reversed by 4-aminopyridine. In contrast, the block of the tibialis anterior muscle induced by the continuous infusion of suxamethonium in the rat could be reversed by 1-2 mg 4-aminopyridine. It seems that there may be a variation in the ability of 4-aminopyridine to antagonize the suxamethonium block depending on the species and/or the type of muscle employed.

Dr. Molgo: Have you seen differences in the current-voltage-relationship of endplate currents in the presence of suxamethonium? Have you seen differences in the rise time of your endplate currents in the presence of the drug?

Dr. Durant: Yes, we have investigated the current-voltage relationship of EPCs in the presence of suxamethonium. The relationship deviated from linearity at negative holding potentials between about -70 mV and -140 mV, EPCs becoming smaller. We have also consistently observed a slower EPC rise time in the presence of suxamethonium.

Dr. McArdle: On the basis of your data Dr. Maeno would you say that 4-aminopyridine may have an effect on the "active zones"?

Dr. Maeno: Electron microscopic pictures show an increase in the number of exocytotic openings. A statistical analysis suggests an increment in the number of quanta readily available for release (n). So, it seems possible that 4-aminopyridine affects indirectly the "active zones". However, this chemical modulator seems to have no effect on the total store of quanta available for release (N).

# Aminopyridines and Skeletal, Smooth and Cardiac Muscle

*Chairman:* K. A. P. Edman

# Effects of 4-Aminopyridine on Contractile Properties of Skeletal Muscle

## K. A. P. Edman and A. R. Khan

Department of Pharmacology, University of Lund,
S-223 62 Lund, Sweden

ABSTRACT

The contractile effects of 4-aminopyridine (4-AP) were studied on isolated muscle fibres of the tibialis anterior and semitendinosus muscles of Rana temporaria (1-4°C) and, in one series of experiments, on curarized isolated lumbrical muscles of the rat (22-23°C).

4-AP potentiated the isometric twitch response of both frog ($\sim$ 0.5 mM) and rat ($\sim$ 0.1 mM) muscles without significantly affecting the tetanus amplitude. The time to peak twitch force was increased in both muscles. The time constant of tension decay measured during the tetanus was not affected by the drug. The twitch potentiation produced by 4-AP was obtained also in the absence of extracellular calcium, i.e. after replacing calcium with lanthanum (0.05 mM) in the Ringer solution in order to maintain membrane excitability. The mechanical threshold, i.e. the level of depolarization at which the contractile response is initiated, was determined by rapidly increasing the external potassium ion concentration to various levels. This threshold was not affected by 4-AP, nor was there any effect of the drug on the time course of the potassium induced contracture. Neither did 4-AP affect the threshold concentration of caffeine required to produce contracture of the muscle fibre. Taken together these findings suggest that 4-AP does not exert any specific effects on the mechanism of release of activator calcium in the excitation-contraction coupling.

The contractile effects of 4-AP were paralleled by an increased duration of the membrane action potential. This latter effect was due to slowing of the repolarization phase, there being no significant change in the maximum rate of rise and overshoot of the action potential. The prolongation of the action potential probably accounts for the enhancement of twitch force and the increase in time to peak twitch tension. By the increase in duration of the action potential activator calcium will be released over a longer time leading to increased concentration of calcium in the myofibrillar space. The lack of effect of 4-AP on the relaxation kinetics (see above) suggests that 4-AP does not to any significant degree affect calcium resequestration.

Membrane depolarization facilitates transport of 4-AP to the site of action of the drug in the fibre membrane. No effect of 4-AP on either action potential or twitch response was obtained after 30 min exposure to the drug if the fibre was left unstimulated during this time. However, on stimulation of the fibre the effects of

4-AP increased steadily with the number of excitation cycles reaching a maximum after about 10 action potentials.

KEYWORDS

4-aminopyridine, skeletal muscle, single muscle fibre, excitation-contraction coupling, contractile potentiation, action potential, membrane potential.

INTRODUCTION

As has been documented in several previous studies (Molgo, Lemeignan and Lechat, 1975 and 1977; Lundh and Thesleff, 1977; Thesleff, 1980) aminopyridines may greatly potentiate the mechanical response of skeletal muscle to indirect stimulation by enhancing the transmittor function in the neuromuscular junction. There is reason to believe that the aminopyridines exert this effect by increasing the inflow of calcium into the nerve terminal thereby causing a larger quantity of acetylcholine to be released from its presynaptic store (Molgo, Lemeignan and Lechat, 1975 and 1977; Lundh and Thesleff, 1977; Lundh, 1978). The present investigation deals with effects of aminopyridine that are produced on the muscle fibre itself, i.e. effects produced beyond the neuromuscular junction. As is now generally accepted calcium plays a key role in the coupling between excitation and contraction, and it is of interest to find out if this function of calcium can also be modified by the aminopyridines. A suitable test object for this kind of study is the intact muscle fibre preparation of the frog, as it enables simultaneous recordings of electrical and mechanical events in the same functional unit. Evidence will be presented to show that the contractile effect of 4-aminopyridine is attributable to prolongation of the membrane action potential.

METHODS

Frog Skeletal Muscle Fibres

Single fibres were dissected from the ventral or dorsal head of the semitendinosus muscle of Rana temporaria. For mounting a small link of stainless steel wire (diameter 0.1 mm) was attached to each tendon as described previously (Edman and Kiessling, 1971).

The fibres were mounted horizontally between a force transducer (see below) and a stainless steel hook, the position of which could be set by means of a micrometer screw. The chamber contained 1.2 ml solution which could be exchanged by introducing fresh solution at the transducer end of the chamber at the same time as suction drain was applied at the other end. A flush time of about 3 s produced an almost complete (> 95%) exchange of the bath solution (Andersson and Edman, 1974).

Stimulation was produced by means of a multielectrode assembly of alternating anodes and cathodes as described previously (Edman and Kiessling, 1971). In some experiments the fibre was stimulated by passing current between two platinum plate electrodes that were placed on either side of the fibre approximately 2 mm from it. Pulses of 0.2 ms duration were used and the stimulation strength was adjusted to be supramaximal. For tetanic stimulation, a 1 s train of pulses with a frequency of 16-22 Hz was used. Generally 2 min intervals were used between twitch and/or tetanus responses.

Contracture was induced by increasing the potassium concentration of the bathing solution or by the addition of caffeine. For this purpose a solution containing caffeine or increased potassium concentration was flushed from a pre-cooled container until plateau contracture tension was attained. Relaxation was produced by re-administration of the normal Ringer solution. The time interval between two successive potassium or caffeine contractures was 20-25 min.

Tension was recorded by an RCA 5734 mechano-electric transducer and in later experiments by means of a semiconductor strain-gauge element (AE801, Aksjeselskapet Mikroelektronikk, Horten, Norway). The signals were displayed on a Tektronix 502A or a 5113N storage oscilloscope and photographed on 35 mm film. Recordings were also made on paper by means of an Elema-Schönander ink-jet writer.

Membrane potentials were recorded intracellularly using conventional glass capillary electrodes as described by Khan and Edman (1979). The solutions used in the frog muscle experiments had the following composition (mM): Ordinary Ringer solution: NaCl 115.5, KCl 2.0, $CaCl_2$ 1.8, Na-phosphate buffer 2.0, pH 7.0. Calcium-free Ringer: NaCl 116.3, KCl 2.0, EDTA 1.0, Na-phosphate buffer 2.0, pH 7.0. Lanthanum containing Ringer: NaCl 117.2, KCl 2.0, $LaCl_3$ 0.05, Tris-(hydroxymethyl)-aminomethane 2.0. The pH was adjusted to 7.0 by addition of $H_2SO_4$ to a final concentration of 0.94 mM.

For potassium contractures the concentration of potassium in the bathing solution was increased to 10, 20, 40, 80 and 117.5 mM. These solutions had constant [K] x [Cl] product and constant tonicity. For details of their composition, see Khan and Edman (1979).

The drugs 4-aminopyridine sulfate and caffeine were dissolved in the above solutions. It was ensured that the pH was 7.0 also in the presence of drug.

The bath temperature varied between 1 and 4°C in the frog muscle fibre experiments but was maintained constant to within ± 0.2°C throughout any particular experiment, even during exchange of solution.

Rat Skeletal Muscle

Thin lumbrical muscles were isolated from the front leg of Sprague-Dawley rats (150-200 g). A small loop of silk thread was attached to each tendon for mounting of the muscle in the experimental chamber. The same muscle chamber was used as in the frog fibre experiments (see above). Stimulation and recording of responses were also performed as described above.

The solution used in the rat muscle experiments had the following composition (mM): NaCl 154.0, KCl 5.6, $NaHCO_3$ 3.6, $CaCl_2$ 1.0, $NaH_2PO_4$ 0.55, $Na_2HPO_4$ 0.9, glucose 5.5, d-tubocurarine 0.5 mg/ml, pH 7.4. This solution was aerated by a mixture of 95% $O_2$ and 5% $CO_2$. 4-aminopyridine sulfate was dissolved in this solution and it was acertained that the pH was 7.4 also in the presence of the drug.

The temperature varied between 22 and 23°C in the different experiments on rat toe muscles.

RESULTS AND DISCUSSION

Fig. 1 shows the effects of 4-aminopyridine on twitch and tetanus responses of a single muscle fibre of the frog. It can be seen that the twitch amplitude is increased, but it is evident that the rate of rise of tension is not changed in proportion; the twitch force continues to rise over a longer time leading to a higher amplitude and a later attainment of peak twitch tension. The maximal tetanic force, on the other hand, is not significantly affected by 4-AP. As is illustrated in Fig. 1 it is possible to potentiate the twitch to approximately

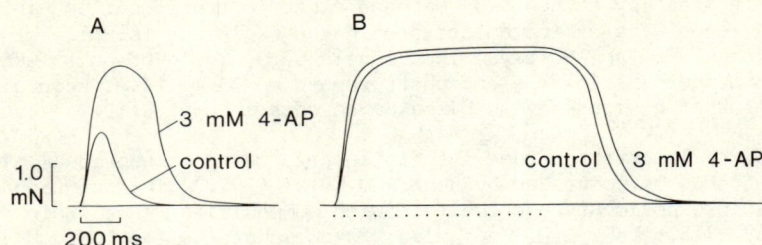

Fig. 1.  Effects of 3 mM 4-aminopyridine on isometric twitch (A) and tetanus (B) of frog single muscle fibre (Khan and Edman, 1979).

90% of the tetanic force at 3 mM 4-AP which produces maximal effect. With the twitch amplitude normally obtained in the control solution 4-AP can thus approximately double the peak twitch force (mean increase: 94 $\pm$ 2 (S.E.) %, n = 11). The increase in time to peak tension was found to average 70 $\pm$ 1% in the same experiments.

It is of interest to consider if 4-AP alters the relaxation kinetics, for this may provide a relevant clue as to whether or not the drug acts on the fibre by inhibiting the calcium reuptake by the sarcoplasmic reticulum. A change in relaxation kinetics can best be studied during the tetanus, for in this case tension starts to decay from the same maximal level both in the presence and absence of 4-aminopyridine. As is shown in Fig. 1 there is merely a slight delay in the onset of tension decay in the presence of 4-AP. This delay is most likely attributable to a longer lasting release of activator calcium (compare the difference

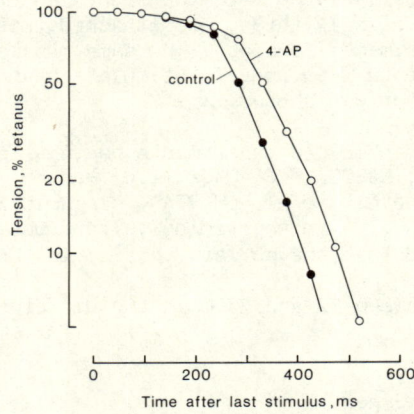

Fig. 2.  Semilogarithmic plotting of isometric relaxation during tetanus of single muscle fibre of the frog in presence and absence of 3 mM 4-aminopyridine. The data are from the same experiment as shown in Fig. 1 and are expressed in per cent of the maximum tetanic force measured with and without drug, respectively.

in time to peak force). The rate of tension decay, however, is very little changed by 4-AP. This is further demonstrated in Fig. 2 which shows a semilogarithmic plotting of the tetanus relaxation phase of the same experiment as illustrated in Fig. 1. A linear regression analysis of the log tension values within the range 5-50% of maximum tetanic tension was performed in altogether five experiments similar to that shown in Fig. 2. The time constant of the exponential decay of tension was determined from this analysis. In the presence of 3 mM 4-AP the time constant was found to be 1.03 $\pm$ 0.07 (mean $\pm$ S.E. paired observations, n = 5) of that obtained in the control Ringer solution, i.e. 4-AP did not significantly alter the relaxation kinetics. A reasonable conclusion from this finding is that 4-AP does not to any substantial degree affect the rate of resequestration of activator calcium by the sarcoplasmic reticulum.

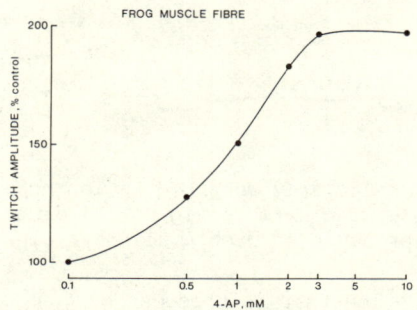

Fig. 3.  Relationship between twitch potentiation and bath concentration of 4-aminopyridine in single muscle fibre of the frog. 3$^o$C.

As is illustrated in Fig. 3 the threshold concentration of 4-AP for twitch potentiation in an isolated frog muscle fibre is between 0.1 and 0.5 mM and maximum effect is attained at about 3 mM. This is about 10x higher concentrations than found to be effective on the transmittor release at the endplate in both frog (Molgo, Lemeignan and Lechat, 1977) and mammalian (Lundh and Thesleff, 1977) muscle. For its "direct" contractile effects 4-AP is effective in somewhat lower concentrations (0.05-0.1 mM) in mammalian skeletal muscle than in frog muscle fibres (Khan and Edman, 1979). Fig. 4 illustrates, for comparison, the contractile effects on curarized toe muscle of the rat. Similar to the situation in frog muscle the rate of force development is only slightly increased, but the force continues to rise over a longer time and a higher twitch amplitude is attained. The tetanic amplitude is unaffected and, as observed in the frog fibres, the re-

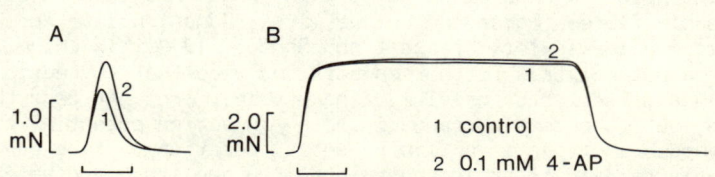

Fig. 4.  Effects of 0.1 mM 4-aminopyridine on isometric twitch and tetanus of curarized lumbrical muscle of the rat (Khan and Edman, 1979).

laxation kinetics during the tetanus is not altered in the presence of 4-AP. Effects similar to those shown in Fig. 4 were obtained by Bowman, Rodger and Savage (1979) in a study on cat tibialis anterior muscle, whereas no effects of 4-AP were observed on the cat soleus muscle. This lack of effect of 4-AP in some muscles (also see Lemeignan and Lechat, 1967 and Bowman, Harvey and Marshall, 1977) could mean that the receptor site for 4-AP is located in a deep layer of the membrane (see below) and that the accessibility of this site varies between different types of muscles.

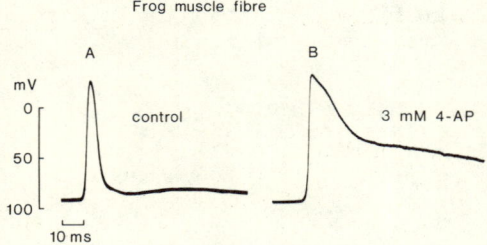

Fig. 5. Intracellularly recorded action potentials of single muscle fibres in normal Ringer (A) and in the presence of 3 mM 4-aminopyridine.

The type of twitch potentiation that is produced by 4-AP (increased twitch amplitude, prolongation of the time to peak tension with no significant change in rate of force development) is suggestive of a longer lasting release of activator calcium from the storage site. It is therefore of interest to see if 4-AP in twitch potentiating concentrations affects the action potential which most likely governs the calcium release. Fig. 5 confirms that 4-AP does indeed exert a marked effect on the action potential under these conditions. There is an increase in duration of the action potential which can be attributed entirely to a slowing of the repolarization phase, there being no significant change in resting potential or in the rate of rise and overshoot of the action potential (Khan and Edman, 1979). It is now well established that this widening of the propagated impulse is due to a quite specific blockade of the fast potassium channel by 4-AP (Pelhate and Pechon, 1974; Yeh, Oxford, Wu and Narahashi, 1976; Gillespie and Hutter, 1975).

The prolongation of the action potential is likely to play an essential role for the twitch potentiation by 4-AP, for there is reason to believe that the action potential gates the calcium release from the storage site when the action potential exceeds a certain level (e.g. Sandow, 1970). In support of this view studies of intracellular calcium transients, using aequorin as an indicator, have shown (Ashley and Ridgway, 1970) that the free calcium concentration increases progressively in amplitude and attains its peak at a later and later time, the longer the depolarizing pulse is made within a certain range. Previous experiments on both single muscle fibres (Edman and Grieve, 1966; Edman, Grieve and Nilsson, 1966) and whole muscle (Taylor, Preisser and Sandow, 1972), in which zinc was used as a twitch potentiator, further support the view that the action potential gates the release of activator calcium. Zinc probably does not pass through the fibre membrane, but it causes a graded increase in action potential duration as does 4-AP. Any such increase in action potential duration by zinc was found to be quantitatively related to an increase in twitch amplitude and an increase in duration of the mechanical activity, i.e. the same kind of changes that are seen with 4-AP. Other results are presented below which further emphasize the parallelism between the changes in action potential duration and twitch response in the presence of 4-AP. It is essential, however, also to consider other possible routes by which 4-aminopyridine may affect the mechanical output of the fibre.

One conceivable mechanism of twitch potentiation would be, as already pointed out, that the calcium pump of the sarcoplasmic reticulum is inhibited, for this would raise the concentration of activator calcium in the myofibrillar space. However, such a mechanism can almost certainly be ruled out in the case of 4-AP, since the relaxation kinetics during the tetanus is unaffected by this agent (see above).

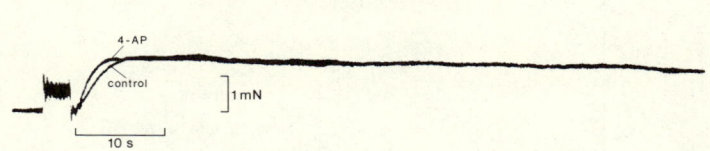

Fig. 6. Two superimposed contractures of frog single muscle fibre induced by 20 mM potassium in the presence and absence of 3 mM 4-aminopyridine. Increase in force level immediately before the onset of contracture caused by flushing of potassium solution.

The possibility to be considered next is whether 4-aminopyridine affects the mechanical threshold (Khan and Edman, 1979), i.e. the membrane potential at which the contractile activity is initiated when the fibre is depolarized. A change in mechanical threshold could arise, for example, if 4-AP in some way labilized the calcium store so that activator calcium were more easily released as the fibre membrane is depolarized. As a means of testing the mechanical threshold, contractures were produced by quickly immersing the fibre in an isotonic solution containing potassium in concentrations varying between 10 and 117.5 mM (see Methods). Fig. 6 illustrates two superimposed contractures at a submaximum potassium concentration, in the presence and absence of 4-aminopyridine. It can be seen that the total amplitude of the contracture is the same in the two situations; the time course of the two contractures is indeed very similar over the long time, more than one minute, that the fibre is activated. Fig. 7 illustrates a complete set of data for determination of the mechanical threshold. A step depolarization to 55-60 mV is required to just initiate contractile activity, and it can be seen that this threshold, or any part of the relationship between force and membrane depolarization is unaffected by 4-AP. Fig. 8 shows that 4-AP is also without effect on the contracture response to caffeine which is known to release activator calcium by acting directly on the calcium store in the sarcoplasmic reticulum (Weber and Herz, 1968; Endo, 1975). Taken together these results suggest that 4-AP does not facilitate the release of activator calcium from the storage site, neither in response to membrane depolarization nor in response to caffeine. The results also provide evidence against the idea that 4-AP increases the sensitivity of the contractile system to activator calcium. Such an effect would be expected to shift the curve relating contractile force to membrane depolarization, and no such shift can be observed.

Enhancement of the calcium influx into the cell has been proposed to play an important role for the action of aminopyridines both in cardiac muscle and at the motor end plate (Molgo, Lemeignan and Lechat, 1975 and 1977; Lundh and Thesleff, 1977; Lundh, 1978; Wollmer, Wohlfart and Khan, 1981). Such an effect is unlikely to be of relevans for the twitch potentiation by 4-AP in skeletal muscle, as the contractile effect of 4-AP also appears in the absence of calcium in the extracellular fluid. Fig. 9 presents an experiment to demonstrate this point. The left trace is the isometric twitch in ordinary calcium containing Ringer. Removal of calcium abolishes the twitch response, since lack of calcium leads to partial depolarization and inexcitability (Edman and Grieve, 1964). Introduc-

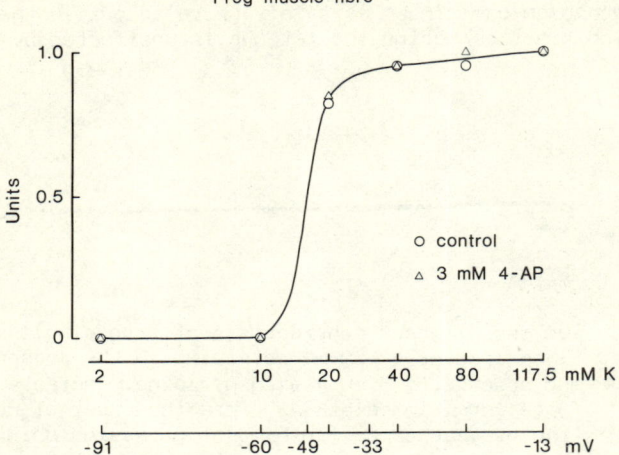

Fig. 7. Relations between contracture tension (units) and extracellular potassium concentration in the presence and absence of 3 mM 4-aminopyridine. Frog single muscle fibres. Each point represents mean value of three different experiments. Lower abscissa shows membrane potential values recorded in the absence of 4-AP in bundles of muscle fibres. Each value on this abscissa represents the mean of 19-40 impalements in at least three different bundles of muscle fibres.

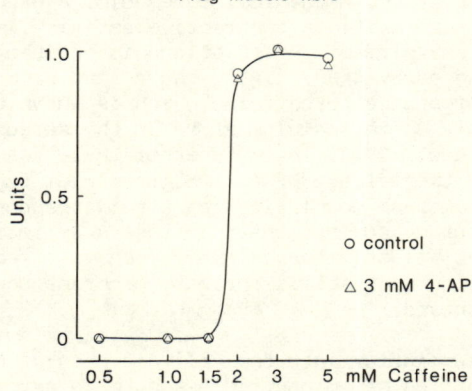

Fig. 8. Relation between peak contracture tension (units) and caffeine concentration in the presence and absence of 3 mM 4-aminopyridine. Frog muscle fibres. Each point represents mean value of three different experiments (Khan and Edman, 1979).

Frog muscle fibre

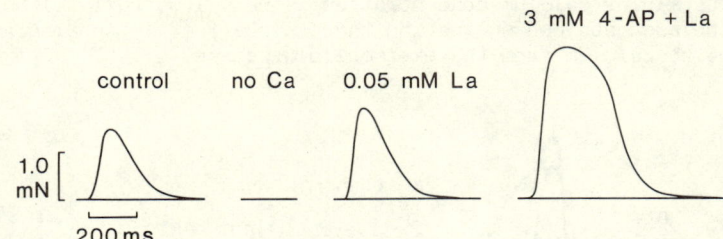

Fig. 9. Effect of 4-aminopyridine on isometric twitch response of frog single muscle fibre after removal of calcium from the extracellular medium and introduction of 0.05 mM lanthanum. Note that: 1. lack of extracellular calcium abolishes twitch response, 2. introduction of lanthanum restores twitch and 3. twitch potentiation is produced in the calcium--lacking, lanthanum-containing medium (Khan and Edman, 1979).

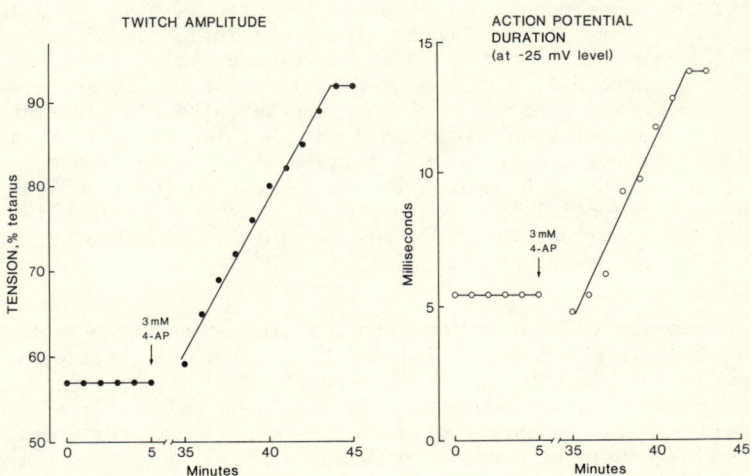

Fig. 10. Development of twitch potentiation (left) and increase in action potential duration (right) after addition of 4-aminopyridine (3 mM) and its relation to the number of times the fibre is electrically stimulated. After the addition of 4-AP the fibre was kept resting for 30 min. Thereafter a single supramaximal stimulus was applied at one-minute intervals. The data in the left and right diagrams are from two different fibre preparations. The action potential recordings in the right diagram were made while the fibre was mechanically inactivated by immersion in a Ringer solution made hypertonic by addition of 200 mM sucrose.

tion of lanthanum restores the twitch, as lanthanum is able to take over calcium's function in the membrane and reestablish membrane polarization and excitability (Andersson and Edman, 1974). Unlike calcium, however, lanthanum probably does not pass into the cell (Lesseps 1967; Langer and Frank, 1972, van Breemen and co-workers, 1972). When 4-aminopyridine is added at this state, i.e. at a point where the extracellular calcium concentration is very low, full twitch potentiation is nevertheless obtained suggesting that this effect is not mediated by enhanced inflow of calcium from the extracellular space.

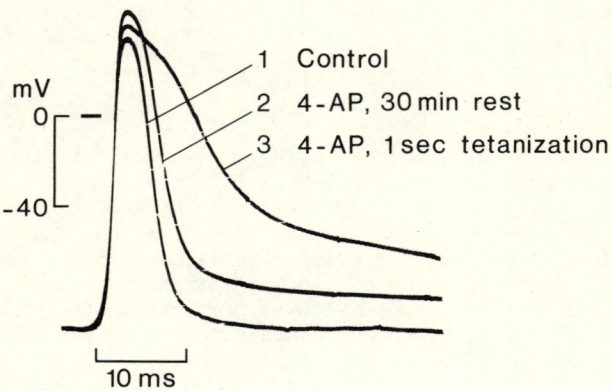

Fig. 11. Superimposed action potentials from a single muscle fibre of the frog to illustrate influence of membrane excitation on the development of 4-AP effect. Record 1: action potential in ordinary Ringer solution. Record 2: action potential after 30 min rest in solution containig 3 mM 4-AP. Immediately thereafter a supramaximal tetanic stimulation (1 sec, 20 Hz) was applied to the fibre. Record 3: action potential recorded one min after the tetanic stimulation. The fibre was mechanically inactivated as described in Fig. 10.

4-Aminopyridine appears to bind strongly to the site where it acts on the fibre, for its effects on both action potential and twitch are only partially reversible (Khan and Edman, 1979). At the neutral pH normally used, 4-aminopyridine has a positive charge and membrane depolarization is found to greatly speed up the effects of 4-AP. This is demonstrated in Fig. 10 which shows the development of twitch potentiation (left) and the increase in action potential duration (right), respectively. The twitch force can be seen to be very little influenced if the fibre is left unstimulated in the 4-AP containing medium for 30 min. The small increase recorded at this time can in fact be attributed to the rest per se. Application of a single stimulus at one-minute intervals causes a steady increase in twitch force, maximum twitch amplitude (about 90 per cent of the tetanic force) being attained after about 10 stimuli. The increase in action potential can be seen to have a similar relation to the number of stimuli applied. No increase in action potential duration is observed after 30 min rest in the aminopyridine solution, but a steady widening of the action potential occurs by each subsequent stimulus until a maximum is reached after about 8 stimuli. That this behaviour does not reflect a peculiar time dependence of the effect is demonstrated in Fig. 11. Illustrated are action potentials recorded 1. under control conditions in ordinary Ringer, 2. after 30 min rest in a solution containing 3 mM 4-AP and 3. one minute after the fibre had been tetanized for 1 sec following trace 2. As can be seen, the one-second tetanization (including about 20 action potentials) suffices to make 4-AP develop its full effect. It can be mentioned in this connection that any other means of depolarization, such as electrotonic pulses or potassium depolarization, has the same influence on the onset of the aminopyridine effect. This dependence on membrane depolarization could mean that 4-AP, in order to act, may have to reach the inner surface of the plasma membrane or, at least, pass into the interior of the membrane.

In conclusion, these results have shown that 4-aminopyridine is able to greatly potentiate twitch force in skeletal muscle by acting directly on the muscle fibres. The twitch enhancement can be attributed to the membrane action of 4-AP which leads to prolongation of the action potential and therefore to a longer lasting release of activator calcium. The evidence obtained on the intact fibre preparation lends very little support for the idea that 4-AP would exert any more specific action on the metabolism of activator calcium or affect the response of the contractile system to calcium.

ACKNOWLEDGEMENT

This study was supported by grants from the Swedish Medical Research Council (project 14X-184) and from the Medical Faculty, University of Lund.

REFERENCES

Andersson, K.-E. and K. A. P. Edman (1974). Effects of lanthanum on the coupling between membrane excitation and contraction of isolated frog muscle fibres. Acta Physiol. Scand., 90, 113-123.

Andersson, K.-E. and K. A. P. Edman (1974). Effects of lanthanum on potassium contractures of isolated twitch muscle fibres of the frog. Acta Physiol. Scand., 90, 124-131.

Ashley, C. C. and E. B. Ridgway (1970). On the relationships between membrane potential, calcium transient and tension in single barnacle muscle fibres. J. Physiol. (Lond.), 209, 105-130.

Bowman, W. C., A. L. Harvey and J. G. Marshall (1977). The actions of aminopyridines on avian muscle. Naunyn-Schmiedeberg's Arch. Pharmacol., 297, 99-103.

Bowman, W. C., I. W. Rodger and A. O. Savage (1979). Effect of 4-aminopyridine on muscle contractility in the cat. Brit. J. Pharmacol. 66, 466-467P.

Edman, K. A. P. and D. W. Grieve (1964). On the role of calcium in the excitation--contraction process of frog sartorius muscle. J. Physiol. (Lond.), 170, 138-152.

Edman, K. A. P. and D. W. Grieve (1966). The relation between the electrical and mechanical activities of single muscle fibres in the presence of zinc. J. Physiol. (Lond.), 185, 29-31P.

Edman, K. A. P., D. W. Grieve and E. Nilsson (1966). Studies of the excitation--contraction mechanism in the skeletal muscle and the myocardium. Pflügers Arch., 290, 320-334.

Edman, K. A. P. and A. Kiessling (1971). The time course of the active state in relation to sarcomere length and movement studied in single skeletal muscle fibres of the frog. Acta Physiol. Scand., 81, 182-196.

Endo, M. (1975). Mechanism of action of caffeine on the sarcoplasmic reticulum of skeletal muscle. Proc. Japan. Acad. 51, 479-484.

Gillespie, J. I. and D. F. Hutter (1975). The action of 4-aminopyridine on the delayed potassium current in skeletal muscle fibres. J. Physiol. (Lond.), 252, 70-71P.

Illés, P. and S. Thesleff (1978). 4-aminopyridine and evoked transmitter release from motor nerve endings. Br. J. Pharmacol., 64, 623-629.

Khan, A. R. and K. A. P. Edman (1979). Effects of 4-aminopyridine on the excitation-contraction coupling in frog and rat skeletal msucle. Acta Physiol. Scand., 105, 443-452.

Langer, G. A. and J. S. Frank (1972). Lanthanum in heart cell culture. Effect on calcium exchange correlated with its localization. J. Cell. Biol., 54, 441-455.

Lemeignan, M. and P. Lechat (1967). Sur l'action anticurare des aminopyridines. C.R. Acad. Sci. (Paris), 264, 169-172.

Lesseps, R. J. (1967). Removal by phospholipase C of a layer of La staining material external to the cell membrane in embryonic chick cell. J. Cell. Biol., 34, 173-183.

Lundh, H. (1978). Effects of 4-aminopyridine on neuromuscular transmission. Brain Res., 153, 307-318.

Lundh, H., O. Nilsson and I. Rosén (1977). 4-aminopyridine - a new drug tested in the treatment of Eaton-Lambert syndrome. J. Neurol. Neurosurg. Psychiat., 40, 1109-1112.

Lundh, H., O. Nilsson and I. Rosén (1979). Effects of 4-aminopyridine in myasthenia gravis. J. Neurol. Neurosurg. Psyhiat., 42, 171-175.

Lundh, H. and S. Thesleff (1977). The mode of action of 4-aminopyridine and guanidine on transmitter release from motor nerve terminals. Eur. J. Pharmacol., 42, 411-412.

Molgo, J., M. Lemeignan and P. Lechat (1975). Modification de la libération du transmetteur à la jonction neuromusculaire de grenouille sous l'action de l'amino-4 pyridine. C. R. Acad. Sci. (Paris), 281, 1637-1639.

Molgo, J., M. Lemeignan and P. Lechat (1977). Effects of 4-aminopyridine at the frog neuromuscular junction. J. Pharmacol. Exp. Ther., 203, 653-663.

Molgo, J., H. Lundh and S. Thesleff (1980). Potency of 3,4-diaminopyridine and 4-aminopyridine on mammalian neuromuscular transmission and the effect of pH changes. Eur. J. Pharmacol., 61, 25-34.

Pelhate, M. and Y. Pichon (1974). Selective inhibition of potassium current in the giant axon of the cockroach. J. Physiol. (Lond.), 242, 90-91P.

Sandow, A. (1970). Skeletal muscle. Ann. Rev. Physiol., 32, 87-138.

Taylor, S. R., H. Preiser and A. Sandow (1972). Action potential parameters affecting excitation-contraction coupling. J. gen. Physiol., 59, 421-436.

Thesleff, S. (1980). Aminopyridines and synaptic transmission. Neuroscience, 5, 1413-1419.

Van Breemen, C., B. R. Farinas, P. Gerba and E. D. McNaughton (1972). Excitation-contraction coupling in rabbit aorta studied by the lanthanum method for measuring cellular calcium influx. Circulat. Res., 30, 44-54.

Weber, A. and R. Herz (1968). The relationship between caffeine contracture of intact muscle and the effect of caffeine on reticulum. J. gen. Physiol., 52, 750-759.

Wollmer, P., B. Wohlfart and A. R. Khan (1981). Effects of 4-aminopyridine on contractile response and action potential of rabbit papillary muscle. Acta Physiol. Scand., (in press).

Yeh, J. Z., G. S. Oxford, C. H. Wu and J. Narahashi (1976). Interaction of aminopyridines with potassium channels of squid axon membranes. Biophys. J., 16, 77-81.

Yong, I. K., M. M. Goldner and D. B. Sanders (1980). Facilitatory effects of 4-aminopyridine on neuromuscular transmission in disease states. Muscle & Nerve, 3, 112-119.

# Effects of 4-Aminopyridine on Cardiac Muscle

T. Yanagisawa* and N. Taira**

*Department of Physiology, G4, University of Pennsylvania School of Medicine, Philadelphia, PA 19104, USA
**Department of Pharmacology, Tohoku University School of Medicine, Sendai, Japan

ABSTRACT

4-Aminopyridine (4-AP) released spontaneously neurotransmitters from both parasympathetic and sympathetic nerves in the isolated, blood-perfused sino-atrial node preparation of the dog. The mechanism of the release of neurotransmitters would be due to the excitation of the autonomic nerves by 4-AP. Under the condition which these effects of neurotransmitters on cardiac muscle were abolished by β-blockers, pindolol or propranolol and/or atropine, 4-AP produced a positive inotropic effect on dog ventricular muscle not on frog ventricular strips. The positive inotropic effect of 4-AP was characterized by the slow relaxation accompanied the prolongation of the action potential.

KEYWORDS

4-Aminopyridine; sinus rate; parasympathetic nerves; sympathetic nerves; nerve excitation; tetrodotoxin; ventricular muscle; relaxation; action potential; calcium

INTRODUCTION

The purpose of this study is to investigate the effects of 4-aminopyridine (4-AP) on the cardiac function. Aminopyridines have been known to produce convulsion in mammals. Recently they have been shown to inhibit the potassium conductance in nerves (Pelhate and Pichon, 1974; Schauf and others, 1976; Yeh and others, 1976) and in skeletal muscle (Gillespie and Hutter, 1975). Aminopyridines have also been shown to facilitate neuromuscular transmission in skeletal muscle (Molgo, Lemeignan and Lechat,1975; Bowman, Harvey and Marshall, 1977; Lundh, Leander and Thesleff, 1977). However, it remains unsettled whether 4-AP would be able to excite the autonomic nerves, which have much influences on cardiac function. To obtain the infromation of the effect of 4-AP on cardiac autonomic nerves, we used the isolated, blood-perfused sino-atrial (SA) node preparation of the dog. Further, we investigated the effect of 4-AP on the contractility of both dog and frog ventricular muscles. To get some insight into the mechanism responsible for the action on myocardial contractility, the effect of 4-AP on the membrane potentials was also investigated.

## MATERIALS AND METHODS

### Isolated, Blood-Perfused Sino-Atrial (SA) Node Preparation of the Dog

The preparation is essentially the right atrium included with SA node and is perfused by the heparinized arterial bood from a donor dog, via the cannulated SA node artery(Chiba, Kubota and Hashimoto, 1972; Kubota and Hashimoto, 1973). This preparation contains parasympathetic and sympathetic nerves which are free from the tonic control of the central nervous system. Blood flow through the cannulated SA node artery was monitored by an electromagnetic flowmeter. Sinus rate was measured by the use of cardiotachometer triggered by atrial bipolar electrograms obtained from the SA node area. The drugs were injected intra-arterially.

### Isometric Contraction and Membrane Potential Studies Using Dog Ventricular Muscle

Hearts were obtained from both untreated dogs and those preteated with reserpin. Trabecular muscles, less than 1 mm in diameter and between 10 — 15 mm in length, were excised from the right ventricle. Muscles were suspended in 20-ml organ baths containing Krebs-Henseleit solution which had the following composition (in mM): NaCl 118; $NaHCO_3$ 24.9; KCl 4.7; $KH_2PO_4$ 1.2; $CaCl_2$ 2.5; $MgSO_4$ 1.2; Glucose 11.1. The solution was equilibrated with 95% $O_2$ and 5% $CO_2$ at a temperature of 37°C to give a pH of 7.4. Muscles were driven with rectangular electric pulses of about 1.2 times the threshold voltage and 5-ms duration at a rate of 0.5 Hz delivered by electronic stimulators. Contractions were measured isometrically with strain-gauge transducers and recorded on a chart with a rectilinear recorder. After 1-hr equilibration drug solutions were added to the baths. The concentration of 4-AP was increased cumulatively.

The following measurements were made on the isometric contraction curves recorded on chart: force of contraction ($F_c$), time to peak force ($t_1$), relaxation time ($t_2$), meanvelocity of force development ($S_1$) and mean velocity of relaxation ($S_2$). Changes in mean velocity of force development (klinotropic effect, $\Delta S_1$) and resting force were also measured.

Membrane potential was recorded with conventional glass microelectrodes filled with 3-M KCl and having a resistance of 8 — 20 M$\Omega$. The output from the microelectrode was fed to an electrometer, displayed on the screen of a dual-beam cathode ray oscilloscope and finally photographed on 35-mm film with an oscilloscope camera. The following measurements were made on the photographic records: the resting membrane potential(RMP), the action potential amplitude (AMP), the maximum rate of rise of the action potential ($\dot{V}_{max}$) and the action potential duration at the 30% (APD30), 50% (APD50) and 90% (APD90) levels of repolarization.

### Isometric Contration and Membrane Potential Studies Using Frog Ventricular Strip

Quiescent strips were prepared from circular cuts through the ventricle of the frog maintained at room temperature (23 °C). Strips averaged 0.3 — 0.5 mm in diameter and 5 — 7 in length. Strips were mounted on the single sucrose gap chamber (Morad and Orkand, 1971; Goldman and Morad, 1977). Standard perfusate was normal Ringer solution, consisting 116 mM-NaCl, 2 mM-$NaHCO_3$, 3 mM-KCl 1 mM-$CaCl_2$. Strips were stmulated at a frequency of 0.2 Hz. Tension of a strip was measured by force transducer and membrane potential was measured by transgap potential of the single sucrose gap technique.

## Drugs

4-Aminopyridine base (Wako, Sigma), nicotine base (Merck), methacholine chloride (Merck), atropine sulphate (Merck), (-)-iosprenaline hydrochloride (Nikken Kagaku), (-)-hyoscyamine sulphate (Merck), (+)-propranolol hydrochloride (ICI, Aryest), tetrodotoxin (Sankyo), (+)-pindolol base (Sandoz) and resrepin (Daiichi Seiyaku). 4-AP base was dissolved in 0.9% saline. The pH of 4-AP solution was adjusted to about 7 by the addition of 1 N HCl.

Values are given in terms of mean ± S.E. The difference between mean values was analysed by Student's $t$-test, and jdged to be significant when $P$ values were lees than 0.05.

## RESULTS

### Effect of 4-AP on the Rate of the Isolated, Blood-Perfused SA Node Preparation

The average basal rate of 8 preparation was 106 ± 6 beats/min and the average blood flow through the sinus node artery was 3.4 ± 0.2 ml/min. 4-AP (1 — 3 µmol) injected into the sinus node artery produced a long-lasting decrease in sinus rate preceded by a transient increase. With 10 µmol of 4-AP the sinus rate decreased after a transient increase but again tended to increase. The peak of this rather long-lasting increase in sinus rate, however, only slightly surpassed the basal rate (Fig. 1a) and a long-lasting decrease ensued.

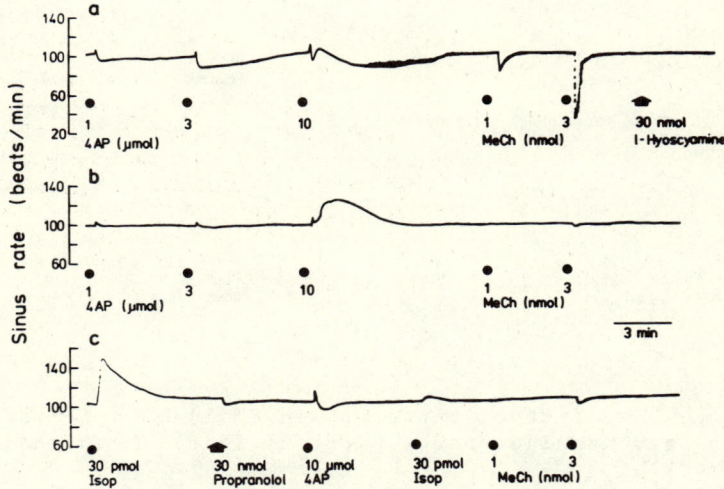

Fig. 1. Effect of 4-AP on the sinus rate (a). Effect of l-hyoscyamine on the 4-AP-induced changes in sinus rate (b). Effect of l-hyoscyamine and propranolol on the 4-AP-induced changes in sinus rate (c). Drugs were injected intra-arterially. Mechachiline (MeCh), Isoprenaline (Isop).

### Effects of Hyoscyamine and Propranolol on the 4-AP-Induced Changes in Sinus Rate

After a single intra-arterial injection of 30 nmol of l-hyoscyamine, which abolished the decrease in sinus rate in response to methacholine (1 — 3 nmol), the long-lasting decrease in sinus rate in response to 4-AP (1 — 10 μmol) was also abolished or reversed to an increase The long-lasting increase in sinus rate in response to 10 μmol of 4-AP was enhanced (Fig. 1b). During the blockade of muscarinic receptors by l-hyoscyamine, the long-lasting increase in sinus rate in response to 10 μmol of 4-AP was abolished by a single intra-arterial injection of propranolol (30 nmol) which fully antagonized the increase in sinus rate in response to isoprenaline (30 pmol) (Fig. 1c).

### Effect of Intra-Arterial Infusion of Tetrodotoxin on the 4-AP-Induced Changes in Sinus Rate

Both the long-lasting decrease and the increase in sinus rate in response to 4-AP were greatly reduced by intra-arterial infusion of tetrodotoxin (0.3 nmol/min) which abolished the decrease and increase in sinus rate in response to nicitine (10 — 30 nmol). The decrease in sinus rate produced by methacholine was not changed by the infusion of tetrodotoxin (Fig. 2).

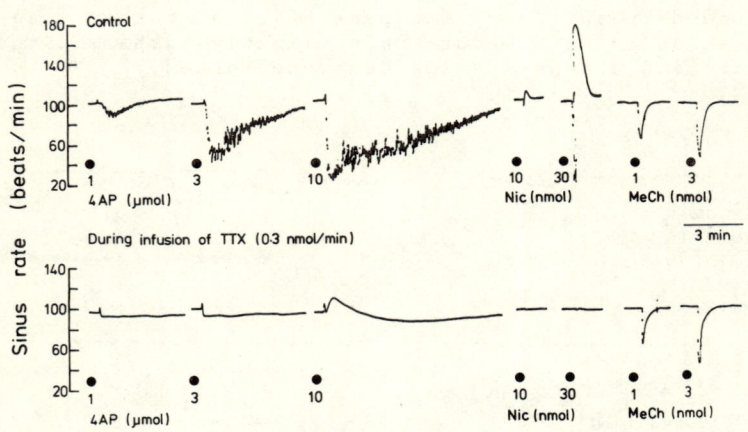

Fig. 2. Effect of tetrodotoxin (TTX) on 4-AP-induced changes in sinus rate. Nicotine (Nic), Methacholine (MeCh).

### Effect of 4-AP on Isometric Contractions of Untreated Ventricular Muscles of the Dog

The mean values of 5 parameters of isometric contractions of 13 untreated ventricular muscles are as follows: force of contraction ($F_c$),

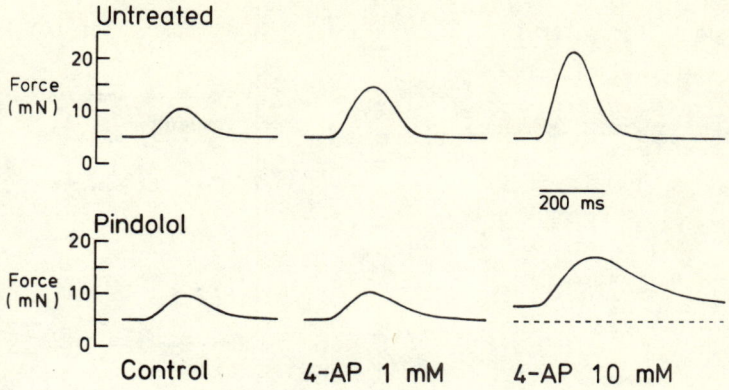

Fig. 3. Effect of 4-AP on isometric contractions of untreated (upper panel) and pindolol-treated (lower panel) ventricular muscles of the dog. A dashed line indicates the resting force in control.

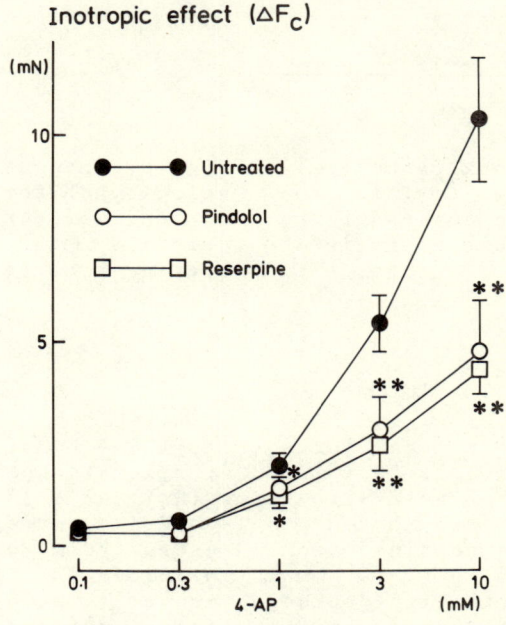

Fig. 4. The positive inotropic effect ($\Delta F_c$) of 4-AP on untreated and pidolol-treated ventricular muscles and on ventricular muscles obtained from reserpine-pretreated dogs. Each symbol is the mean values and vertical bars are S.E. * $P < 0.05$, ** $P < 0.01$ compared with corresponding values of untreated muscles.

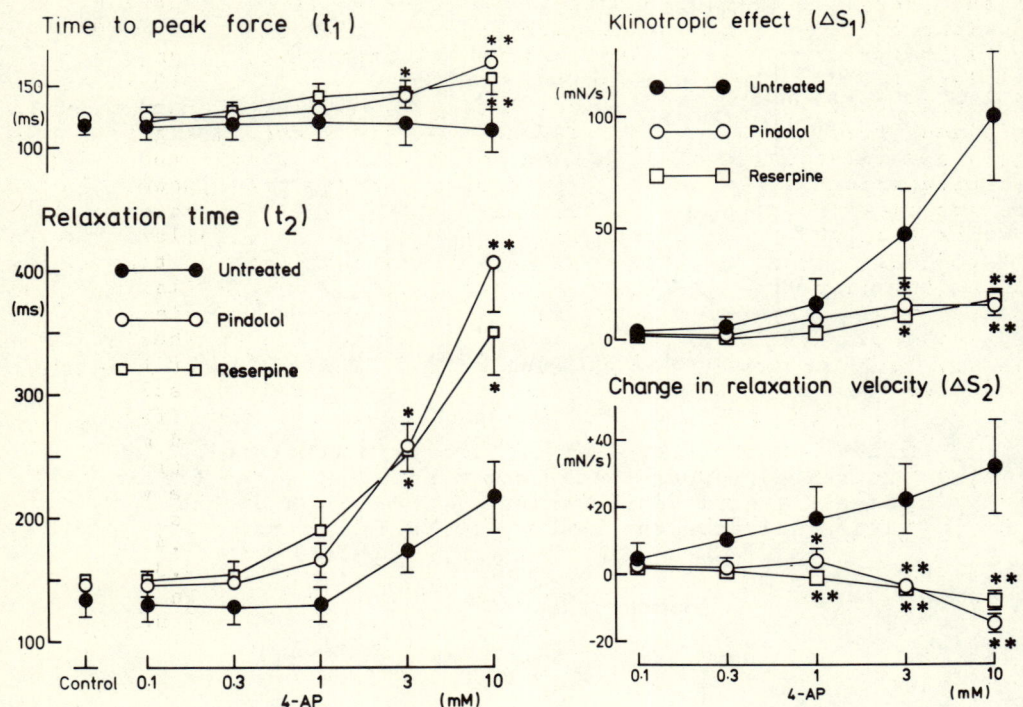

Fig. 5. Time to peak force ($t_1$) and relaxation time ($t_2$) in isometric contraction curves of the dog ventricular muscles as influenced by 4-AP.

Fig. 6. Changes caused by 4-AP in velocity of force development (klinotropic effect) and relaxation velocity of the isometrically contracting trabeculae.

$5.7 \pm 1.3$ mN; time to peak force ($t_1$), $118 \pm 8$ ms; mean velocity of force development ($S_1$), $50 \pm 19$ mN/s; relaxation time ($t_2$), $134 \pm 14$ ms; mean velocity of relaxation time ($S_2$), $45 \pm 17$ mN/s. Fig. 1 shows the effect of 1 and 10 mM 4-AP on isometric contractions of an untreated muscle. Results obtained from 13 untreated muscles are summarized in Figs. 4, 5 and 6. 4-AP (0.1 — 10 mM) produced a positive inotropic effect in a concentration-dependent manner (Fig. 4). The time to peak force ($t_1$) was not changed by these concentrations of 4-AP and the relaxation time ($t_2$) was prolonged by 3 and 10 mM 4-AP (Fig. 5). 4-AP produced a positive klinotropic effect and increased the relaxation velocity (Fig. 6). With 10 mM 4-AP there occured a slight but not significant increase in resting force ($0.1 \pm 0.1$ mN)

### Effects of 4-AP on Isometric Contractions of Pindolol-Treated Ventricular Muscles and of Ventricular Muscles Obtained from Reserpine-Pretreated Dogs

In the absence of 4-AP (control) the 5 parameters of isometric contractions of 12 ventricular muscles exposed to pindolol ($3 \times 10^{-8}$ M) for 1 hr were not significantly different from those of untreated muscles. Fig. 1 (lower panel) shows the effect of 1 and 10 mM 4-AP on isometric contrations of a pindolol-treated muscle. Summarized results obtained from 12 pindilol-treated muscles are shown in Figs. 4, 5 and 6. In pidolol-treated muscles, too, 4-AP (0.1 — 10 mM) produced a positive inotropic effect in a concentration-dependent manner. However, the positive inotropic effect of 4-AP on pindolol-treated muscles was smaller than that on untreated muscles (Fig. 4). Dissimilarly to untreated muscles 4-AP produced slight prolongation of the time to peak force ($t_1$) in pindolol-treated muscles (Fig. 5). Similarly to untreated muscles 4-AP increased the relaxation time ($t_2$) in pidolol-treated muscles (Fig. 5). However, the prolongation of the relaxation time by 4-AP in pindolol-treated muscles was much greater than that in untreated muscles (Fig. 5). Dissimilarly to untreated muscles 4-AP (0.1 — 10 mM) scarcely produced a positive klinotropic effect (Fig. 6) and decreased the relaxation velocity in pindolol-treated muscles (Fig. 6). The effects of 4-AP on isometric contractions of ventricular muscles (n = 13) obtained from dogs pretreated with reserpine were essentially similar to those on pindolol-treated muscles (Figs. 4, 5 and 6). 4-AP at 10 mM produced an increase in resting force by $1.4 \pm 0.3$ mN ($P$ 0.01) in muscles treated with pidolol and by $1.5 \pm 0.3$ mN ($P$ 0.01) in those obtained from dogs pretreated with reserpine. In pindolol-treated muscle the addition of atropine ($1 \times 10^{-6}$ M) did not influence the effect of 4-AP on the isometric contractions.

## Effect of 4-AP on the Membrane Potential of Pindolol-Treated Ventricular Muscles

In Fig. 7 are shown superimposed tracings of action potentials obtained by a single impalement of a single cell in a pidolol-treated muscle in the absence and presence of 4-AP. Mean control values of the resting membrane potential and various parameters of the action potential of 11 pindolol-treated ventricular muscle in the absence of 4-AP (control) are shown in Fig. 8. It is obvious that the action potential duration (APD) is prolonged by 4-AP in a concentration-dependent manner. 4-AP did not significantly alter the resting membrane potential. The action potential amplitude was slightly increased but the maximum rate of rise of the action potential was reduced at the concentration of 3 and 10 mM 4-AP (Fig. 8). The phase 1 repolarization was slowed by 4-AP (1 — 10 mM) (Fig. 7). As clearly seen in Figs. 7 and 8, the most prominent effect of 4-AP on the transmembrane potential of pindolol-treated muscles was a concentration -dependent increase in action potentail duration at the 30, 50 and 90% levels of repolarization.

## Effect of 4-AP on the Frog Ventricular Strip

In untreated frog ventricular stips 4-AP (0.3 — 1 mM) produced a negative inotropic effect with shortening of the action potential duration (Figs. 9 and 10). However at the concentration of 3 — 10 mM of 4-AP, a positive inotropic effect with the prolongation of the action potential became obious (Figs. 9 and 10). In atropine-treated ($1 \times 10^{-6}$ M) strips 4-AP (0.3 — 10 mM) produced a positive inotropic effect with the prolongation of the action potential. This positive inotropic effect of 4-AP was completely abolished by the further addition of pro-

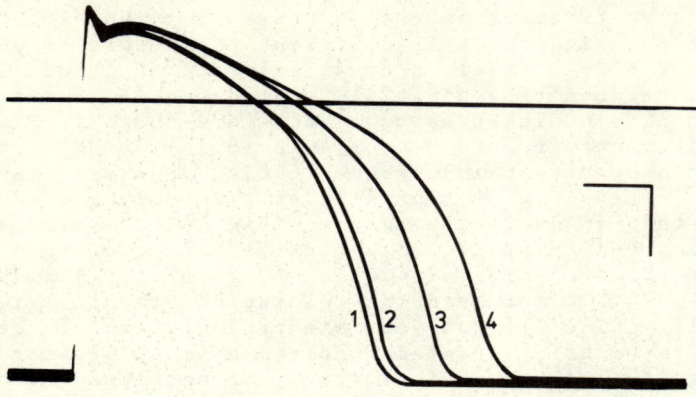

Fig. 7. Effect of 4-AP on the action potential of a pindolol-treated ventricular muscle of the dog. Horizontal line indicats 0 mV, the horizontal bar is 50 ms and the vertical bar is 20 mV. 1, Control; 2, 1 mM; 3, 3 mM; 4, 10 mM 4-AP.

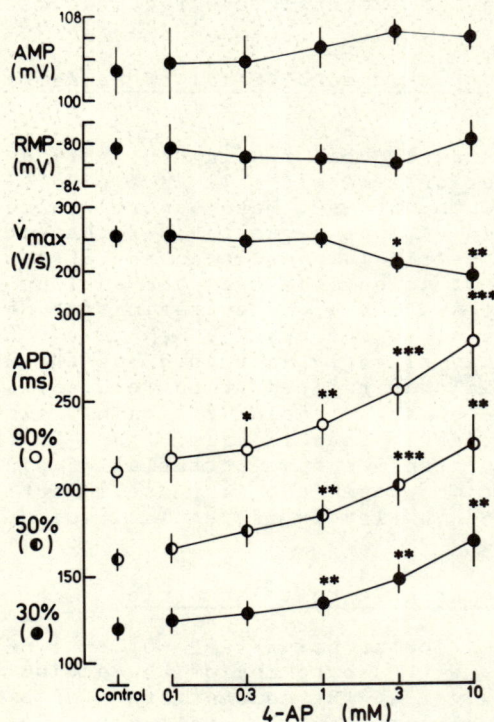

Fig. 8. Effect of 4-AP on the membrane potential of pindolol-treated muscles. Significantly different from control values: * $\underline{P} < 0.05$, ** $\underline{P} < 0.01$, *** $\underline{P} < 0.001$.

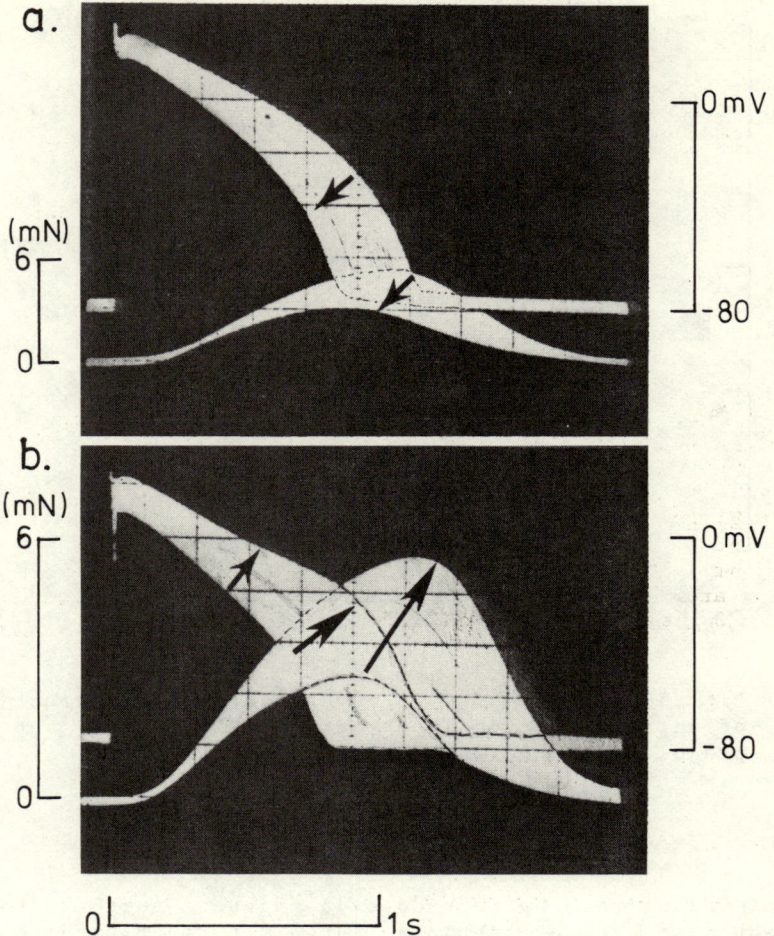

Fig. 9. Effect of 4-AP on the contraction and the membrane potential of an untreated frog ventricular strip. a. Form control to 1 mM 4-AP. b. From 1 mM to 3 mM 4-AP.

pranolol ($1 \times 10^{-6}$ M) in Ringer solution. In the presence of both atropine and propranolol 4-AP did not change the membrane potential greatly.

DISCUSSION

The Isolated, Blood-Perfused SA node Preparation

In the study using the isilated blood-perfused preparation of the dog, 4-AP injected into the sinus node artery produced a long-lasting decrease in sinus rate. Its abolition by (-)-hyoscyamine indicates that the decrease was mediated by cholinergic mechanism. Reduction of the

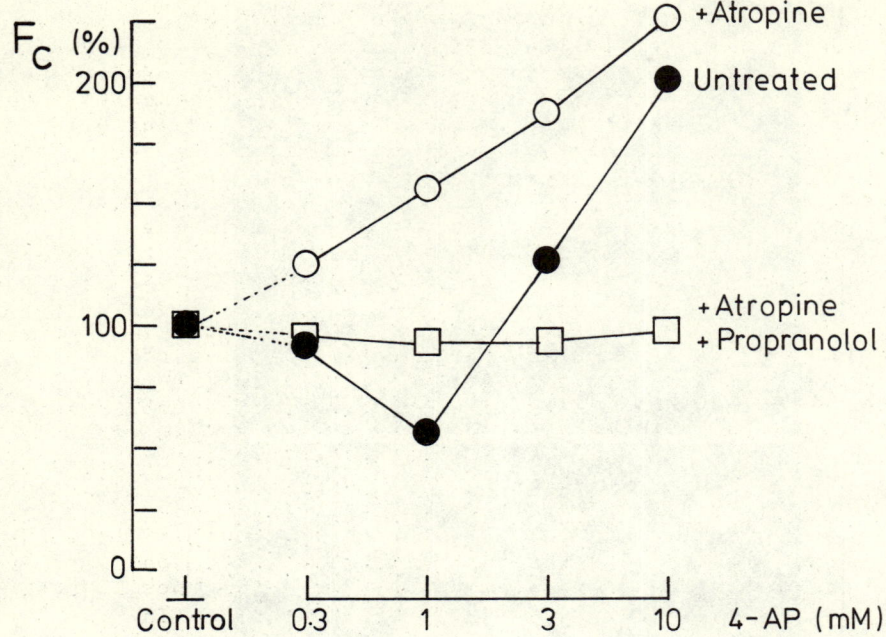

Fig. 10. Effect of 4-AP on the force of contractions of untreated, atropine-treated and atropine- and propranolol-treated frog ventricular strips.

decrease in sinus rate by tetrodotoxin suggests further that a cholinergic mechanism becomes operative largely through excitation of parasympathetic nerve fibers. With a large dose of 4-AP there appeared a rather long-lasting increase in sinus rate which became manifest under the blockade of muscarinic receptors. Since the increase was abolished by propranolol, this was entirely due to an adrenergic mechanism. The reduction of this response by tetrodotoxin suggests that the release of catecholamines by 4-AP would involove the excitation of adrenergic fibers. Evidence obtained in this study is thus sufficient to prove that 4-AP is able to excite both parasympathetic cholinergic and sympathetic adrenergic nerve fibers in the isolated, blood-perfused SA node preparation of the dog. Since the preparation was free from the tonic control of the central nervous sysstem, the observed effect of 4-AP cannot be taken as the facilitatory effect of 4-AP on autonomic neuroeffector junctions in SA node cells. In this respect the present results differ distinctly from the facilitatory effect of 4-AP as obserbed in the neuromuscular junction in the skeletal muscle (Molgo, Lemeignan and Lechat, 1975; Bowman, Harvey and Marshall, 1977; Lundh, Leander and Thesleff, 1977) and adrenergic neuroeffector junctions in the rabbit vas deferens (Johns and others, 1976), in cat spleen (Kirpeker, Kirpeker and Prat, 1977) and in rat portal vein (Leander, Arner and Johansson, 1977). Therefore, possible mechanisms underlying the excitant action of 4-AP should be argued. Reduction by tetrodotoxin of the action of 4-AP may suggest its facilittatory effect on sodium conductance. Such an effect of 4-AP was supposed on guinea pig ventricular strips (Lemeignan and others, 1975) and on chick immature muscle fibers (Thomson and Dryden, 1980). However, in Myxicola giant axons (Schauf and others, 1976) and squid giant axons (Yeh and others, 1976), 4-AP has no effect on sodium conductance. It is difficult to dicide whether this mechanism is reponsible the excitant effect of 4-AP on autonomic nerves. Autonomic nerve fibers in this preparation are unlikely to fire spontaneously, thus the long-lasting action of 4-AP as reported here implies repetitive firing of autonomic nerve fibers. It is difficult to consider that the inhibition of delayed outward current as supposed in invertebrate giant axons (Pelhate and Pichon, 1974) and frog skeletal muscle (Gillespie and Hutter, 1975) is responsible to the repetitive firing of the autonomic nerves. 4-AP may reduce the backgroung potassium conductance in autonomic nerve fibers and depolarize the membrane so as to lead repetitive firing. Such a depolarization of postsynapic membrane of the ganglion of the cockroach (Hue and others, 1978) was reported.

## The Study Using Ventricular Muscles of the Dog

In this study 4-AP produced a positive inotropic effect on untreated ventricular muscles. This effect was associated with a positive klinotropic effect and an increase in relaxation velocity. Inthese respects the effects of 4-AP$_{on}$ isometric contractions of untreated muscles resemble those of catecholamines (Reiter, 1972). Unlike catecholamines, however, 4-AP did not shorten the time to peak force and at 3 and 10 mM prolonged the relaxation time. The positive inotropic effect of 4-AP was reduced and the positive klinotropic effect was nearly abolished in muscle in which β-adrenoceptors were blocked by pindolol and in those obtained from dogs in which endogenous catecholamines had been depleted by pretreatment with reserpine. In these muscles the relaxation velocity was rather decreased by 4-AP. As elucidated in our previous study (Yanagisawa, Satoh and Taira, 1978), the release of endogenous catecholamines appears in all probability to result from the excitation by 4-AP of adrenergic nerve fibers in ventricular muscles. Thus, it is reasonable to conclude that the positive inotropic effect of 4-AP is due partly to the release of endogenous catecholamines by 4-AP. The remaining positive inotropic effect is attributable to the direct action of 4-AP on ventricular muscle. In muscles treated with pindolol or those obtained from dogs pretreated with reserpine the highest concentration of 4-AP (10 mM) produced an increase in resting force. Catecholamines are known to facilitate relaxation (Brady, 1964; Reiter, 1972; Morad, Sanders and Weiss, 1981). Thus, the absence of the effect of 4-AP in increasing the resting force in untreated muscles can also be explained on the basis of the relaxant action of catecholamines.

The positive inotropic effect as the direct action of 4-AP on ventricular muscle was associated with marked prolongation of the relaxation time and a decrease in relaxation velocity. As the direct action of 4-AP ther was slight prolongation of the time to peak force but the klinotropic effect was nearly absent. Thus, the direct positive inotropic effect of 4-AP appears to be mainly due to interference with the process of relaxation. The retardation of the relaxation process by 4-AP suggests that the intracellular concentration of Ca$^{2+}$ may somehow remain high for a longer period than under the normal condition. This would also be conceivable as a possible mechanism for the increase in resting force produced by the highest concentration of 4-AP (10 mM) in muscle treated with pindolol or those obtained from reserpine-pretreated dogs. As proposed to interpret the facilitaion by 4-AP of neuroeffector transmission, four possibilities are conceivable as to mechanisms for the direct positive inotropic action of 4-AP on cardiac muscle.

Firstly 4-AP would prolong the duration of the action potential and allow the slow calcium channel to open longer and more $Ca^{2+}$ to enter (Johns and others, 1976; Bowman, Harvey and Marshall, 1977; Kirpeker, Kirpeker and Prat, 1977; Leander, Arner and Johansson, 1977; Lundh, Leander and Thesleff, 1977). Secondly 4-AP might release $Ca^{2+}$ from their binding or storage sites (Harvey and Marshall, 1977). Thirdly 4-AP might slow binding of intracellular $Ca^{2+}$ to intracellular structures (Lundh, Leander and Thesleff, 1977). Forthly 4-AP directly increases calcium conductance (Lundh and Thesleff, 1977). In nerve terminal the first possibility has been considered in association with the prolongation of the outward-going delayed potassium current.

In the present study, 4-AP prolonged the action potential duration of pindolol-treated ventricular muscles. This may be due to the inhibition of outward-going potassium current as is the case with nerve fibers (Hue, Perhate and Chanelet, 1973; Pelhate and Pichon, 1974). Ochi and Nishiye (1974) observed that when applied intracellularly to guiea pig papillary muscles, tetraethylammonium, which inhibits the outward-going delayed potassium current in nerve (Armstrong, 1971), prolonged the action potential. In mammalian ventricular muscles, Morad and Trautwein (1968) have shown that prolongation of the action potential at the membrane potential over -25 mV tend to maintain force developed (tonic component). Thus, the first posiibility may appear to explain the positive inotropic effect and prolongation of relaxation time by 4-AP. However, in pindolol-treated ventricular muscles the prolongation of the action potential duration at 50% repolarization level (at the membrane potential about -30 mV) in the presence of 10 mM 4-AP was only 64 ms (about 40% of control), as opposed to the prolongation of the relaxation time by 259 ms (about 190% of control). Thus, it is difficult to ascribe the retardation of the relaxation process to the prolongation of the action potential. Consequently, it is unlikely that the positive inotropic action of 4-AP was produced by increased or prolonged entry of $Ca^{2+}$ into the muscle cells during the prolonged action potentials. As to the direct enhancement of calcium channel by 4-AP (forth posibilty), 4-AP did not affect the slow inward current in guinea pig papillary muscle (Ochi, Hino and Yanagisawa, unpublished data). Alternatively, it appears rather likely that 4-AP would release $Ca^{2+}$ from their binding or storage site or slow binding of intracellular $Ca^{2+}$ to intracellular structures. At present it is difficult to disern which of two alternatives is more likely. In the present study the resting membrane potential was not affected by 10 mM 4-AP which produced an increase in resting force in pindolol-treated muscles. This also suggests that the mechanical effect of 4-AP would not be secondary to the change in the membrane potential.

## The Study Using Frog Ventricular Strip

The effect of 4-AP on untreated frog ventricualr strip is essentially produced by the release of neurotransmitter as we have seen in the study using the isolated, blood-perfused SA node preparation. Intrestingly, under the blockade of both muscarinic and β-adrenergic receptors, 4-AP could not produce a positive inotropic effect nor a prolongation of action potential. The difference in the ability of 4-AP to augment contractility in frog and dog ventricular muscles cannot be ascrtained from the results presented in this paper.

REFERENCES

Armstrong, C. M. (1971). Interaction of tetraethylammonium ion derivatives with the potassium channels of giant axons. J. Gen. Physiol., 58, 413-437.
Bowman, W. C., A. l. Harvey, and I. G. Marshall (1977). The actions of aminopyridines on avian muscle. Naunyn-Schnideb. Arch. Pharmacol., 297, 99-103.
Brady, A. L. (1964). In O. Krayer (Ed.), Pharmacology of Cardiac Function, Oxford; Pergamon Press, pp. 15-23.
Chiba, S., K. Kubota and k. Hashimoto (1972). Double peaked positive chronotropic response of the islated blood-perfused S-A node to caffeine. Tohoku J. Exptl. Med., 107, 101.
Gillespie, J. I., and O.F. Hutter (1975). The actions of 4-aminopyridine on the delayed potassium current in skeletal muscle fibres. J. Physiol. (lond.),252, 70P-71P
Goldman, Y., and M. Morad (1977). Measurement of transmembrane potential and current in cardiac muscle: A new voltage clamp method. J. Physiol. (Lond.), 268, 613-654.
Kubota, K., and K. Hashimoto (1973). Selective stimulation of the parasympathetic preganglionic nerve fibres in the exciesd and blood-perfused SA node preparation of the dog. Naunyn-Schmiedeb. Arch. Pharmacol., 278, 135.
Hue, B., M. Perhate, and J. Chanelet (1973). Effects de la 4-aminopyridine (4-AP) sur l"activite de la fibre nerveuse geante isolee d"Insecte (Periplaneta americana). J. Physiol. (Paris), 67, 346A.
Hue, B., M. Pelhate, J.-J. Callec, and J. Chanelet (1978). Postsynaptic effects of 4-aminopyridine in the sixth abdominal ganglion of the coCkroach. Eurp. J. Pharmacol., 49, 327-329.
Johns, A., D. S. Golko, P. A. Lauzon, and D. M. Paton (1976). The potentiating effects of 4-aminopyridine on adrenergic transmission in the rabbit vas deferens. Eurp. J. Pharmacol., 38, 71-78.
Kirpekar, M., S. M. Kirpeker, and J. C. Prat (1977). Effect of 4-aminopyridine on release of noradrenaline from the perfused cat spleen by nerve stimulation. J.Physiol. (lond.), 272, 517-528.
Leander, S., A. Arner, and B. Johansson (1977) Effects of 4-aminopyridine on mechanical activity and noradrenaline release in the rat portal vein in vitro. Eurp. J. Pharmacol., 46, 351-361.
Lemeignan, M., M. C. Auclair, A. Rodallec, and P. Lechat (1975) Analyse electrophysiologique des effects de l'amino-4 pyridine sur le lambeau ventriculaire isole de coeur de cobaye. Arch. int. Pharmacodyn., 216, 165-176.
Lundh, H., S. Leander, and s. Thesleff (1977) Antagonism of the paralysis produced by botulinum toxin in the rat. The effects of tertaethylammonium, guanidine and 4-aminopyridine. J. Neurol. Sci., 32, 29-43.
Lundh, H., and S. Thesleff (1977) The mode of action of 4-aminopyridine and guanidine on transmitter release from motor nerve terminals. Eurp. J. Pharmacol., 42, 411-412.

Molgo, j., M. Lemeignan, and P. Lechat (1975). Modification de la liberation du transmetteur a la jonction neuromusclaire de Grenouille sous l'action de l'amino-4-pyridine. C. R. Acad. Sci. (Paris) Serie D 281, 1637-1639.

Morad, M., and R Orkand (1971). Excitztion-contraction coupling in frog ventricle: Evidence from voltage clamp studies. J. Physiol. (Lond.), 219, 167-189.

Morad, M, C. Sanders, and J. Weiss (1981). The inotropic actions of adrenaline on frog ventricular muscle: Relaxation versus potentiating effects. J. Physiol. (Lond.), 311, 585-604.

Morad, M., and W. Trautwein (1968). The effect of the duration of the action potential on contraction in the mammalian heart muscle. Pflugers Arch., 299, 66-82.

Ochi, R., and H. Nishiye (1974). Effect of intracellular tetraethylammonium ion on action potential in the guinea-pig's myocardium. Pflugers Arch., 348, 305-316.

Pelhate M., and Y. Pichon (1974). Selective inhibition of potassium current in the giant axon of cockroach. J. Physiol. (Lond.), 242, 90P-91P.

Reiter, M. (1972) Differences in the inotropic cardiac effects of noraderenaline and dihydro-ouabain. Naunyn-Schmiedeb. Arch. Pharmacol., 275, 243-250.

Schauf, C. L., C. A. Colton, j. S. Colton, and F. A. Davis(1976). Aminopyridines and sparteine as inhibitors of membrane potassium conductance: Effects on Myxcola giant axons and the lobster neuromuscular junction. J. Pharmacol. Exp. Ther., 197, 414-425.

Thomson, C. M., and W. F. Dryden (1980). Development of membrane conductance of chick skeletal muscle in culture. II Effect of aminopyridines. Can. J. Physiol. Pharmacol., 58, 606-611.

Yanagisawa, T., K. Satoh, and N. Taira (1978) Excitation of autonomic nerves by 4-aminopyridine in the isolated, blood-perfused sinoatrial node preparation of the dog. Eurp. J. Pharmacol., 49, 189-192.

Yanagisawa, T., and N. Taira (1979). Positive inotropic effect of 4-aminopyridine on dog ventricular muscle. Naunyn-Schmiedeb. Arch. Pharmacol., 307, 207-212.

Yeh, J.Z., G.S. Oxford, C. H. Wu, and T. Narahashi (1976). Interactions of aminopyridines with potassium channels of squid axon membrane. Biophys. J., 16, 77-86.

# Effects of 4-Aminopyridine on Isometric Force [Ca++] Relations in Mammalian Slow and Fast Twitch Skinned Muscle Fibres

R. Fink and D. G. Stephenson

Department of Zoology, La Trobe University, Bundoora,
Victoria 3083, Australia

4-aminopyridine (4-AP) has been used as a powerful blocking agent of the potassium conductance in the membrane of skeletal muscle fibres (Gillespie & Hutter, 1975; Fink & Wettwer, 1978) but not much is known about interactions of 4-AP with the contractile apparatus. In a comparative study we tested therefore 4-AP in respect to its effects on Ca- activation of contraction of fast and slow twitch mammalian skeletal muscle. For this purpose single muscle fibres from the slow twitch muscle Soleus and the fast twitch muscle extensor digitorum longus (EDL) of the rat (Rattus norvegicus) were mechanically skinned under parafin oil by standard microdissection procedures. The preparations were attached to an Aksjeselskapet AE 875 force transducer and the sarcomere length was determined from the first order diffraction maximum produced by a He-Ne laser. The fibres were activated at room temperature (20-22°C) in Ca- buffered solutions containing (mmole . $l^{-1}$): Na$^+$ 36; K$^+$ 127; Mg$^{++}$1; TES$^-$17; ATP 8; creatine phosphate 10; creatine kinase 15U.ml$^{-1}$; Na N$_3$ 1; pH 7.10 ± 0.01. 50 mmole. $l^{-1}$ total EGTA was used to buffer Ca$^{++}$. The concentration of 4-AP in solutions varied between 10 μmole . $l^{-1}$ and 5 mmole . $l^{-1}$, and the pH was adjusted to 7.10 ± 0.01 with HCl. From the results it appears that the sensitivity of the contractile apparatus in slow twitch muscle fibres was significantly increased in the presence of 4-AP concentrations in the range of 1-5 mmole . $l^{-1}$. Thus, the sigmoid curve relating isometric steady state force and free Ca$^{++}$ level was shifted by about 0.1 log units towards lower Ca-concentrations. This apparent increase in Ca$^{++}$-sensitivity cannot be explained by spurious effects of 4-AP on the Ca-EGTA-buffer. However, the maximum peak tension was not altered, and the frequency of the observed force oscillations for submaximal activation (<60% maximum force) (Stephenson & Williams, 1981) was similar in the presence and absence of 4-AP. This shift of the Ca-mediated tension activation curve by 4-AP was reversible. In comparison with the slow twitch fibres 4-AP did not significantly change the sensitivity of the contractile apparatus of fast EDL fibres to Ca$^{++}$. Peak tension in these fast twitch fibres was also not affected. Experiments were also performed on human dystrophic muscle fibres. 4-AP did not appear to influence the Ca$^{++}$- sensitivity in preparations with Ca-activation curves characteristic of the fast twitch type fibres. The effect of 4-AP on slow mammalian twitch fibres is similar to that found in the presence of local anaesthetics.

Fink, R & Wettwer, E. (1978) Pflügers Arch. 374, 289-292.
Gillespie, J.I. & Hutter O.F. (1975) J. Physiol., Lond. 252, 70-71P.
Stephenson, D.G. & Williams, D.A. (1981) J. Physiol. (in press).

---

This work was supported by the NH/MRC and the National Heart Foundation (Australia).

# 4-Aminopyridine and Outward Membrane Currents in Rat Uterine Smooth Muscle at Various Stages of Pregnancy

J. P. Savineau, J. Mironneau and Ch. Mironneau

Institut de Biochimie Cellulaire et Neurochimie du CNRS,
Université de Bordeaux II, 1 rue Camille St-Saëns,
33000 Bordeaux, France

It is well-known that periodical changes in resting membrane potential occur during pregnancy in rat myometrium. Measurements of intracellular ionic concentrations indicated that the ionic content of smooth muscle cells remained constant suggesting that the resting membrane displacement was caused by a change in membrane conductance, especially the potassium conductance. 4-aminopyridine (4-AP), a potent inhibitor of the potassium channels in many excitable tissues was used in the present work in order to clarify the evolution of the potassium outward current during different stages of gestation.

Small strips (100 µm in diameter, 3-4 mm in length) from the longitudinal smooth muscle layer of the pregnant rat myometrium were used. These muscular strips were current and voltage-clamped by means of a double sucrose gap apparatus.

In strips isolated from 19-21 days-pregnant rats (where the resting membrane potential was $-47 \pm 1.5$ mV, n=40), the potassium conductance was characterized by a steady-state outward current when a depolarizing pulse was applied to the membrane. A semilogarithmic plot of the tail current showed that the steady-state potassium current developed according to two components : i) the first one which had the largest amplitude presented a fast and only voltage-dependent activation; it was blocked by TEA (20 mM) and by 4-AP (20 mM); ii) the second one which was lower and slower was calcium-sensitive; it was blocked by TEA (20 mM) but unaffected by 4-AP.

In strips isolated from 14-16 days-pregnant rats (where the resting membrane potential was $-60 \pm 3$ mV, n=30), a depolarizing pulse (+30 mV) elicited a fast transient outward current. This current was fully activated after 45 msec and partially inhibited the initial inward current. This fast outward current was specifically suppressed by externally applied 4-AP and the maximal inhibition was obtained at about 20 mM. At the end of gestation (19-21 days) where the fast outward current was absent, a hump of outward current mixed with the initial inward current could be observed when the membrane was hyperpolarized by a conditioning prepulse. This hump of outward current was also very sensitive to 4-AP. The activation-voltage dependence of the fast outward current in mid-pregnancy (14-16 days) was very similar to that of the fast component of the steady-state outward current in the last stage of gestation (19-21 days) and thus could not represent an additional separate conductance system.

It is suggested that during the gestation the potassium conductance of the uterine membrane is governed by two sets of channels : i) a first set of fast potassium channels is available from -80 mV and very sensitive to 4-AP; ii) a second set of potassium channels is insensitive to 4-AP and could be activated by the internal calcium concentration.

# Effects of 4-Aminopyridine on Membrane Currents in the Pace-maker Voltage Range of Sheep Cardiac Purkinje Fibres

P. P. Van Bogaert

Laboratorium voor Fysiologie, Universiteit Antwerpen, RUCA,
Groenenborgerlaan 171, B-2020 Antwerpen, Belgium

4-Aminopyridine, applied in quantities varying from 0.1 to 0.5 mM, is known to selectively abolish the majority of the early outward current, $i_{qr}$, activated in sheep cardiac Purkinje fibres by voltage clamp pulses positive to -30 mV.
The increase in action potential duration, the depolarization of the resting potential and the induction of spontaneous activity by 1 to 5 mM 4-AP indicate that this drug also affects membrane currents responsible for the electrical behaviour of this preparation at more negative potentials. This was investigated with the voltage-clamp technique using two intracellular micro-electrodes in short sheep Purkinje strands.
With 5 mM 4-AP added to a normal solution, buffered at pH 7.4 with 20 mM HEPES ( T = 36.5° C ), the steady-state current-voltage relation flattens and loses its typical N-shape. The time-dependent current, responsible for the pacemaker activity is reduced in amplitude, and its voltage dependency is shifted 16 + 2.2 mV towards less negative potentials. In the presence of 2 to 4 mM $BaCl_2$, the back-ground inward-rectifying $K^+$ current is largely suppressed while the time-dependent pace-maker current is still recorded. With 5 mM 4-AP, this time-dependent pace-maker current is reversibly reduced in amplitude and the same depolarizing shift of its voltage-dependency is observed.
On the other hand, 4-AP has no effect on the currents recorded in the presence of 20 mM Cesiumchloride while it is still effective with smaller amounts of Cesiumchloride i.e. 1 or 2 mM : i.e. the steady-state current-voltage relation is flattened.
According to these results, 4-AP has a dual effect on membrane currents recorded in the pace-maker voltage range.
First, 4-AP decreases an inward rectifying back-ground $K^+$ current and second, it affects the time-dependent pace-maker current. This latter effect is the only one observed in barium containing solutions when the back-ground current is eliminated. On the other hand, the influence of 4-AP on the back-ground current is observed, in isolation, in the presence of small amounts of Cesiumchloride where the pace-maker current is abolished. With 20 mM Cesiumchloride, the pace-maker current is absent and the inward rectifying $K^+$ current is largely decreased. This could explain the absence of effects of 4-AP in these conditions. This dual action of 4-AP can explain the observed modifications in resting potential level, action potential configuration and the induction of spontaneous activity in normal Tyrode solutions.

# Is the Cardiotonic Effect of Aminopyridines and Aminopyrimidines in vitro A Consequence of Increased Extracellular pH?

## M. Shahid and I.W. Rodger

Department of Physiology and Pharmacology, University of Strathclyde, Glasgow G1 1XW, UK

In a recent study we reported (Rodger & Shahid, 1981) that raised extracellular pH increased the contractile force of isolated cardiac muscle. We have now compared the effects of the strongly basic substances 4-aminopyridine (4-AP) and 2,4,6-triaminopyrimidine (TAP) with those of increased pH on tension responses and cyclic AMP levels in rabbit isolated electrically-driven (1 Hz) papillary muscles.

Both 4-AP base and TAP base (.08 - 1.0 mg/ml) elicited concentration-dependent increases in contractile force. As the force of contraction increased, however, so too did the extracellular pH rising from a resting level of 7.2 to 9.6 at the highest concentration used. In contrast, Pymadin® (4-AP hydrochloride) or neutralised TAP (pH = 7.3) were devoid of inotropic activity and did not significantly alter the pH of the bathing medium. Increasing the pH of the bathing solution from 7.0 up to 9.6 in the absence of either drug induced inotropic responses almost identical to those elicited by either 4-AP or TAP. These responses were highly reproducible and readily reversed to control tension levels on re-immersion in solution at pH 7. In an attempt to minimise pH alterations that might occur within the cells we used the intracellular buffer creatinol-O-phosphate. Addition of creatinol-O-phosphate ($10^{-5} - 10^{-3}$ M) failed to reduce the inotropic responses to 4-AP base, TAP base or increased pH.

The levels of cyclic AMP measured within the cells were not significantly changed by 4-AP base, 4-AP HCl or increased pH.

| C-AMP (pmol/mg) | pH | | | 4-AP (base) | | 4-AP HCl | |
|---|---|---|---|---|---|---|---|
| | 7 | 8 | 9 | 0.1 mg/ml | 1 mg/ml | 0.1 mg/ml | 1 mg/ml |
| | 0.72 ± .06 | .68 ± .07 | .68 ± .06 | .76 ± .05 | .85 ± .08 | .62 ± .07 | .68 ± .06 |

The results suggest, therefore, that the inotropic effect of aminopyridines and aminopyrimidines is a direct consequence of increased extracellular pH. The mechanism underlying the inotropic effect of high pH remains unknown but clearly it does not involve cyclic-AMP. As we postulated previously it is possible that a rise in pH may act to facilitate translocation of membrane $Ca^{2+}$ and/or increase the release of $Ca^{2+}$ from sources within the cell.

### REFERENCE

RODGER, I.W. & SHAHID, M. (1981) Effects of increased pH on contractile force of rabbit isolated papillary muscles. Br. J. Pharmac. in press

DISCUSSION OF THE SIXTH SESSION.

Dr. Pelhate: Dr. Edman, I should like to ask you if you have tried voltage clamp on the muscle fibre?

Dr. Edman: No, we have not pursued that type of measurement. Reference to such work is given in our paper.

Dr. Glover: Dr. Edman, have you seen the paper by Maetani and co-workers in the Hiroshima J. of Medical Science? They showed that in the mouse diaphragm $Zn^{2+}$, $Uo^{2++}$ and 4-aminopyridine prolong action potentials without modifying contractility. Could you comment on this finding?

Dr. Edman: I feel that their finding has to be confirmed, as a true dissociation of the effects of 4-aminopyridine on action potential and twitch force is very unlikely. Their electrical recordings were made on a number of surface fibres, whereas the mechanical response was recorded from the whole muscle. One has to make sure that the number of excitable fibres remains constant throughout such an experiment. A single muscle fibre would be the preparation of choice for such a study.

Dr. Shahid: With regard to the question concerning extracellular pH, there have been studies carried out on sarcoplasmic reticulum fragments which suggest that raised pH increases the release of $Ca^{2+}$ from the structure.

Dr. Edman: It is quite true that pH changes affect the state of activation of muscle. An intracellular pH change may alter both release and reuptake of activator $Ca^{2+}$ and alter the sensitivity of the contractile system to $Ca^{2+}$ (for further discussion see Edman and Mattiazzi, J. Muscle Res. Cell Motil., 1981). I cannot see, however, that we need to consider any pH effect in the experiments that I have reported here. The pH of the extracellular solution was carefully checked to be 7.0 both in the presence and in the absence of 4-aminopyridine. Furthermore, the effects of 4-aminopyridine on both action potential and twitch were maintained for hours after the aminopyridine solution had been removed and replaced by control Ringer solution. This would seem to rule out that 4-aminopyridine acts by virtue of a pH change. The contractile effects of a pH change are readily reversible.

Dr. Foldes: One may obtain some insight on the probable muscular effect of 4-aminopyridine by observing its interactions with dantrolene and verapamil. In the completely curarized rat phrenic nerve-hemidiaphragm preparation the concentrations of dantrolene and verapamil required to block tension output during direct stimulation are very similar to those required to block the twitch tension in the absence of curare during indirect stimulation. This indicates that dantrolene and verapamil act primarily on the muscle fibre. The inhibitory effects of dantrolene can be antagonized by 4-aminopyridine, those of verapamil, a compound that blocks $Ca^{2+}$ channels cannot. This suggests that 4-aminopyridine has a postjunctional effect and that this effect is probably due to the increased release of $Ca^{2+}$ from the sarcoplasmic reticulum during direct stimulation.

Dr. Edman: The direct depressant effect of dantrolene can be demonstrated in the isolated single muscle fibre preparation (Edman, J. Physiol., 1979, 291, 143) and there is reason to believe that dantrolene reduces the tension output by diminishing the $Ca^{2+}$ release in response to the action potential. Dantrolene does not, however, affect the duration of the action potential. 4-aminopyridine restores some of the depressed tension in the dantrolene treated fibre (Khan and Edman, 1979). This potentiating effect of 4-aminopyridine is explainable by the widening of the action potential, as this leads to longer lasting release of activator $Ca^{2+}$. As I indicated before, 4-aminopyridine probably does not exert any direct action on the calcium store to facilitate the release of activator $Ca^{2+}$.

Dr. McArdle: Does 4-aminopyridine restore the twitch in muscle fibres treated with dantrolene? Does 4-aminopyridine affect skinned muscle fibres or does 4-aminopyridine induce electrogenic activity in the longitudinal sarcoplasmic reticulum?

Dr. Edman: 4-aminopyridine restores some of the twitch force after it has been depressed by dantrolene in the single fibre (Khan and Edman, 1979). This in line with the idea that 4-aminopyridine potentiates the twitch force by prolonging the action potential. As to your second question, 4-aminopyridine may have an effect on skinned fibres as proposed by Dr. Fink in this Symposium. This does not mean, however, that the drug exerts a direct effect on the contractile machinery in the intact fibre. In fact, there is evidence against this idea, as I pointed out before.

Dr. Durant: Previous workers have demonstrated, using the squid giant axon, that repetitive depolarization caused 4-aminopyridine to dissociate from the $K^+$ channels witch it was blocking. In your study you demonstrated that a tetanic stimulus was necessary before the muscle action potential became prolonged. Can you explain this difference?

Dr. Edman: The finding you refer to in the squid axon suggests that in this tissue the affinity of the receptor sites for 4-aminopyridine is critically dependent on the membrane charge. This does not seem to be the case in skeletal muscle. Here instead the membrane charge appears to provide a barrier for the transport of 4-aminopyridine preventing it from reaching the receptor site.

Dr. Fink: Hutter and Gillespie used alkaline pH to increase the internal concentration of 4-aminopyridine, another possibility would be to directly inject the drug into the fibre (Fink and Wettwer, 1978). Have you tried these procedures to speed up the onset of the 4-aminopyridine effect?

Dr. Edman: As is demonstrated in our paper, membrane depolarization greatly speeds up the development of the 4-aminopyridine effect in frog muscle fibres. Indeed, full twitch potentiation can be attained within 1 s by applying a tetanizing pulse train after 4-aminopyridine has been added to the bath. This supports the idea that the normal membrane charge provides the barrier which prevents the positively charged 4-aminopyridine molecule from reaching its locus of action in the membrane. Removal of this barrier for no more than 100-200 ms, that is the time covered by 10 action potentials is evidently sufficient to enable 4-aminopyridine to reach its site of action in full concentration.

Dr. Bowman: Marshall and Harvey showed that the quaternary derivative 4-aminopyridinemethiodide, is equipotent with 4-aminopyridine in prolonging frog muscle action potentials. Therefore, according to your theory it should increase frog muscle twitch tension. Is it worth testing as confirmatory evidence of your theory? The result would be interesting because this drug has very little action in facilitating transmitter release and probably does not penetrate the blood-brain barrier. Agoston, Savage, Rodger and myself found in the anaesthetized cat that 4-aminopyridine increased the directly evoked twitches of fast contracting twitch muscles such as flexor digitorum longus, but had little, or no, effect on slow-contracting twitch muscles (soleus). Lechat found no effect on rabbit tibialis and Marshall and Harvey only a weak effect on the chick biventer cervicis. There seems therefore to be not only a species difference but also a muscle difference within the same species. It would therefore be interesting to know whether 4-aminopyridine increases the twitches of the rat soleus and of frog multiple-innervated fibres.

Dr. Edman: The aminopyridinemethiodide would certainly be of interest to compare on the twitch response as it would probably have a lower ability than 4-aminopyridine to pass through the fibre membrane. The evidence obtained from intact muscle fibres suggests, however, that 4-aminopyridine does not exert any effect on the kinetics of activator $Ca^{2+}$ in the excitation-contraction coupling or on the sensitivity of the contractile system to $Ca^{2+}$. My prediction is therefore that the methiodide derivative would produce the same contractile effects as 4-aminopyridine in concentrations that are equipotent in prolonging the action potential. The species difference of the 4-aminopyridine effect and the observed difference in the effect between muscles within the same species are interesting and should be further investigated. An essential point to find out is whether the differences between muscles and species concern the effects on action potential and twitch response to the same extent. This question would need to be studied in single fibre preparations, if possible. Once conceivable explanation for the observed differences between various muscles would be, as I indicated in my talk, that the site of action of 4-aminopyridine is located in a deep structure of the membrane and that the accessibility of this site varies between different types of muscles.


Dr. Shahid: Dr. Yanagisawa, what effect does 4-aminopyridine in concentrations greater than 10 mM have on your preparation? Have you studied the effect of 4-aminopyridine on the duration of the action potential under different physical conditions such as stimulation frequency, temperature, etc.?

Dr. Yanagisawa: In untreated muscles 10 mM 4-aminopyridine produced a positive inotropic effect with increases of the velocity of force development and relaxation velocity and without changes in the resting tension. In pindolol treated muscles and in muscles obtained from reserpine treated animals 10 mM 4-aminopyridine produced less positive inotropic effect than in untreated muscles. The positive inotropic effect of 4-aminopyridine is characterized by a slow relaxation. I did not try to change the stimulation frequency nor the temperature.

Dr. Schiavone: You stated that 4-aminopyridine enhances spontaneous NA release in the heart and that this effect involves the release of $Ca^{2+}$ from intracellular stores. In our studies of NA release in the cat spleen such a mechanism is suggested by the observation that 1) in the perfused spleen 10 mM 4-aminopyridine enhances spontaneous NA release during $Ca^{2+}$-free perfusion; 2) in spleen slices, 4-aminopyridine enhances the response to nicotine in $Ca^{2+}$-free medium. However, since $La^{2+}$ blocks the response to nicotine and 4-aminopyridine we suspect that this putative effect may be dependent upon the influx of small amounts of extracellular $Ca^{2+}$. In your cardiac preparation I wonder if the effect of 4-aminopyridine on spontaneous release was similarly dependent on extracellular $Ca^{2+}$?

Dr. Yanagisawa: The spontaneous release of neurotransmitters will partly be due to the excitation of autonomic nerves but the release that remains in the presence of TTX must be related to other mechanisms.

Dr. Khan: In your cardiac muscle preparation I wonder if 4-aminopyridine exerts its effects primarily on the $Ca^{2+}$ metabolism and if the prolongation of the action potential is secondary to this effect? Alternatively 4-aminopyridine, like in other excitable membranes, could block the $K^+$ channel and the positive inotropic effect could be secondary to this action.

Dr. Yanagisawa: I believe that the effect of 4-aminopyridine on the action potential duration would be related to the inhibition of the outward membrane current in the heart. However, there is no evidence that outward current consists of a single component.

Dr. Tazieff-Depierre: Does 4-aminopyridine act in the absence of extracellular $Ca^{2+}$ as is the case with purified scorpion toxin II? In the perfused isolated heart preparation it is well-known that contraction disappears in the absence of extracellular $Ca^{2+}$ and in the presence of EGTA. If you to such a preparation add scorpion toxin II the preparation again starts to beat, suggesting that the toxin releases $Ca^{2+}$. I would like to know if you have tried the same kind of experiments with 4-aminopyridine to show that part of its action can be correlated to $Ca^{2+}$ release.

Dr. Yanagisawa: I did not try such an experiment.


Dr. Bergmann: Dr. Fink, it is rather surprising that you find that human dystrophic muscle behaved like fast-twitch muscle. I would have expected it to resemble slow muscle. Did you try to stimulate dystrophic muscle several times before applying $Ca^{2+}$ and 4-aminopyridine?

Dr. Fink: Since Duchenne muscular dystrophy is a rather rare disease we only get a few biopsies per year. The fibres used in the experiments described in my talk were obtained from a patient with Duchenne muscular dystrophy at an early stage and has clearly fast-twitch fibre characteristics. Later we got only one fibre from a patient with Beckers muscular dystrophy which behaved like a slow fibre. Unfortunately, this fibre did not survive long enough to test the effect of 4-aminopyridine carefully. It would be highly interesting if we, in our skinned fibre preparations, found that a fast fibre, during muscular dystrophy, changes to slow twitch fibre characteristics. Concerning the stimulation, we activated our fibre several times to maximal tension in the initial testing procedure and during the experiments.

Dr. McArdle: Is the differential effect of 4-aminopyridine on the extensor digitorum longus muscle versus the soleus muscle related to initial sarcomere length? Have you examined the effects of 4-aminopyridine in denervated muscle?

Dr. Fink: We tested the effects of 4-aminopyridine at different sarcomere lengths between 2.4 - 3.0 $\mu$m. In this range the characteristic differential effect of 4-aminopyridine was apparent. Experiments over a wider range as well as experiments on denervated muscles are planned for in future investigations.

Dr. Edman: As indicated in my paper there is reason to believe that increased sensitivity of the contractile system to $Ca^{2+}$ does not underly the twitch enhancement produced by 4-aminopyridine in the intact muscle fibre. With regard to the effects you showed on the contractile force-$Ca^{2+}$-concentration relationship in the skinned fibre one obvious reason for a shift of this relationship would be that the free $Ca^{2+}$ concentration is altered when 4-aminopyridine is added to the medium. Can you exclude such a complication?

Dr. Galvan: This is a question to Dr. Savineau, have you tried holding the membrane at -100 mV and depolarizing it to -40 mV? I believe that you under that condition might elicit a pure fast outward current.

Dr. Savineau: Yes, the fast outward current is zero at -80 mV. Thus, when the membrane potential of the uterus is clamped at -80 mV in mid-pregnancy as well as in the last stage of pregnancy and then depolarized to +50 mV, a pure fast and large outward current is elicited. This fast and outward current in smooth muscle cells of rat myometrium can be described by Hodgkin-Huxley equations (with activation and inactivation parameters).

Dr. Galvan: I should like to ask Dr. van Bogaert why he thinks the time dependent inward relaxations are so slow?

Dr. van Bogaert: The time constant of pace-maker current relaxation varies between a maximal value of 2 s and minimal values of a few 100 ms. This current is very slow indeed, but not exceptional, because very slow currents have been described in a similar voltage range in other preparations, e.g. invertebrate neurons (Partridge and Stevens, J. Physiol., 1976) and in skeletal muscle (Adrian, Chandler and Hodgkins, J. Physiol., 1970).

Dr. Edman: Have you found any effect of 4-aminopyridine on the contractile output of this specialized part of the myocardium?

Dr. van Bogaert: I did not measure contractile changes in this preparation. In situations where the contractility is markedly increased by replacing $Ca^{2+}$ by $Sr^{2+}$ a slow contraction can be seen by visual inspection. No such change was observed with 4-aminopyridine. Neither were there indirect signs of altered contractility as a dislocation of the microelectrode in the presence of 4-aminopyridine.

## Discussion

Dr. Glover: Dr. Shahid, when Professor Bowman recently visited Australia he told me of your results and I briefly looked at the possible role of pH changes in the effect of 4-aminopyridine in the rabbit atrium. I agree that the addition of 4-aminopyridine ($10^{-3}$ M) increases the pH of the Ringer-Locke solution bubbled with $O_2$ from about 8.3 to about 8.9 and that an increase in pH by itself has a positive inotropic effect. However, when I used 5% $CO_2$ in $O_2$ the pH was in the range of 6.0-7.0 and was little altered by the addition of 4-aminopyridine. The control contractions were certainly smaller at the lower pH, but 4-aminopyridine still increased the force of contraction by about 100%.

Dr. Bergmann: What is the pKa value of 2,4,6-triaminopyridine? This will determine how much the pH will be shifted.

Dr. Shahid: I am not quite sure about the exact pKa value for 2,4,6-triaminopyridine but it is roughly about 7.5 - 8 and certainly much less than the pKa value for 4-aminopyridine.

Dr. Yanagisawa: Have you ever checked the effect of atropine on the positive inotropic effect of 4-aminopyridine? Have you checked the effect of propranolol on the changes of c-AMP content of the papillary muscles in response to 4-aminopyridine?

Dr. Shahid: Atropine does not modify the positive inotropic response of 4-aminopyridine. No, we have not performed this particular experiment since 4-aminopyridine does not significantly modify the intracellular c-AMP concentration and since propranolol in our system does not reduce the inotropic effect of 4-aminopyridine.

Dr. Schiavone: Was the change in pH associated with the addition of aminopyridines to the medium sufficient to account for the cardiotonic effect of this agent?

Dr. Shahid: In our system it seems that the cardiotonic effects of 4-aminopyridine and of 2,4,6-triaminopyridine are a consequence of their ability to raise the extracellular pH.

Dr. Molgo: Do you have ruled out the possibility that by modifying the pH of the extracellular medium in the presence of propranolol and 4-aminopyridine there is a modification in the release of neurotransmitters that could account for the positive inotropic effect reported? The activity of propranolol may vary with pH as that of other local anaesthetic agents. Have you studied if propranolol blocks β-receptors in a pH dependent way?

Dr. Shahid: This is something we considered when we were examining the influence of propranolol in the presence of high pH. The only reasonably way that we could test if propranolol still blocked β-adrenal receptors at high pH was to perform cumulative dose-response curves to isoprenaline in the presence and absence of propranolol at different pH. From such a study we found that propranolol exerted a β-blocking action irrespective of extracellular pH.

# Clinical Applications of Aminopyridines

*Chairman:* F. F. Foldes

# Therapeutic Applications of Aminopyridines in Diseases of Neuromuscular Transmission

## H. Lundh

Department of Neurology, University Hospital, 221 85
Lund, Sweden and Department of Pharmacology, University of
Lund, 223 62 Lund, Sweden

ABSTRACT

4-Aminopyridine is a potent drug to increase transmitter release from motor nerves and reverse muscle paralysis in human diseases of neuromuscular transmission as demonstrated in vitro in intercostal muscle specimens from patients with myasthenia gravis and the Eaton-Lambert syndrome. The drug is also effective in vivo in the treatment of these disorders, but its therapeutic usefulness is limited by severe side effects from the central nervous system like ataxia, psychotic delusions and epileptic fits. At present its use can only be justified in cases of Eaton-Lambert syndrome with a carcinoma and in severely disabled myasthenia gravis patients not responding to conventional treatments. It is suggested that 3,4-diaminopyridine might prove to be a more favourable drug with less side effects.

KEYWORDS

4-Aminopyridine; 3,4-diaminopyridine; human intercostal muscle; myasthenia gravis; Eaton-Lambert syndrome; clinical side effects.

INTRODUCTION

In the medical treatment of diseases of neuromuscular transmission drugs that act presynaptically like guanidine, theophylline, ephedrine and germine diacetate are not very useful because of poor therapeutic response except for guanidine in the myasthenic syndrome of Eaton-Lambert (Lambert, 1966) and in botulism (Cherington and Ryan, 1968, 1970). Unfortunately, guanidine has recently been almost abandoned even in these conditions as it has been known to produce serious side effects on bone marrow (Lambert and Howard, 1972; Cherington, 1976; Henriksson and others, 1977). It therefore caused great expectations among neurologists when it was learnt that the aminopyridines also increase nerve evoked transmitter release and act much more potently than previously studied drugs (Molgó, Lemeignan and Lechat, 1975, 1977, 1979; Lundh, Leander and Thesleff, 1977; Lundh, 1978).

Myasthenia gravis and the myasthenic syndrome of Eaton-Lambert are the two major chronic human diseases caused by blockade at the neuromuscular junction. In myasthenia gravis endplate potential amplitude is reduced because of decreased acetylcholine sensitivity of the muscle membrane due to an autoimmune attack against the receptors (Grob, 1976), and in the Eaton-Lambert syndrome by diminished transmitter release from the nerve terminal of unknown cause (Elmqvist and Lambert, 1968; Lambert and Elmqvist, 1971).

## METHODS

A biopsy of external intercostal muscle was removed from a patient with myasthenia gravis during thoracotomy for thymectomy. From the muscle specimen several neuromuscular preparations were dissected, and examined by conventional intracellular glass capillary microelectrode techniques in normal rat Ringer's solution with 2 mM $Ca^{2+}$ and phosphate buffer. The effects of the addition of 4-aminopyridine (4-AP) (Sigma, USA) and 3,4-diaminopyridine (3,4-DAP) (Aldrich, USA) were studied. To stimulate the intramuscular nerve an electromyography needle was used.

In vivo observations were made on patients with Eaton-Lambert syndrome and myasthenia gravis, and neuromuscular functions were examined by clinical tests and by recordings of the compound muscle action potential (CMAP) with surface electrodes on orbital, thenar and hypothenar muscles in response to single and repetitive stimulation of the corresponding motor nerve.

4-AP was prepared for human usage as previously described (Lundh, Nilsson and Rosén, 1979).

## EFFECTS IN VITRO ON INTERCOSTAL MUSCLE

Endplate potentials (epps) and miniature endplate potentials (mepps) were studied in intercostal muscle specimens from a patient with generalized myasthenia gravis. At most endplates in these preparations neuromuscular transmission was blocked and epp amplitude in the range of 1 to 4 mV in normal Ringer's solution with no added blocking substance. In the majority of fibres (23 of 31) no mepps could be seen even when focal epps with a rise time of less than 2 ms were recorded and with a noise level of the recording circuit of approximately 100 µV. In 8 of 31 fibres studied mepps were observed with a mean amplitude of $0.2\pm0.08$ mV ($\pm$S.D.) and a mean frequency of $3.3\pm1.72$, and in these fibres epp amplitude was in the range of 3 to 7 mV.

The addition of 4-aminopyridine (4-AP) (5-30 µM) or 3,4-diaminopyridine (3,4-DAP) (2-6 µM) increased epp amplitude in a dose-dependant manner, and at all endplates studied 30 µM 4-AP or 6 µM 3,4-DAP reversed the neuromuscular block and induced muscle action potentials and muscle twitches (Fig. 1). Mepp amplitude and frequency were not influenced, and resting membrane potential was not changed after drug addition, indicating that the drugs have no postsynaptic effects in these muscles.

In vitro observations on muscle biopsies from a patient with Eaton-Lambert syndrome made by other investigators (Sanders and others, 1980) have shown that 4-AP strongly increases epp amplitude and reverses muscle paralysis also in that disease.

## EFFECTS IN VIVO IN EATON-LAMBERT SYNDROME

The myasthenic syndrome of Eaton-Lambert is often associated with carcinoma of the bronchus but also appears in patients without any cancer. Clinically it is characterized by proximal muscle weakness in limbs and trunk causing difficulties in arm movements and walking and typically the patient has problems in rising from a sitting position or mounting a staircase. It is differentiated from other muscle diseases by its electromyographic picture showing a much reduced compound muscle action potential (CMAP) which is markedly facilitated by repetitive nerve stimulation

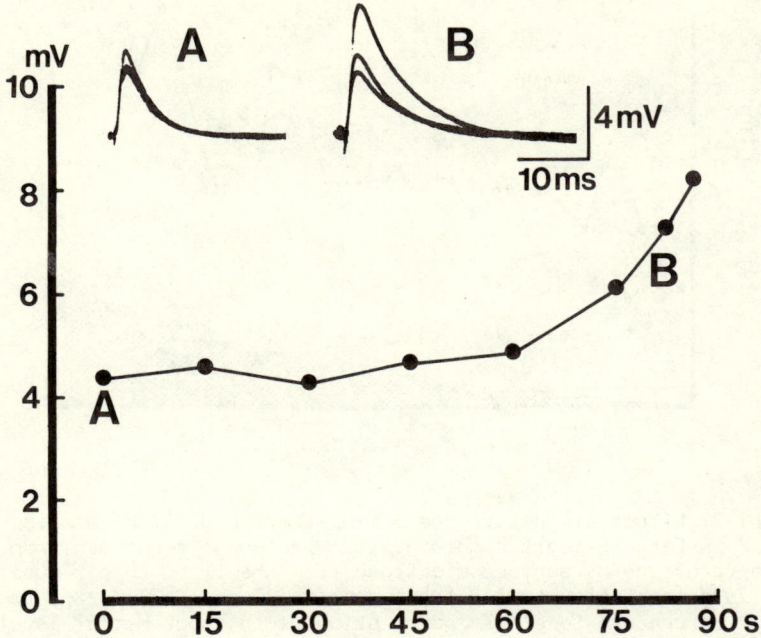

Fig. 1. Effect of 3,4-DAP on epps at one single endplate in a human intercostal muscle from a patient with myasthenia gravis. At time zero (A) recording is made in normal Ringer's solution and perfusion with a bathing solution containing 6 µM 3,4-DAP was started. As indicated epp amplitude increased and after 90s epps could no longer be recorded because of muscle twitches. Each point represents epp amplitude in response to nerve stimulation at 0.5 Hz, and A and B demonstrate at the points indicated superimposed epps at 10 Hz nerve stimulation.

(Fig. 3, upper traces). Anticholinesterases have poor therapeutic effects except for edrophonium, a single injection of which may cause long-lasting dramatic clinical improvement (Henriksson and others, 1977; Nilsson, 1981), probably by a presynaptic action different from its cholinesterase inhibitory properties. Guanidine has long been considered the drug of choice in Eaton-Lambert syndrome (Elmqvist and Lambert, 1968; Cherington, 1976), but its use has now been restricted because of its toxicity to bone marrow and kidney (see introduction).

In 1977 (Lundh, Nilsson and Rosén, 1977) we started to use 4-AP in the treatment of Eaton-Lambert syndrome. Intravenous injection of 4-AP chloride to a patient with bronchogenic carcinoma and a typical myasthenic syndrome restored neuromuscular transmission. The drug was initially administered by repeated small doses over a two hour time period, and when 23 mg (0.33 mg/kg body weight) had been given the CMAP in response to single maximal nerve stimulus had increased to normal level (Fig. 2), and during repetitive nerve stimulation the CMAP had changed to an almost normal electrophysiological response (Fig. 3).

The drug was effective when given orally, and with continuous oral medication by 20 mg 4-AP sulphate four to five times a day (maximum 1.42 mg/kg and day) neuromuscular transmission stayed normal during all day. The patient's muscle strength

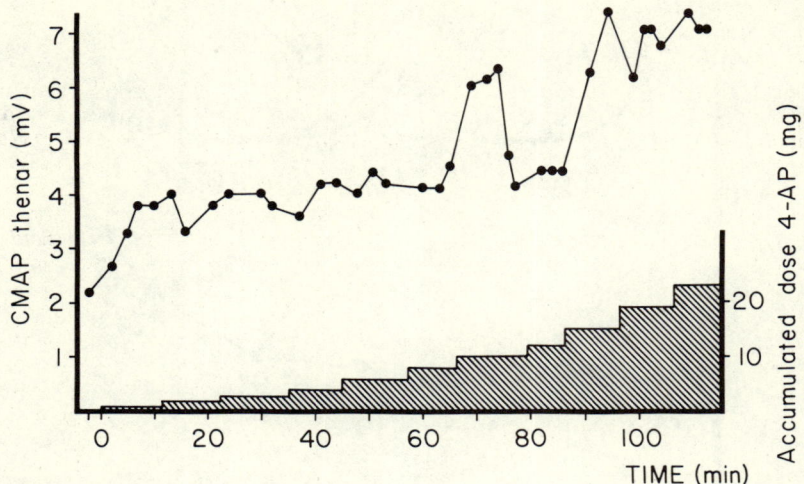

Fig. 2. Effect of intravenous administration of 4-AP chloride on CMAP in Eaton-Lambert syndrome. Stimulation of right median nerve and recording by surface electrode from the right thenar muscles. It is demonstrated that a total dose of 23 mg (0.33 mg/kg) restored CMAP i response to single nerve stimulus to about normal level.

was restored, and it was possible for him to rise from a chair and walk without difficulty. When the drug was withdrawn after three weeks muscle weakness reappeared, and the CMAP decreased to levels below that recorded before treatment.

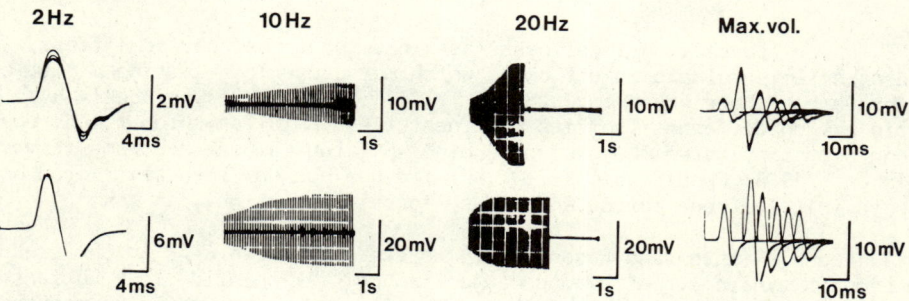

Fig. 3. Effects of 4-AP on electrophysiological recordings during repetitive nerve stimulation in thenar muscles in Eaton-Lambert syndrome. Upper trace before treatment at indicated frequencies of nerve stimulation, and lower traces after i.v. injection of 4-AP chloride (23 mg; 0.33 mg/kg). Trace to the right shows responses at 2 Hz stimulation before and 5, 10, 15 seconds, etc. after a 10 second-period of maximal voluntary contraction.

## EFFECTS IN VIVO IN MYASTHENIA GRAVIS

The abnormal muscular fatigability in myasthenia gravis is clinically manifested as cranial nerve palsies and limb weakness, and electrophysiologically as an abnormal decline in amplitude of the CMAP during repetitive nerve stimulation (Fig. 4 and 5; upper traces). Being an autoimmune disease the use of immunosuppressive drugs is a logical treatment and corticosteroids and azathioprine are effective (Grob, 1976). However, the early enthusiastic reports on the use of corticosteroids have now changed into a more cautious attitude, when the side-effects of long-term high-dose corticosteroid therapy in this disease have been presented (Osterman and others, 1978). Therefore, anticholinesterases have regained their position as the drugs of first choice, but in most patients these compounds do not relieve symptoms completely. Presynaptically acting drugs like guanidine have proved of little value (Brown and Johns, 1969) despite of earlier reports of its beneficial effects (Minot, Dodd and Riven, 1939; Desmedt, 1956)

At present the clinical management of myasthenia gravis often presents difficult problems, and potential new supplementary drugs should be studied with interest. We have tried 4-AP in several patients with myasthenia gravis, and single-dose injections intravenously to six patients caused marked improvement of clinical status (Table 1) and neuromuscular transmission (Fig. 4 and 5). The therapeutic effect was sustained during continuous oral administration (two patients) in doses equal to those used in the Eaton-Lambert syndrome (see above). The restorative effect on muscle fatigue was equally strong in cranial nerve innervated muscles (Fig. 5) as in limb muscles (Fig. 4).

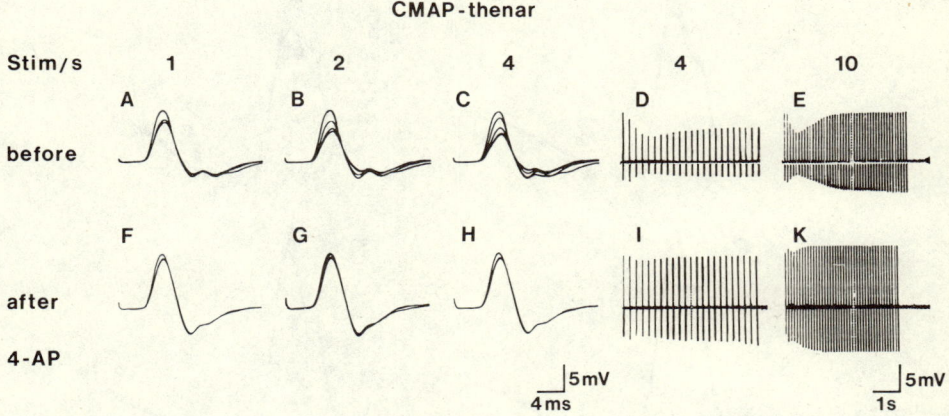

Fig. 4. Effects of 15 mg 4-AP intravenously on CMAP in a patient with myasthenia gravis. Recordings are made from the right thenar muscles and the median nerve is stimulated at the frequencies indicated. Records A-E are before and F-K after 4-AP injection.

The combined use of neostigmine and 4-AP was synergistical (Table 1) as has been shown in animal experiments with postsynaptic blockade produced by pancuronium (Miller and others, 1978) and in man during neuromuscular blockade induced by pancuronium (Miller and others, 1979).

TABLE 1 Clinical tests of muscle strength in a patient with myasthenia gravis before (control) and 10 minutes after intravenous injection of 4-AP (10 mg) and neostigmine (0.5 mg) respectively. Effects of the addition of 4-AP (10 mg) 10 minutes after 0.5 mg neostigmine are also shown

|  | Repetitive hand dynamometer values | Max. number of repeated head bends | Ptosis seconds |
|---|---|---|---|
| Test 1 | Right hand |  |  |
| control | 20,20,18,20 | 12 | 22 |
| 4-AP | 35,30,30,35 | 28 | 50 |
|  |  |  |  |
| Test 2 | Left hand |  |  |
| control | 30,30,35,30 | 13 | 30 |
| Neostigmine | 50,50,45,45 | 24 | 70 |
| Neostigmine+4-AP | 50,55,55,55 | 25 | >180 |

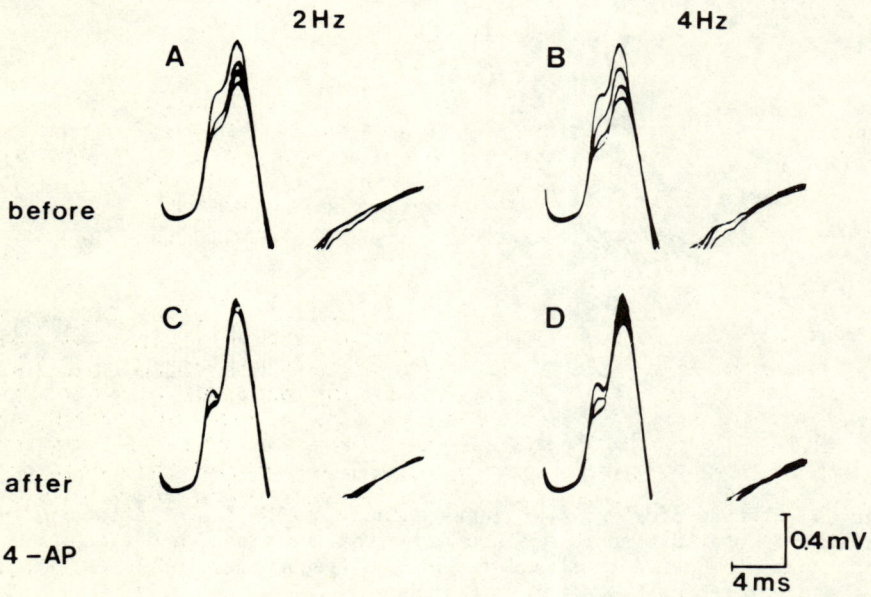

Fig. 5. Effects of 4-AP on a cranial nerve innervated muscle in a patient with myasthenia gravis. Records of CMAP with a surface electrode over the infraorbital muscle in response to repetitive stimulation of the facial nerve at 2 and 4 Hz before (A,B) and after (C,D) intravenous injection of 20 mg 4-AP.

PHARMACOKINETICS

For oral treatment we prefer to use 4-AP sulphate since the chloride is more hygroscopic and difficult to dose.

The pharmacokinetics of 4-AP is unknown, but serum levels have been determined (Ball and others, 1979). Clinical observations and electrophysiological recordings have shown that the effect of a single drug dose disappears within two to four hours after its maximum. Therefore, 4-AP like cholinesterase inhibitors has to be administered several times a day.

CLINICAL SIDE EFFECTS

In all patients examined the intravenous injection of 4-AP caused the immediate appearance of perioral paraesthesia, which disappeared after a few minutes. This side-effect is well-known during guanidine treatment (Henriksson and others, 1977), but did not appear in anyone of our patients treated with continuous 4-AP medication (two with myasthenia gravis and one with Eaton-Lambert syndrome), but paraesthesias of hands and feet have been reported with 4-AP (Murray and Newsom-Davis, 1981).

The intravenous injection of 4-AP in four of six myasthenia gravis patients led to a sensation of unsteadiness on walking during half to two hours. Two of the three patients treated continuously orally were out of bed and both showed disturbance of gait with minor ataxia at clinical tests when they were taking 120 mg 4-AP a day. The third patient was bound to bed as she required mechanical respiratory assistance, and this patient developed paranoid delusions when on 120 mg 4-AP/ day, and one day later at 100 mg 4-AP/ day she got epileptic fits.

Both myasthenia gravis patients on oral medication complained of nervousness, and two of the six patients who received intravenous injection of 10 and 20 mg 4-AP respectively, experienced marked anxiety for a few hours after the injection. The patient with Eaton-Lambert syndrome receiving oral treatment did not complain of anxiety but reported increased wakefulness with difficulty in sleeping and also a disturbing sensitivity to light.

Minor side effects like nausea and stomach pain may appear, and have been considered caused by either the use of the pure alcaline compound or autonomic nervous system actions of the drug (Fastier and McDowall, 1958) like sweating and abdominal cramping (Sanders and others, 1980; Murray and Newsom-Davis, 1981).

We have noticed a small increase of blood pressure (10-30 mm Hg systolic) in some patients after intravenous injection of 20 mg 4-AP tested as an anticurare agent following surgical operations (Lundh, Carlsson and Thesleff, unpublished observations).

DISCUSSION

4-AP is a potent drug to increase transmitter release from motor nerves and to reverse muscle paralysis in human intercostal muscles obtained from patients with myasthenia gravis and the Eaton-Lambert syndrome (see also Kim, Goldner and Sanders, 1980; Sanders and others, 1980). The drug has also been proved capable of antagonizing muscle weakness in vivo in patients with these diseases. 4-AP acts presynaptically, and in neuromuscular disorders with diminished transmitter release like the Eaton-Lambert syndrome, it increases acetylcholine release at each nerve impulse and restores neuromuscular transmission. Although 4-AP acts by enhancing transmitter release it improves neuromuscular transmission and the clinical status in the postsynaptic disorder myasthenia gravis. The reason for this is probably that 4-AP increases normal transmitter release not only in response to single nerve impulses but also during repetitive nerve activity at frequencies used during physiological muscle action (Lundh, 1978).

4-AP has now been used successfully in the treatment of Eaton-Lambert syndrome in many patients published and unpublished in Europe and North America (Lundh, Nilsson and Rosén, 1977; Agoston and others, 1978; Sanders and others, 1980; Murray and Newsom-Davis, 1981), and it has also been tried in human botulism (Ball and others, 1979). In myasthenia gravis it has been used as a supplementary drug in conditions with poor response to conventional therapy like congenital myasthenia (Murray and Newsom-Davis, 1981) and some cases with myasthenic crisis (Lundh, unpublished). We have used 4-AP treatment in patients with generalized myasthenia gravis with respiratory failure not responding satisfactorily to anticholinesterases, corticosteroids and azathioprine, alas with poor effect on respiratory muscles.

Adverse clinical side effects such as unsteadyness on walking and anxiety appeared in the majority of patients examined. During continuous medication severe side effects like ataxia, disturbances of mental function and epileptic fits seem to occur frequently when using the high doses (100-120 mg/day) often required to obtain clinical effects on neuromuscular functions (see also Ball and others, 1979; Murray and Newsom-Davis, 1981). These side effects are probably caused by the central nervous system stimulant actions of 4-AP, demonstrated in animal experiments as convulsions (Lemeignan, 1970; Lundh, Leander and Thesleff, 1977), facilitation of synaptic transmission in the spinal cord (Lemeignan, 1972, 1973; Jankowska and others, 1977), and augmentation of cerebral metabolism in parts of the brain (Edvinsson, Hardebo and Lundh, 1981).

The therapeutic usefulness of 4-AP seems to be severely limited by its adverse side effects. Also, the chronic toxicity and pharmacokinetics of the drug has not been examined in animals or man, which further restricts its usability. At present its use can only be justified in seriously disabled patients with Eaton-Lambert syndrome in combination with a carcinoma and in myasthenia gravis patients not responding to other types of treatment. The observations in animal experiments that 3,4-diaminopyridine is less convulsant (Lechat and others, 1968) but 6-7 times more potent to improve neuromuscular transmission (Molgó, Lundh and Thesleff, 1980) suggest that 3,4-diaminopyridine might be more favourable than 4-AP in the treatment of disorders of neuromuscular transmission. Tests of this new drug in humans are in preparation in the hope that it will cause less central nervous system disturbances.

ACKNOWLEDGEMENTS

Figures 2,3 and 4 and Table 1 are reproduced after Lundh, Nilsson and Rosén (1977, 1979).

The work presented in this study has been supported by grants from the Medical Faculty, University of Lund, Sweden. Technical assistance was provided by Miss B. Hansson.

REFERENCES

Agoston, S., T. van Weerden, P. Westra, and A. Broekert (1978). Effects of 4-aminopyridine in Eaton Lambert syndrome. Br. J. Anaesth., 50, 383-385.
Ball, A. P., R. B. Hopkinson, I. D. Farrell, J. G. P. Hutchinson, R. Paul, R. D. S. Watson, A. J. F. Page, R. G. F. Parker, C. W. Edwards, M. Snow, D. K. Scott, A. Leone-Ganado, A. Hastings, A. C. Ghosh, R. J. Gilbert. Human Botulism caused by

Clostridium botulinum type E: The Birmingham outbreak. Quart. J. Med. New Series XLVIII, 191, 473-491.
Brown, J. C. and R. J. Johns (1969). Clinical and physiological studies of the effect of guanidine on patients with myasthenia gravis. John Hopkins Med. J., 124, 1-8.
Cherington, M. (1976). Guanidine and germine in Eaton-Lambert syndrome. Neurology (Minneapolis), 26, 944-946.
Cherington, M. and D. W. Ryan (1968). Botulism and guanidine. New Engl. J. Med., 278, 931-933.
Cherington, M. and D. W. Ryan (1970). Treatment of botulism with guanidine. New Engl. J. Med., 282, 195-197.
Desmedt, M. J.-E. (1956). Guanidine et myasthénie grave. Revue Neurologique, 94, 154-158.
Edvinsson, L., J. E. Hardebo and H. Lundh (1981). Action of 4-aminopyridine on cerebral circulation. Acta Neurol. Scand., 63, 122-130.
Elmqvist, D. and E. H. Lambert (1968). Detailed analysis of neuromuscular transmission in a patient with the myasthenic syndrome sometimes associated with bronchogenic carcinoma. Mayo Clinic Proceedings, 43, 689-713.
Fastier, F. N. and M. A. McDowall (1958). A comparison of the pharmacological properties of three isomeric aminopyridines. Aust. J. exp. Biol. med. Sci., 36, 365-372.
Grob, D. (1976). Myasthenia gravis. Ann. N. Y. Acad. Sci., Vol. 274.
Henriksson, K. G., O. Nilsson, I. Rosén and H. H. Schiller (1977). Clinical, neurophysiological and morphological findings in Eaton Lambert syndrome. Acta Neurol. Scand., 56, 117-140.
Jankowska, E., A. Lundberg, P. Rudomin and E. Sykova (1977). Effects of 4-aminopyridine on transmission in excitatory and inhibitory synapses in the spinal cord. Brain Research, 136, 387-392.
Kim, Y. I., M. M. Goldner and D. B. Sanders (1980). Facilitatory effects of 4-aminopyridine on neuromuscular transmission in disease states. Muscle and Nerve, 3, 112-119.
Lambert, E. H. (1966). Defects of neuromuscular transmission in syndromes other than myasthenia gravis. Ann. N.Y. Acad. Sci., 135, 367-384.
Lambert, E. H. and D. Elmqvist (1971). Quantal components of endplate potentials in the myasthenic syndrome. Ann. N. Y. Acad. Sci., 183, 183-199.
Lambert, E. H. and F. M. Howard (1972). Complications of guanidine treatment. Presented to the Myasthenia Gravis Foundation. December 1972.
Lechat, P., G. Deysson, M. Lemeignan and M. Adolphe (1968). Toxicité aigue composeé de quelques aminopyridines in vivo (Souris) et in vitro (cultures cellulaires). Ann. Pharmac. Fr., 26, 345-349.
Lemeignan, M. (1970). Etude du mécanisme de l'action convulsivant de l'amino-4 pyridine. Thèse d'Etat, Faculté des Sciences de Paris.
Lemeignan, M. (1972). Analysis of the action of 4-aminopyridine on the cat lumbar spinal cord. I. Modification of the afferent volley, the monosynaptic discharge amplitude and the postsynaptic evoked responses. Neuropharmacology, 11, 551-558.
Lemeignan, M. (1973). Analysis of the effects of 4-aminopyridine on the lumber spinal cord of the cat. II. Modifications of certain spinal inhibitory phenomena, post-tetanic potentiation and dorsal root potentials. Neuropharmacology, 12, 641-651.
Lundh, H. (1978). Effects of 4-aminopyridine on neuromuscular transmission. Brain Research, 153, 307-318.
Lundh, H., S. Leander and S. Thesleff (1977). Antagonism of the paralysis produced by botulinum toxin in the rat. J. Neurol. Sci., 32, 29-43.
Lundh, H., O. Nilsson and I. Rosén (1977). 4-Aminopyridine - A new drug tested in the treatment of Eaton-Lambert syndrome. J. Neurol. Neurosurg. and Psych., 40, 1109-1112.
Lundh, H., O. Nilsson and I. Rosén (1979). Effects of 4-aminopyridine in myasthenia gravis. J. Neurol. Neurosurg. and Psych., 42, 171-175.
Miller, R.D., P. Dennissen, F. van der Pol, S. Agoston, L. Booij and J. Crul (1978). Potentiation of neostigmine and pyridostgmine by 4-aminopyridine in the rat. J.

Pharm. Pharmac., 30, 699-702.
Miller, R. D., L. H. D. J. Booij, S. Agoston and J. F. Crul (1979). 4-Aminopyridine potentiates neostigmine and pyridostigmine in man. Anestesiology, 50, 416-420.
Minot, A. S., K. Dodd and S. S. Riven (1939). Use of guanidine hydrochloride in treatment of myasthenia gravis. J. A. M. A., 113, 553-559.
Molgó, J., M. Lemeignan and P. Lechat (1975). Modification de la libération du transmetteur à la jonction neuromusculaire sous l'action de l'amino-4 pyridine. C. R. Acad. Sci. Paris, Ser. D., 281, 1637-1639.
Molgó, J., M. Lemeignan and P. Lechat (1977). Effects of 4-aminopyridine at the frog neuromuscular junction. J. Pharmacol. Exp. Therap., 203, 653-663.
Molgó, J., H. Lundh and S. Thesleff (1980). Potency of 3,4-diaminopyridine and 4-aminopyridine on mammalian neuromuscular transmission and the effect of pH changes. Europ. J. Pharmacol., 61, 25-34.
Murray, N. M. F. and J. Newsom-Davis (1981). Treatment with oral 4-aminopyridine in disorders of neuromuscular transmission. Neurology (Ny), 31, 265-271.
Nilsson, O. (1981). Personal communication.
Osterman, P. O., L. Hammarström, A. K. Lefvert, G. Matell, E. Smith, J. Säfvenberg and E. Wedlund (1978). Prognostic factors and side effects of high single dose alternate day prednisone (HSDADP) treatment of myasthenia gravis (MG). Presented to the IVth International Congress on Neuromuscular Diseases. Montreal September 1978.
Sanders, D. B., Y. I. Kim, J. F. Howard and C. A. Goetsch (1980). Eaton-Lambert syndrome: a clinical and electrophysiological study of a patient treated with 4-aminopyridine. J. Neurol. Neurosurg. and Psych., 43, 978-985.

# Use of 4-Aminopyridine in Human Botulism

A. P. Ball*, M. Snow* and R. Paul**

*Department of Communicable and Tropical Diseases, East Birmingham Hospital, Birmingham, UK
**Department of Neurophysiology, Walsgrave Hospital, Coventry, UK

ABSTRACT

4-aminopyridine was used to treat 4 patients with severe paralytic botulism due to Clostridium botulinum type E toxin. An immediate but transient improvement in peripheral muscle power and motor action potential amplitude was observed. Severe ventilatory paralysis was essentially unaffected. Prolonged intravenous infusion produced sustained improvement in peripheral muscle power during therapy and an apparent continued decrease in paralysis thereafter, but was complicated by convulsions shortly after termination of infusion.

KEYWORDS

Human botulism; 4-aminopyridine; neuro-muscular transmission; reversal of paralysis; convulsive phenomena.

INTRODUCTION

Botulism is a rare disease in the UK, only 25 cases with 14 resultant deaths having been reported in the last 60 years. In the USA during the same period an average of 10 outbreaks have occurred per year (Horwitz and others, 1977), but the original very high mortality has fallen to less than 30% overall. Food borne human botulism is caused by the ingestion of pre-formed neurotoxin (BoTox) in food contaminated by Cl. botulinum. There are seven different types of Cl. botulinum, types A, B, and E usually being involved in human disease. Each produces an antigenically distinct high molecular weight protein toxin, subunits and polymers of which vary in neurotoxicity (Sacks and Covert, 1974). It has been recognised for some time (Burgen, Dickens and Zatman, 1949) that the site of action of BoTox is at the pre-terminal cholinergic motor neuro-fibril proximal to the myoneural junction: its effect being the blockade of acetylcholine (Ach) release. Recent in vitro studies have shown that the transmission defect is due to a failure of evoked Ach quantal release, caused by a reduction in calcium-ion sensitivity of the release mechanism (Cull-Candy, Lundh and Thesleff, 1976). Further studies by this team showed that tetraethylammonium and guanidine could potentiate Ach release in vitro in BoTox exposed neuro-fibrils, possibly by reducing intracellular calcium binding (Lundh and others, 1976). However, parallel clinical studies with guanidine demonstrated that although peripheral paralysis, caused by BoTox, was improved or reversed, severe respiratory paralysis was largely unaffected (Cherington, 1974; Cherington, Greenberg and Soyer, 1973). As acute ventilatory failure and the complications of long-term assisted ventilation are the major determinants of continued mortality, the unexplained lack of effect on respiratory muscle is a major limitation of guanidine therapy of human botulism.

Subsequently, 4-aminopyridine (4-AP) was shown to be twenty times more active in vitro than guanidine, to be effective at physiological calcium concentrations and to transiently reverse severe paralysis in BoTox treated rats (Lundh, Leander and Thesleff, 1977). Studies in the patho-physiologically related Eaton-Lambert syndrome in man demonstrated that 4-AP was capable of reversing human neuro-muscular blockade (Lundh, Nilsson and Rosen, 1977; Agoston and others, 1978). This suggested its use in botulism. In 1978, 4 patients with severe paralytic botulism due to Cl. botulinum type E were treated with 4-AP. The present report details the results obtained in that study (Ball and others, 1979).

PATIENTS AND METHODS

All 4 patients were severely paralysed, requiring assisted ventilation within 6 hours of the onset of symptoms. Administration of high dose trivalent anti-toxin had no effect on the paralysis. By day 4, severe respiratory paralysis continued in all patients, peripheral muscle power varying from minimal in patient B to transient movement against resistance in patient D. None had received additional neuro-muscular blocking agents to facilitate assisted ventilation. Urinary retention and intestinal ileus was present, indicating parasympathetic dysfunction, and, in addition, the presence of systolic hypotension (60-70 mm Hg) and absence of vasomotor reflexes suggested sympathetic dysfunction.

On days 4/5 the patients received single intravenous (IV) bolus doses of 4-AP (0.35 - 0.5 mg/Kg), either alone or with neostigmine (3 patients) and atropine (2 patients). Second doses were administered to 2 patients and infusion therapy (total dose 4-AP: 90 mg) was investigated in a further 2.

The results were assessed both clinically and by electromyography. The latter recordings were made using a Medelec MS6 machine, stimulating the right lateral popliteal nerve, with a concentric electrode being placed in the ipsilateral Extensor digitorum brevis muscle. The amplitude of the first supra-maximal motor action potential was measured. Blood pressure and pulse rate variations were recorded via a transducer throughout therapy.

RESULTS OF SINGLE AND DOUBLE DOSE ADMINISTRATION OF 4-AP

Clinical

The clinical results were similar in all patients. Within the first 5 minutes the following features were observed:
1. Immediate arousal
2. Return of bowel sounds (hyperactive and associated with discomfort in 2 patients
3. Elevation of systolic blood pressure by 20 mm Hg, and increase in heart rate of 5-12 beats per minute.

A marked progressive improvement in peripheral muscle power was noted within 5-10 minutes, persisting for 2-4 hours and then returning to the pre-treatment level. The maximum effect was present in the extrinsic ocular and limb muscles, and in 2 patients power in these muscles was virtually normal during treatment. However, clinical observation and measurement of spontaneous tidal and minute volumes demonstrated only minimal effect on the respiratory muscles. No adverse effects were detected during single and double dose 4-AP therapy.

Electromyographic Studies

Complete records of evoked muscle motor action potentials before and throughout therapy were possible in 2 patients, the recording electrode being displaced from the motor unit by muscular activity during therapy in the others. Motor nerve conduction velocities were normal (greater than 40 metres/second) in all four patients prior to 4-AP therapy.

Patient C received a single 0.35 mg/Kg IV bolus of 4-AP, together with atropine 1.2 mg and neostigmine 0.08 mg/Kg. The resultant improvement in motor action potential amplitude is shown in Fig. 1.

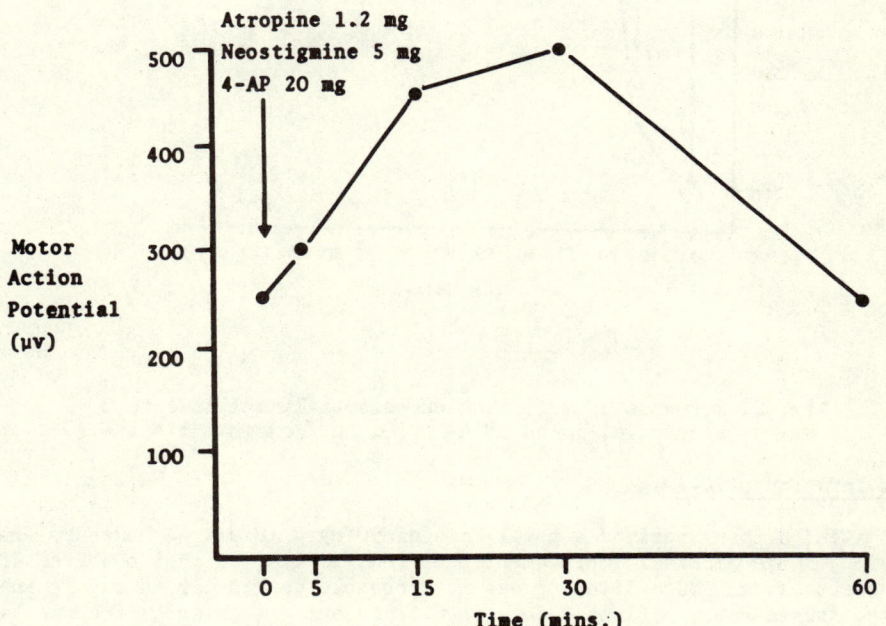

Fig. 1. Response of motor action potential amplitude in patient C (dose 4-AP: 0.35 mg/Kg by IV bolus).

Patient D demonstrated a similar improvement after a 0.5 mg/Kg IV bolus. Patient A initially received a 0.35 mg/Kg bolus of 4-AP alone with a response of lesser magnitude, but, following administration of 0.08 mg/Kg neostigmine (25 minutes later) an increase in amplitude similar to that of patient C was observed. The effect of 4-AP in these patients lasted for between 45-120 minutes. Patient A initially received atropine and neostigmine alone with minimal effect on motor action potential amplitude. He then received two doses of 4-AP (0.5 mg/Kg by IV bolus) at 15 and 65 minutes respectively. There was an immediate and dramatic response, action potential amplitude increasing from 400 to over 1100 microvolts after the first dose and to 1400 microvolts following the second. These effects are shown in Fig. 2.

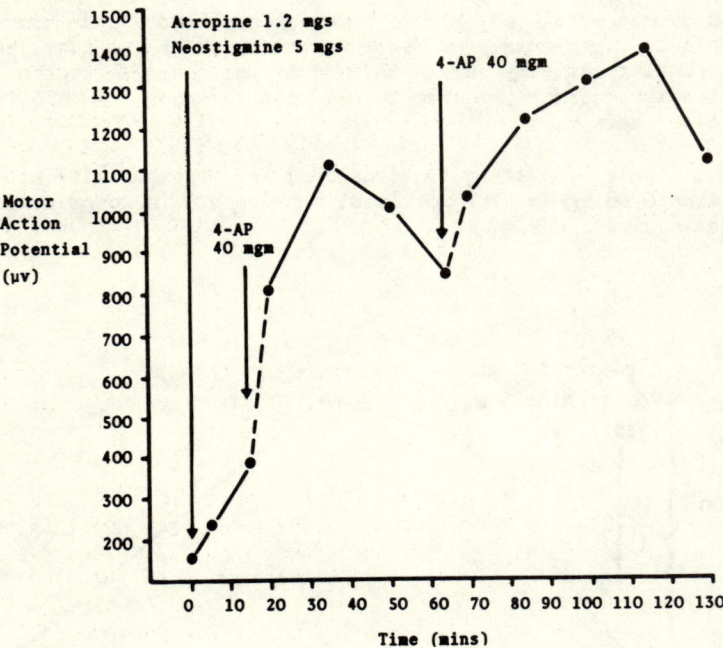

Fig. 2. Response of motor action potential amplitude to 2 sequential doses of 4-AP (0.5 mg/Kg) in patient A

Constant Infusion of 4-AP

Patients A and C then received a total dose of 90 mg 4-AP over 4 hours by constant IV infusion. Rapid clinical improvement occurred, similar to that observed after single dose therapy. EMG monitoring was not possible due to marked restlessness. During the fourth hour, patient C developed transient twitching of the face and right arm. This passed off within 5 minutes and infusion was continued. However, within one hour of the termination of infusion both developed generalised fits, requiring large intravenous doses of diazepam (60-80 mg) for control. No further convulsive phenomena were noted and no other immediate adverse effects of therapy were observed.

There was little improvement in respiratory muscle power in either patient.

CONCLUSIONS

Treatment with 4-AP produced a considerable increase in evoked motor action potential amplitude, this effect being reflected by a dramatic improvement in peripheral muscle power. However, for reasons which remain unknown, the respiratory muscles were essentially unaffected. BoTox has traditionally been thought to act entirely peripherally and to have no effect on the central nervous system. However a central effect might explain the disparity of the effect of 4-AP on peripheral and respiratory muscle. All of the presently reported patients had abnormal EEGs prior to 4-AP therapy.

The duration of clinical effect following 4-AP therapy exceeded that of the EMG response in all patients, and, in those treated by IV infusion, there was a suggestion of some permanent improvement in peripheral muscle power following treatment.

Therapy with 4-AP was curtailed by the occurrence of convulsions in the patients receiving a total dose of 90 mg over 4 hours. It therefore seems unlikely that the lack of response of respiratory muscles might be overcome by further increase in dosage. Analogues of 4-AP with reduced central neurotoxicity but retained or greater effect on the Ach release mechanism might be of increased efficacy and should be evaluated when the opportunity arises. At present the benefits of 4-AP therapy are outweighed by potential toxicity.

ACKNOWLEDGEMENT

Figures 1 and 2 are reproduced from the Quarterly Journal of Medicine with the kind permission of the Editor.

REFERENCES

Agoston, S., van Weerden, T., Westra, P., and A. Broekert (1978) Brit. J. Anaesth. 50, 383-385
Ball, A.P., Hopkinson, R.B., Farrell, I.D., Hutchison, J.G.P., Paul, R., Watson, R.D.S., Page, A.J.F., Parker, R.G.F., Edwards, C.W., Snow, M., Scott, D.K., Leone-Ganado, A., Hastings, A., Ghosh, A.C. and R.J.Gilbert (1979) Quart. J. Med, 48, 473-491
Burgen, A.S.V., Dickens, F., and L.J. Zatman (1949) J. Physiol. 109, 10-24
Cherington, M., Greeberg, H., and A. Soyer (1973) Clin. Toxicol. 6, 83-89
Cherington, M. (1974) Arch. Neurol. 30, 432-437
Cull-Candy, S.G., Lundh, H., and Thesleff, S. (1976) J.Physiol., 260, 177-203
Horwitz, M.A., Hughes, J.M., Merson, M.H. and E.J. Gangarosa (1977) J. Infect. Dis., 136, 153-159
Lundh, H., Cull-Candy, S.G., Leander, S., and S. Thesleff (1976) Brain Research, 110, 194-198
Lundh, H., Leander, S., and S. Thesleff (1977) J. Neurol. Sci., 32, 29-43
Lundh, H., Nilsson, O., and I. Rosen (1977) J. Neurol. Neurosurg. Psychiatr., 40, 1109-1112
Sacks, H.S., and S.V.Covert (1974) Appl. Microbiol., 28, 374-382

# Therapeutic Applications of 4-Aminopyridine in Anaesthesia

## S. Agoston, D. R. A. Uges and R. L. Sia

Research Group of the Institutes of Anaesthesiology and
Clinical Pharmacology, State University of Groningen, Oostersingel
59, Groningen, The Netherlands

### ABSTRACT

The results of clinical studies with 4-AP in anaesthetized patients and healthy human volunteers are reviewed. The anti-curare effect of 0.3 mg/kg 4-AP when given alone appeared to be weak. However, in combination with neostigmine or pyridostigmine, 4-AP considerably potentiated the antagonistic effects of these anti-cholinesterases. Due to this synergism the dose of neostigmine and pyridostigmine required for 50 percent antagonism could be reduced by 70 and 80 percent respectively. 4-AP appeared to be useful in reversing neuromuscular blockade due to presynaptic effects of antibiotics or in situations where the conventional antagonists are of little or no use. In human volunteers 4-AP significantly shortened the duration of sleep and facilitated the return to full physical normality following diazepam/ketamine anaesthesia. In anaesthetized patients this compound was shown to reverse central respiratory depression induced by opiates. Human pharmacokinetic studies with 4-AP revealed a long elimination half-life (4 hr), large distribution volume at steady state (200 L/70 kg) and high total plasma clearance (11 ml/kg/min). Urinary elimination of the unchanged compound accounted for 90 percent of the administered dose.

### KEYWORDS

4-Aminopyridine; anaesthetics; opiates; muscle relaxants; pharmacokinetics.

### INTRODUCTION

The first reports of the facilitatory actions of the 2-, 3- and 4-aminopyridines (4-AP) on transmission at various synapses (Fastier and McDowal, 1958; Lemeignan and co-workers, 1969; Molgo and co-workers, 1975) were soon followed by the clinical application of 4-AP by Bulgarian anaesthetists (Paskov, Stojanov and Micov, 1973). Since then much experimental work has been done in order to clarify the pharmacological profile and define the clinical usefulness of this compound, which was originally known and used as a bird repellant in the U.S.A.

4-AP is thought to facilitate synaptic transmission in both the central and peripheral nervous systems by a $Ca^{++}$-dependent increase of transmitter release. Consequently, in the central nervous system (CNS) it may facilitate transmission in both excitatory and inhibitory pathways and augment central and peripheral synaptic activity at cholinergic and adrenergic (and probably also other) synapses at the same time. From such a drug a multitude of possibly useful clinical effects can be expected, which initially encouraged its careful application in various clinical disciplines. However, such a lack of specificity may also complicate and ultimately limit its clinical use - due to increased risks of unwanted effects or interactions.

The accumulated clinical experience with 4-AP so far includes its therapeutic application in myoneural disorders such as myasthenia gravis (Lundh, Nilsson and Rosén, 1979), the Eaton-Lambert syndrome (Lundh, Nilsson and Rosén, 1977) and Huntington's chorea (Wesseling and Lakke, 1980), and its use in clinical anaesthesia for reversal of neuromuscular blockade resulting from the use of non-depolarizing muscle relaxants and certain antibiotics (Burkett and co-workers, 1979; Booij, Miller and Crul, 1978). In this lecture we briefly review our own clinical experiences obtained during the last few years with 4-aminopyridine and also report on its pharmacokinetic profile in man.

## NEUROMUSCULAR JUNCTION

At the neuromuscular junction 4-AP increases the release of acetylcholine. This presynaptic action is helpful in reversing the neuromuscular effects of certain aminoglycoside-type antibiotics and non-depolarizing muscle relaxants. The reversal of a neuromuscular block, produced by a combination of pancuronium and lincomycin, by 4-AP (Fig. 1) was shown by Booij, Miller and Crul in 1978.

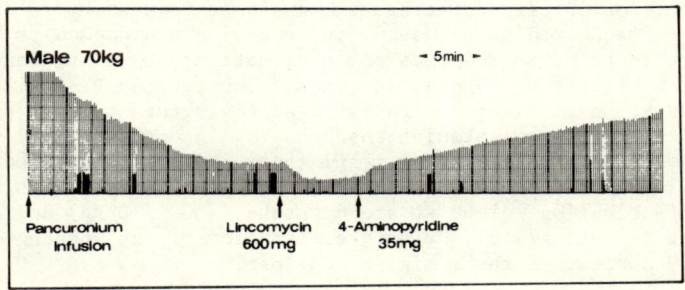

Fig. 1. 4-Aminopyridine reversal of a combined pancuronium/
lincomycin neuromuscular blockade in man.
(From: Booij, Miller and Crul, 1978).

When given alone, 4-AP has only a modest anticurare effect (Fig. 2). In this patient a constant 90% twitch height depression was produced and maintained with pancuronium bromide. After stopping the infusion spontaneous recovery to 20% of control was allowed and then 230 µg/kg 4-AP was injected in a 2 min period. As a result the recovery rate visibly increased; however, there was less than 80% recovery by 15 min, and therefore neostigmine 12 µg/kg was given together with atropine, which resulted in a prompt and complete restoration of the neuromuscular transmission within a few minutes

Under similar conditions neostigmine, the most commonly used antagonist, usually completes reversal in less than 10 min. Without the use of an antagonist, however, the spontaneous recovery of a partial pancuronium blockade may last as long as 50 min.

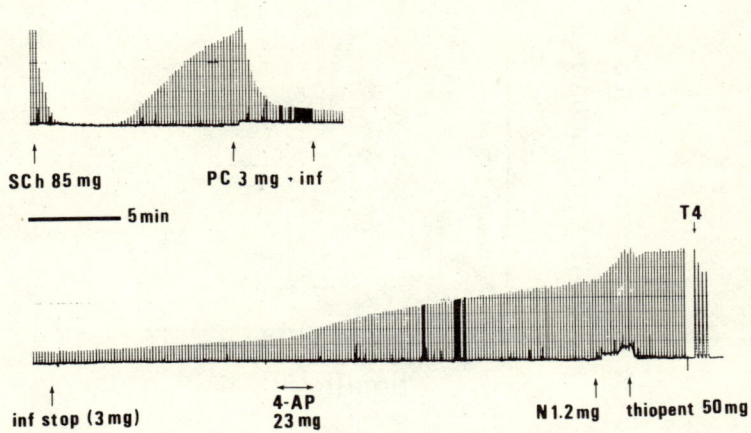

Fig. 2. Reversal of pancuronium (Pc)-induced neuromuscular blockade by 4-aminopyridine (4-AP) and neostigmine (N).
(From: Sohn and Uges, 1980).

In order to speed up recovery perhaps higher doses of 4-AP could be used. However, in our experience 0.3 mg/kg appeared to be the highest safe dose. Higher doses were frequently associated with central nervous system stimulation resulting in post-operative restlessness and confusion. In order to achieve a fast and complete reversal 4-AP might be combined with one of the routinely used reversal agents like neostigmine or pyridostigmine. In view of their different mechanisms of action one would expect the effects of such a combination to be synergistic. Consequently the dose of one or both drugs in such a combination could be diminished without loss of antagonistic activity and with a considerably smaller risk of side effects.

The synergism between 4-AP and the cholinesterase inhibitors was demonstrated in a clinical study (Miller and co-workers, 1979) in which a steady state neuromuscular blockade of 90% was produced and maintained by the infusion of pancuronium bromide. Unlike the previous study, in this investigation spontaneous recovery was not allowed; the antagonist was given during the continuous infusion of the relaxant. Under these experimental conditions the dose of 350 µg/kg 4-AP when given alone appeared to be ineffective. A dose of 500 µg/kg produced only 24% antagonism and also resulted in central nervous system excitation at the same time. When, however, the - by itself ineffective - dose of 350 µg/kg 4-AP was combined with neostigmine or pyridostigmine, tremendous potentiation of their effects could be demonstrated. In combination with the above dose of 4-AP the doses of neostigmine and pyridostigmine producing 50% antagonism could be reduced by 70 and 80% respectively.

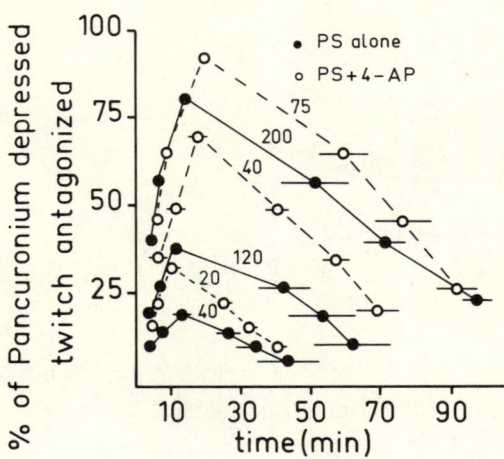

Fig. 3. Plot of time and percentage of pancuronium induced depression of twitch tension antagonized. The numbers present the doses of pyridostigmine (PS) in µg/kg. The dose of 4-AP was 350 µg/kg. Three patients were studied at each dose.
(From: Miller and co-workers, 1979).

## CENTRAL NERVOUS SYSTEM (CNS)

The analeptic effects of 4-AP were already suggested in the early reports of the Bulgarian investigators (Paskov, Stojanov and Micov, 1973). Before our own human studies focused on the CNS effects of 4-AP we made two relevant observations in animal experiments. In 1979 Folgering, Rutten and Agoston studied the effects of 4-AP on ventilation in cats by measuring the quantified phrenic nerve activity as an indication of the central respiratory drive. In this study 4-AP 1 mg/kg increased spontaneous phrenic nerve activity by approximately 30% (Fig. 4).

This effect could be abolished within 2-3 min by high doses of atropine (1 mg/kg) indicating the involvement of cholinergic mechanisms. In this study the increase in the phrenic nerve activity was also observed when the peripheral chemoreceptors were either suppressed by hyperoxia or bypassed by injecting 4-AP to the vertebral artery. Furthermore, while the phrenic nerve activity increased following the administration of 4-AP, the simultaneously-recorded femoral nerve activity remained constant indicating that the changes in phrenic nerve activity were not due to an unspecific effect of 4-AP on spinal motorneurones.

The other observation was made in monkeys during experiments designed to investigate the antagonistic effect of 4-AP on tubocurarine-induced neuromuscular block. In these experiments the monkeys were anaesthetized with high doses of ketamine. However, the animals frequently became awake following the administration of 4-AP in spite of the continuing ketamine infusion.

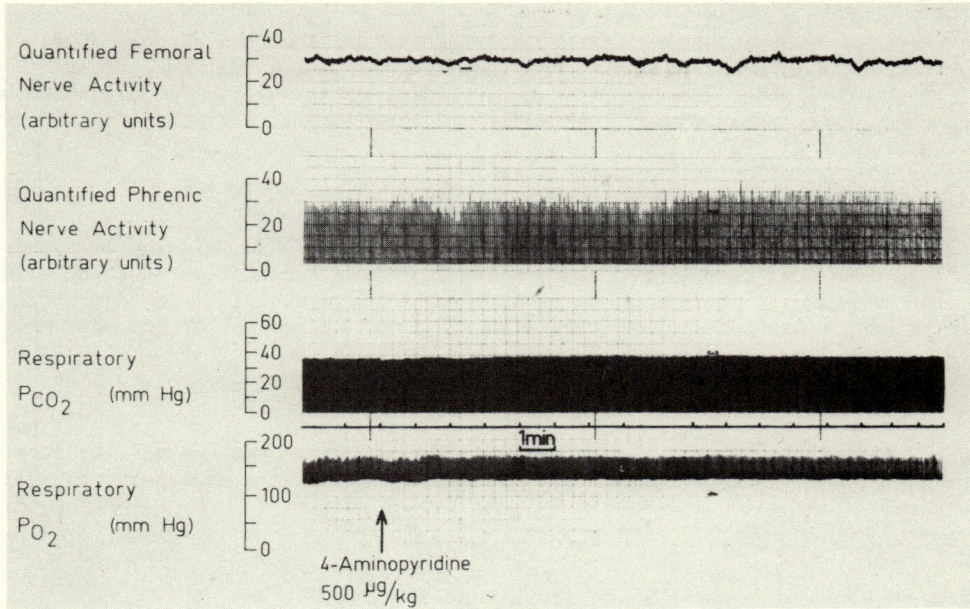

Fig. 4. Simultaneous recording of quantified femoral and phrenic nerve activity - respiratory $P_{CO_2}$ and $P_{O_2}$ in the cat before and after 0.5 mg/kg 4-AP. (From: Folgering, Rutten and Agoston, 1979).

These observations prompted us to study the interaction of ketamine and 4-AP in human volunteers (Agoston and co-workers, 1980). The volunteers were subjected on two occasions, at least 1 week apart, to a ketamine-diazepam anaesthetic lasting

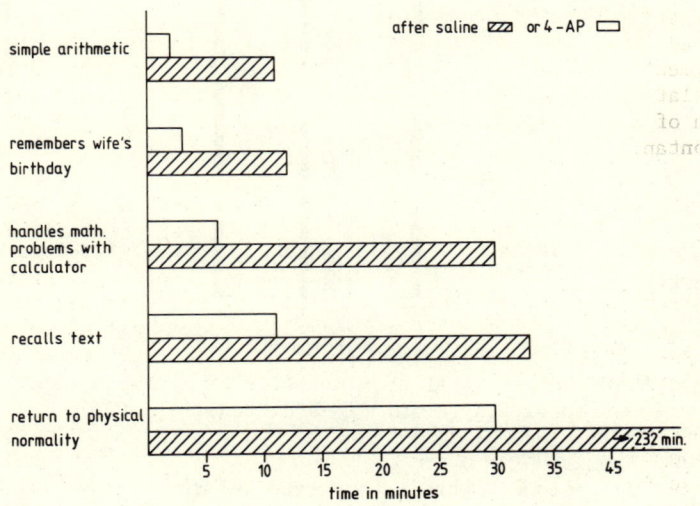

Fig. 5. Time required for the successful completion of tests after saline or 4-AP (from: Agoston and co-workers, 1980).

1 hr. At the end of the anaesthetic either 4-AP 0.3 mg/kg or the same volume of saline was administered, and the subsequent rate of recovery from the anaesthetic was monitored. Each volunteer was repeatedly challenged with a battery of tests in order to obtain information about the graded return to a normal awake-state. Logical thought, short and long-term memory and general physical coordination were among the parameters assessed. The results of these experiments showed a considerable shortening of the mean times required for the successful completion of the tests employed, following the administration of 4-AP.

The observed antagonism between ketamine and 4-AP in man and the serious consequences of the abuse of the precursor of ketamine, phencyclidine (or "angel dust") in drug addicts prompted us to investigate the interaction of phencyclidine and 4-AP in monkeys. Increasing doses of phencyclidine were administered until a state of stupor was reached and then either 0.3-0.9 mg/kg 4-AP or the same volume of saline was injected i.v. and the recovery from the CNS depressant effects of phencyclidine were observed. In these experiments 4-AP appeared not to antagonize the stuporous state produced by phencyclidine in the monkeys.

In a clinical study Sia and Zandstra (1981) have demonstrated the ability of 4-AP to reverse opiate-induced respiratory depression in patients undergoing general anaesthesia (Fig. 6).

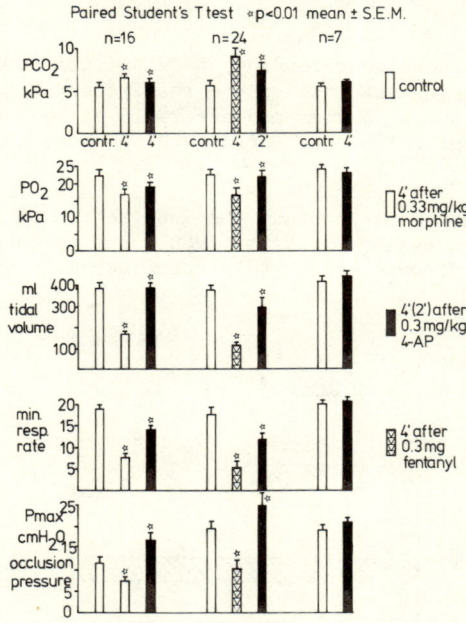

Fig. 6. Effects of 4-AP upon morphine or fentanyl depressed respiration (from: Sia and Zandstra, 1981).

The $P_{CO_2}$, $P_{O_2}$, tidal volumes, respiratory rate and the occlusion pressure were measured before, four min after the administration of either morphine or fentanyl, and 2 and 4 min following the administration of 4-AP. All patients who received one of these opiates showed apnoea, followed by a slow and shallow respiratory pattern. After the administration of 4-AP there was a statistically significant improvement in all parameters. The tidal volume was doubled and approached the control values after the administration of 0.3 mg/kg 4-AP. Significant improvement was also seen in occlusion pressure. The occlusion pressure has been found, also by other investigators (Derene and co-workers, 1976), to be a reliable index of respiratory drive in anaesthetized patients. From these studies it appears that 4-AP stimulates respiratory activity when this is severely depressed, since in the control group of patients, who received 4-AP alone, the drug did not appear to produce any significant changes upon the parameters studied.

PHARMACOKINETICS

The growing clinical interest in 4-AP prompted further studies to elucidate its pharmacokinetic profile in man. Sensitive gas-liquid chromatographic (Evenhuis and co-workers, 1981) or "high-performance" liquid chromatographic (Uges and Bouma, 1981) procedures for determination of 4-AP in human and animal biological fluids were developed and used in our pharmacokinetic studies. Nine volunteers (Uges and co-workers, in press) received 20 mg 4-AP either by the intravenous route or orally in the form of enteric coated or non-coated tablets. In these studies 4-AP concentrations were determined in saliva, plasma and urine. Each of the volunteers was studied on three different occasions. Fig. 7 is a computer-plot of the saliva concentration curves obtained from one volunteer following intravenous and oral doses.

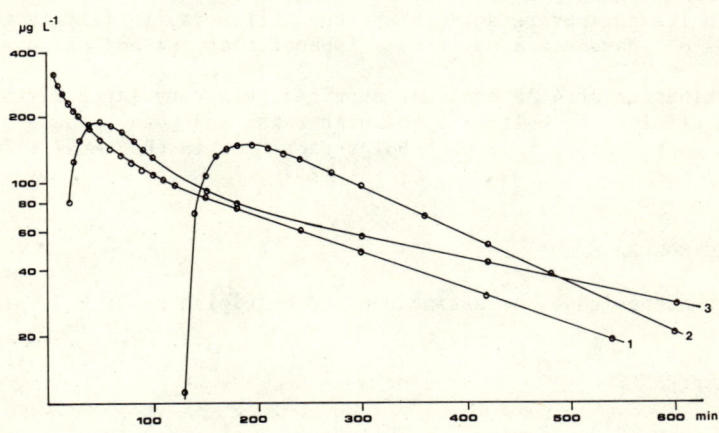

Fig. 7. Saliva concentrations of 4-AP following i.v. (1), oral administration enteric coated (2) and non-coated tablets (3).
(From: Uges and co-workers, 1981).

Interestingly, the saliva concentrations appeared to be higher than the concomitant serum concentrations; however, the intra-individual correlation between serum and saliva was found to be very good - with a coefficient of r=0.98 in all the investigated cases. The kinetic analysis of the serum concentrations following intravenous administration fitted a 3-phase model best in 5 subjects and a 2-phase model in 4 subjects.

The kinetics of 4-AP are further characterized by a large distribution volume at steady state approximating 200 L in an average sized adult, a long elimination half-life of about 4 hr and a high total plasma clearance of 11 ml/kg/min. Most of the drug (about 90% of the administered dose) appears unchanged in urine within 24 hr. The administration of 10 mg 4-AP in coated tablets 3 times a day resulted in serum levels of 30 µg/L. This concentration is regarded as therapeutically relevant in the majority of patients on long-term treatment with 4-AP (Wesseling, 1981).

## SUMMARY AND CONCLUSIONS

Many of the various actions of 4-AP could be useful in daily anaesthetic practice and also in some neurological diseases. Its presynaptic effects, resulting in an increase of acetylcholine release, are used by anaesthesiologists to antagonize partial neuromuscular blockade not only following non-depolarizing muscle relaxants but also in cases when the standard antagonists are of little or no use - such as in cases of neuromuscular block due to, or potentiated by, certain antibiotics. The potentiation of the effects of neostigmine and pyridostigmine by 4-AP makes it possible to use smaller than usual doses of these compounds when combined with 4-AP. The use of small doses in combination most probably will minimize or eliminate the unwanted effects that these drugs may have when given alone in greater dosage.

The analeptic effects of 4-AP reversing opiate-induced respiratory depression would by no means justify its use as an opiate antagonist, but this effect together with its anticurare actions and the ability to facilitate recovery from certain types of anaesthesia may prove of benefit at the end of surgery.

The pharmacokinetics of 4-AP are characterized by a very large distribution volume, long elimination half-life and high renal and total plasma clearance, suggesting a contributory role of tubular secretion in the renal elimination of this drug.

## ACKNOWLEDGEMENT

We gratefully acknowledge the assistance and criticism of Dr F.J. Richardson.

## REFERENCES

Agoston, S., Salt, P.J., Ermann, W., Hilkemeijer, T., Bencini, A. and Langrehr, D. (1980). Antagonism of ketamine-diazepam anaesthesia by 4-aminopyridine in human volunteers. Br. J. Anaesth., 52, 367-370.

Booij, L.H.D.J., Miller, R.D. and Crul, J.F. (1978). Neostigmine and 4-aminopyridine antagonism of lincomycin-pancuronium neuromuscular blockade in man. Anesth. Analg., 57, 316-321.

Burkett, L., Bikhazi, G.B., Thomas jr., K.C., Rosenthal, D.A., Wirta, M.G. and Foldes, F.F. (1979). Mutual potentiation of the neuromuscular effects of antibiotics and relaxants. Anesth. Analg., 58, 107-115.

Derene, J.P., Contoure, J., Iscoe, S., Whitelaw, W.A. and Milic, E. (1976). Occlusion pressures in men rebreathing $CO_2$ under methoxyfurane anesthesia. J. Appl. Physiol., 40, 805-814.

Evenhuis, J., Agoston, S., Salt, P.J., de Lange, A.R., Wouthuyzen, W. and Erdmann, W. (1981). Pharmacokinetics of 4-aminopyridine in human volunteers. A preliminary study using a new GLC method for its estimation. Br. J. Anaesth., 53, 567-570.
Fastier, F.N. and McDowal, M.A. (1958). A comparison of the pharmacological properties of the three isomeric aminopyridines. Aust. J. Exp. Biol. Med. Sci., 36, 365-372.
Folgering, H., Rutten, J. and Agoston, S. (1979). Stimulation of phrenic nerve activity by an acetylcholine releasing drug: 4-aminopyridine. Pflügers Arch., 379, 181-185.
Lemeignan, M., Chanelet, J. and Saade, N.E. (1969). Etude de l'action d'un convulsivant spécial (la 4-aminopyridine) sur les nerfs de vertébrés. C.R. Soc. Biol. (Paris), 163, 359-365.
Lundh, H., Nilsson, O. and Rosén, J. (1977). 4-Aminopyridine - a new drug tested in the treatment of Eaton-Lambert syndrome. J. Neurol. Neurosurg. Psychiatry, 40, 1109-1112.
Lundh, H., Nilsson, O. and Rosén, J. (1979). Effects of 4-aminopyridine in myasthenia gravis. J. Neurol. Neurosurg. Psychiatry, 42, 171-175.
Miller, R.D., Booij, L.H.D.J., Agoston, S. and Crul, J.F. (1979). 4-Aminopyridine potentiates neostigmine and pyridostigmine in man. Anesthesiology, 50, 416-420.
Molgo, J., Lemeignan, M. and Lechat, P. (1975). Modifications de la libération du transmitteur à la jonction neuromusculaire de grenouille sans l'action de l'amino-4-pyridine. C.D. Acad. Sci. (Paris), D. 281, 1637-1639.
Paskov, D.S., Stojanov, E.A. and Micov, V.V. (1973). New anticurare and analeptic drug Pimadin (4-aminopyridine hydrochloride) and its use in anaesthesia. (In Russian). Eksper. Khir. Anestesiol., 18, 48-52.
Richardson, F.J. (1980). Personal communication.
Sia, R.L. and Zandstra, D.F. (1981). 4-Aminopyridine reversal of morphine-induced respiratory depression in human. Br. J. Anaesth. in press.
Sohn, Y.J. and Uges, D.R.A. (1980). Pharmacokinetics and side effects of 4-aminopyridine. Anesthesiology - Int. Congr. Series no. 538. Proceedings of the 7th World Congress of Anaesthesiologists. Excerpta Medica, Amsterdam-Oxford-Princeton.
Uges, D.R.A. and Bouma, P. (1981). Liquid chromatographic determination of 4-aminopyridine in serum, saliva and urine. Clin. Chem., 27, 437-440.
Uges, D.R.A., Sohn, Y.J., Greijdanus, B., Scaf, A.H.J. and Agoston, S. (1981). Pharmacokinetics of 4-aminopyridine in man. Clin. Pharm. Ther. in press.
Wesseling, H. and Lakke, J.P.W.F. (1980). Observations with 4-aminopyridine in Huntington's chorea. IRCS Medical Sciences, 8, 332-333.
Wesseling, H. (1981). Personal communication.

# Effects of 3,4-Diaminopyridine in Cynomolgus Monkeys Poisoned with Type A Botulinum Toxin

## G. E. Lewis and R. M. Wood

U.S. Army Medical Research Institute of Infectious Diseases,
Fort Detrick, Frederick, Maryland 21701, USA

4-Aminopyridine (4-AP) appears to be useful in the treatment of disorders involving defects in synaptic transmission. 4-AP has been shown to antagonize the blockade of nerve impulse-invoked transmitter release produced by type A botulinum toxin in rats and by type E botulinum toxin in man (LUNDH et al., 1977; BALL et al., 1979). Convulsive side-effects have been reported with the use of high doses (> 1 mg/kg) of 4-AP. A similar, but more potent and thought-to-be-less convulsive compound, 3,4-diaminopyridine (3,4-DAP) was evaluated in nonhuman primates as an intravenously (i.v.) administered antagonist of botulinum toxin-induced paralysis. Six male cynomolgus monkeys (4.1 to 6.0 kg) were poisoned i.v. with 100 to 350 mouse $LD_{50}$/kg of type A botulinum toxin. Onset of signs of botulism paralleled those reported in man and correlated with the dosage of toxin, ranging in time of first appearance from 10.5 to 31 hours. 3,4-DAP was administered as multiple doses of 1.1 to 2.6 mg/kg and/or as a continuous i.v. drip of 0.78 to 0.95 mg/kg per hour. Treatment was intentionally delayed from 3 to 6 hours after appearance of the first signs of botulism. The interval between the first and second treatment was 2 to 5 hours. All poisoned monkeys responded favorably within 2 to 10 minutes after treatment with 3,4-DAP at 1.1 to 2.6 mg/kg. Muscle tone returned, ptosis was reduced or negated, respiratory patterns improved unequivocally; prostrate animals were able to stand; and mobility was restored in all treated monkeys. Within 2 hours after initial treatment, signs of paralysis again appeared. Treatment with a second dose induced a response considerably less dramatic than that observed after the initial dose. Continuous i.v. administration of 3,4-DAP did not prevent the return or progression of paralysis. At the dosage rates used, 3,4-DAP was not convulsive, prolonged survival, but did not prevent death.

BALL, A. P., HOPKINSON, R. B., FARRELL, I. D., HUTCHINSON, J. G. P., PAUL, R., WATSON, R. D. S., PAGE, A. J. F., PARKER, R. G. F., EDWARDS, C. W., SNOW, M., SCOTT, D. K., LEONE-GANADO, A., HASTINGS, A., GHOSH, A. C., and GILBERT, R. J. (1979) Q. J. Med. 48, 273.
LUNDH, H., LEANDER, S. and THESLEFF, S. (1977) J. Neurobiol. Sci. 32, 29.

DISCUSSION OF THE SEVENTH SESSION.

Dr. Grafe: Dr. Lundh, do you have experience with anticonvulsants in the treatment of 4-aminopyridine induced side effects? Did you try 4-aminopyridine in patients suffering from amyotrophic lateral sclerosis?

Dr. Lundh: The answer to the first question is no. I have tested 4-aminopyridine on two patients with amyotrophic lateral sclerosis with single dose injections and observed no effect. However, to decide if 4-aminopyridine has an effect in that disease continuous treatment for some period is needed.

Dr. Westra: Did your patients complain about deep aching pain after 4-aminopyridine at the site of injection as we observed in all our volunteers?

Dr. Lundh: Yes, in some patients. When this pain appeared it lasted for a few hours. Its appearance was independent of the pH of the injection solution and was also observed when diluted solutions were used.

Dr. Bowman: Did you use atropine when you gave 4-aminopyridine orally and if not, did you observe any gastro-intestinal or other autonomic side-effects?

Dr. Lundh: We did not use atropine and did not observe gastro-intestinal side-effects. Stomach pain has, however, been reported by others. Also, abnormal sweating has been observed in some patients by other investigators.


Dr. Molgo: I should like to ask Dr. Ball if he thinks that specific antitoxins may enhance the effect of 4-aminopyridine in human botulism?

Dr. Ball: Possibly, certainly if pre-treatment with antitoxin prevents progression of paralysis. However, there was a 4-5 days time interval between the administration of antitoxin and 4-aminopyridine in our patients. I am unaware of any data on that combination in man.

Dr. Foldes: Did you consider the possibility that the dose of 4-aminopyridine that appeared to be optimal for peripheral skeletal muscles represented an overdose for respiratory muscles? Would it be advisable to administer 4-aminopyridine in botulism intoxication as continuous intravenous infusion adjusting the rate of infusion to obtain optimal effects on respiration? When attempting to improve the therapeutic effects of 4-aminopyridine with the simultaneous use of neostigmine it should be administered in small (0.25 mg) increments, again using the respiratory response as a guide for the administration of additional doses. I would also like to ask if it would be worthwhile to use diazepam, or a similar compound, prophylactically to prevent the CNS effects of 4-aminopyridine.

Dr. Lundh: May I just add after Dr. Foldes question that after intravenous injection of 4-aminopyridine to myasthenic patients the first effect observed, before any effect on neuromuscular transmission, is an increase in respiratory depth and frequency.

Dr. Thesleff: One should consider the possibility that botulinum poisoning induces changes in the central nervous system. My reason for suggesting this is that we have in animals, in which peripheral muscles were poisoned with botulinum toxin, failed to restore function by 4-aminopyridine. This was not because 4-aminopyridine was ineffective in antagonizing the neuromuscular block but because of some central nervous system effect of the poisoning.

Dr. Ball: Tradiionally, botulinum toxin is considered to have no effect on the CNS. However, we demonstrated a consistent EEG abnormality in our patients prior to treatment with 4-aminopyridine. Our EEG department considered this abnormality to be specific and correlated to hypoxia and other factors. Although these findings are unsupported by others *in vitro* or *in vivo* experiments it may be that the disparity between the effects of 4-aminopyridine on peripheral and respiratory mus-

## Discussion

cle is related to an unrecognized central effect of the toxin.

Dr. Westra: Did the sedative and anticonvulsant agent diazepam prevent your patients from convulsing after the large doses of 4-aminopyridine which you used?

Dr. Ball: Diazepam was used to control convulsions, not to prevent their occurrence. Our patients developed status epilepticus and required large doses of diazepam for control. These doses were given over a time-course of 5-10 minutes and the effect was dose-related.

Dr. Galvan: In our experiments on brain slices we found that pretreatment with phenytoin (50 uM) completely prevented all obvious effects of 4-aminopyridine. In contrast if phenytoin was added during 4-aminopyridine induced seizure activity there was only a dampening effect. I suggest one should protect against seizures by prior administration of phenytoin.

Dr. Ball: We have no experience of the use of phenytoin in prevention. You will appreciate that these were early studies and although we were aware of the possibility of convulsions we were not expecting fits of such a magnitude and severity.

Dr. Brandom: Did 4-aminopyridine administration cause an improvement in the profound hypotension demonstrated in these patients? Would there be an advantage to use pyridostigmine rather than neostigmine?

Dr. Ball: Yes, we did observe an increase, on average, of about 20 mm Hg in systolic pressure in the patients. There was also an increase in the heart-rate of between 5-12 beats/minute. We have no experience in the use of pyridostigmine and therefore cannot comment. Neostigmine was used on advice from our anaesthetists and those with experience of 4-aminopyridine.

Dr. Lundh: Do you think that 4-aminopyridine at all is indicated in the treatment of botulism. I mean, do the effects on limb muscles and on cranial nerve innervated muscles justify its use despite its lack of effect on respiratory muscles?

Dr. Ball: Probably not, as the objective in treatment is to restore ventilation and in our patients 4-aminopyridine was not effective in this respect. Increasing doses by infusion were equally ineffective on respiratory muscle and produced neurotoxicity. We had hoped that following our studies further human studies would be made with either 4-aminopyridine or 3,4-diaminopyridine but no other studies have sofar been reported in human botulism. I should like to add that in botulinum intoxicated patients treated by infusion of 4-aminopyridine we had the impression of a degree of permanent improvement. It is known that guanidine in high concentrations will inactivate botulinum toxin. Perhaps 4-aminopyridine may have such an effect *in vitro*, either by direct toxin inactivation or by reducing toxin binding to the release mechanism. However, these are unsupported anecdotal observations.

Dr. Bowman: In a patient who cannot breath, the respiratory drive is likely to be high even though the muscles cannot respond. Possibly after 4-aminopyridine, the initial high release of ACh cannot be continuously matched by mobilization of transmitter and so breathing does not improve as much as limb muscle function. A second point is that the clinical response might outlast the EMG response, because part of the effect may be due to an action on contractility rather than on transmission. Even though the effect on contractility may be secondary to an effect on the muscle action potential, you might not pick up the muscle action potential effect (as distinct from the transmission effects) with an EMG recording.

Dr. Lundh: Dr. Agoston, in what type of anaesthesia is it of benefit to get the patient to wake up quickly?

Dr. Agoston: 4-aminopyridine only facilitates recovery from anaesthesia. It does not terminate suddenly the sleep in anaesthetized patients. However, it shortens considerably the recovery of consciousness and counteracts respiratory depression due to both muscle relaxants and some anaesthetics at the same time. Therefore it seems to be a very useful tool to assure smooth post-anaesthetic recovery of the patient.

Dr. Rowan: Have you found any metabolites in the urine?

Dr. Agoston: No, although we were looking for them, we were unable to demonstrate any biotransformation products with the available assays.

Dr. Barnard: In regard to the question of the elimination, and the duration of action of aminopyridines, is it known whether these can be substrates for monoamine oxidase? Are any animal experiments known in which an inhibitor of that enzyme has been tested for its effect on any of the responses to aminopyridines?

Dr. Agoston: To my knowledge there are no available experimental data concerning the interaction with monoamine oxidase.

Dr. Molgo: Do you know if there is some development of tolerance with 4-AP when given to man?

Dr. Agoston: The total clinical experience with 4-aminopyridine, especially following long-lasting administration, is rather limited. Therefore it would not be appropriate to answer this question now. So far I have not heard of any case who developed tolerance to 4-aminopyridine effects.

Dr. Durant: In the studies you carried out with phencyclidine in monkeys, did you study neuromuscular transmission?

Dr. Agoston: No, we studied only the CNS effects.

Dr. Thesleff: Previously we learned that 3,4-diaminopyridine might be more advantageous to use than 4-aminopyridine since it is more potent and less convulsant. Do you or anyone present have some experience from the use of 3,4-diaminopyridine in man?

Dr. Agoston: No, but one of the first things I intend to do after this meeting is to start such a study as soon as the circumstances will allow.


Dr. Bowman: In response to Dr. Lewis' presentation I should like to emphasize that we should not abandon aminopyridines just because of tachyphylaxis with repeated doses. We should do research to find out why the drug stops working. It is hard to believe that it stops blocking $K^+$ channels. Perhaps the ACh supply is the limiting factor and maybe electron microscopy of vesicles would through some light on the subject. Is ACh synthesis a limiting factor? Maybe a mixture of choline and aminopyridine would be an improvement although that may be unlikely. We should do more research to find out how to maintain the aminopyridine effect.

Dr. Marshall: I should like to ask Dr. Lewis what was the dose of botulinum toxin in monkeys in relation to the sort of dose that might be found in man in situations similar to that reported by Dr. Ball? Do you have any comparative results for 4-aminopyridine and 3,4-diaminopyridine in your experimental situation?

Dr. Lewis: The credit for our use of 3,4-diaminopyridine belongs to Professor Thesleff. It is my hope that clinical trials in human patients will shift to the use of 3,4-diaminopyridine. Regarding Dr. Bowman's question I absolutely agree with your comments. We have no intent of abandoning 3,4-diaminopyridine and indeed we have considerable hopes for its use in combination with specific antitoxin for the treatment of botulism. Our study has answered only a few questions while posing any more. It will be important to conduct extensive basic and applied research. We do not know if the nerve terminal becomes tolerant to 3,4-diaminopyridine because choline is exhausted, if acetylcholine is depleted and/or if calcium is accumulated. It is also possible that the use of aminopyridines may cause a rapid turn-over of membrane and indeed speed up the intoxication of the nerve terminal by exposing more toxin receptors and thus an accelerated incorporation of botulinal toxin. The use of antitoxin should prevent additional toxin binding. In reply to Dr. Marshall I should like to say that the dose of toxin administered to the monkeys was derived by extrapolation from previous work in rhesus monkeys. Our monkeys received 2.5 - 9 times the $LD_{50}$ dose/kg body weight for a rhesus monkey. I am not aware of any direct measurements of the $LD_{50}$ dose/kg body weight in the patients treated by Dr. Ball.

# Further Miscellaneous Actions of Aminopyridines and Related Compounds

# Short Communications

*Chairman:* W. C. Bowman

# Potassium Channel Block by S-Methyl-thiouronium, A Pharmacological Analogue of 4-Aminopyridine

F. N. Fastier*, M. Pelhate** and B. Hue**

*Pharmacology Department, Otago University, P.O. Box 913, Dunedin, New Zealand
**Laboratoire de Physiologie, U.E.R. Médecine, 49045 Angers, France

The close pharmacological resemblance between 4-aminopyridine (4-AP) and S-methylthiouronium (SM) was first observed by FASTIER & MCDOWALL (1). They showed that 4-AP, like SM and other small amidinium cations, can produce sustained rises of blood pressure in anaesthetized cats, constriction of perfused rat blood vessels, and increased maximal contractions of isolated rat diaphragms. Both SM (2) and 4-AP (3) promote the release of acetylcholine at neuromuscular junctions. Both increase the maximal contractions of curarized rat diaphragms without increasing oxygen consumption (4). Both enhance the response of some smooth muscle preparations to stimulant actions of catecholamines and of acetylcholine (5,6). These analogies led CHITCHAROENTHUM & FASTIER to suggest (7) that SM, like 4-AP (8,9), can block $K^+$ channels in excitable membranes. SM has therefore been tested for this property on the isolated cockroach giant axon and 6th abdominal ganglion. Although it proved to be less than one-hundredth as potent as 4-AP, SM acted qualitatively like it. In a 2 mM concentration it decreased the $K^+$ current by some 20-30% without affecting the $Na^+$ current and the effect was voltage-frequency dependent as with 4-AP. SM also clearly facilitated synaptic transmission.

The low potency of SM was not unexpected in view of the results obtained through comparing the effects of SM and 4-AP on such preparations as the isolated rat diaphragm, where SM is less than one-tenth as potent as 4-AP, though much more potent in turn than such other small cations as tetraethylammonium, diethylammonium and piperidinium (7). Potency in $K^+$ channel blocking may be influenced by such molecular features as ability to form hydrogen bonds, incomplete ionization and flatness resulting from delocalization of charge (5).

References: (1)FASTIER FN & McDOWALL MA (1958), Aust.J.Exper.Biol.Med.Sci. 36, p.365. (2)BLACKMAN JG & SKELSEY M (1965), Proc.Univ. Otago Med.Sch. 43, p.15. (3)MOLGO J, LEMEIGNAN M & LECHAT P (1979), Europ.J.Pharmacol. 53, p.307. (4)BERESFORD R, BILLS GNB, FASTIER FN & MILNE RJ (1979), Brit.J.Pharmacol.Exp.Ther. 65, p.63. (5) FASTIER FN (1962), Pharmacol.Rev. 14, p.37. (6)THESLEFF S (1980), Neuroscience 5, p.1413. (7)CHITCHAROENTHUM M & FASTIER FN (1980), Proc. Univ. Otago Med.Sch. 58, p.33. (8) PELHATE M & PICHON Y (1974), J.Physiol. 242, 90P. (9)MEVES H & PICHON Y (1975), J.Physiol. 251, 60P.

# Differences in Actions of 4-Aminopyridine and 4-Methyl-2-Aminopyridine

## W. E. Glover

School of Physiology and Pharmacology, University of New South Wales, P.O. Box 1, Kensington, NSW, 2033, Australia

Studies mainly with 4-methyl-2-aminopyridine (4M2AP) led von Haxthausen (1955) to conclude that aminopyridines had sympathomimetic effects. While 4M2AP shares convulsant and other actions with aminopyridines (Fastier & McDowall, 1958) it differs in the following important respects.

1. In rat diaphragm and chick biventer cervicis preparations 4M2AP increased responses to nerve stimulation and acetylcholine (ACh) but depressed responses to direct stimulation. In presence of neostigmine, the effect of 4M2AP on responses to nerve stimulation and ACh was greatly reduced. This suggests that 4M2AP facilitates neuromuscular transmission by inhibition of cholinesterase rather than augmentation of ACh release (Kiloh, Harvey & Glover, 1981).

2. In isolated rabbit atria 4AP had a positive inotropic effect unaffected by propranolol and a negative chronotropic effect abolished by atropine. In isolated cat atria 4AP decreased both force and rate and these effects were reversed by atropine. In contrast, 4M2AP increased rate and force in both species and these effects were greatly reduced by propranolol. It is concluded that both compounds have a direct positive inotropic effect but in addition 4AP increases spontaneous release of ACh while 4M2AP releases noradrenaline (Nor) (Glover, 1981).

These and results of other workers (see Thesleff, 1980) show that in general 4AP, but not 4M2AP, facilitates nerve stimulated release of transmitter irrespective of whether it is ACh or Nor. In addition, 4AP increases spontaneous release of ACh from autonomic and frog motor nerves, while 4M2AP selectively increases spontaneous noradrenaline release. 4AP could enhance nerve stimulated release either by prolonging action potentials or acting directly on $Ca^{++}$ channels. In squid giant axon 4M2AP has little effect on $K^+$ conductance (P.W. Gage personal communication). This could explain its lack of effect on evoked release of ACh; alternatively, 4AP may have a direct action on $Ca^{++}$ channels not shared by 4M2AP. Inhibition of $K^+$ conductance could likewise contribute to spontaneous release of ACh by 4AP but not to release of Nor by 4M2AP. More likely, 4AP and 4M2AP facilitate $Ca^{++}$ influx or modify intraneuronal $Ca^{++}$ concentration; if so, the selectivity of their actions reflects differences in the handling of $Ca^{++}$ in the respective nerve terminals.

Fastier, F.N. and McDowall, M.A. (1958). Aust. J. exp. Biol. 36, 491-498.
Glover, W.E. (1981). Eur. J. Pharmacol. (in the press).
Haxthausen, E. von (1955). Arch. exp. Path. Pharmakol., 226, 163-171.
Kiloh, N. Harvey, A.L. and Glover, W.E. (1981). Eur. J. Pharmacol., 70, 53-57.
Thesleff, S. (1980). Neuroscience 5, 1413-1419.

# Effects of Aminopyridines in Avian Muscular Dystrophy

P. J. Barnard, E. A. Barnard and E. S. Allan

Department of Biochemistry, Imperial College of Science and Technology, London SW7, UK

Aminopyridines are known to increase enormously neurally-evoked transmitter release from motor nerves, and neuromuscular transmission has been restored by 4-aminopyridine (4-AP) after paralysis produced by botulinum toxin in the rat and improved in human myasthenia gravis (1). Since a neurogenic origin may be implicated in inherited muscular dystrophy, and since activation at nerve terminals might possibly improve innervation in muscle regeneration, we have investigated some of the effects of aminopyridines in the dystrophic chicken model. This mutant reproduces many of the physical, biochemical and morphological features of the human disease (2), affecting the fast-twitch skeletal muscles at an early age. We have measured the effects of these drugs by the use of four indices established (2) as a measure of the progress of the disease; these are the levels of plasma creatine phosphokinase (CPK) and pyruvate kinase (PK), and the physical disability as shown by the "Flip Number" (the ability of the chick to rise from the supine in five consecutive attempts) and also by the degree of wing stiffness, as shown by the wing apposition, i.e. the minimum separation of the passively-raised wings.

Ten birds in each series were injected intraperitoneally with 4-AP at 0.1 mg/kg or with 3,4-diaminopyridine (DAP) at 7.5 mg/kg, daily, for 56 days. Treatment with 4-AP led to significant reductions in plasma enzyme levels compared to the water-injected controls, the mean reduction being 47% for CPK and 42% for PK plasma concentrations. The physical parameters were also improved, the treated animals showing an improved performance at every assay. DAP produced a still greater reduction in serum enzyme levels (mean reductions of 61% in CPK and 52% in PK). The mean Flip Number in DAP-treated dystrophic birds was 8 times that of the dystrophic control birds at day 56 and 3 times in 4-AP birds.

The effectiveness of both drugs showed a steady decline with time, and further experiments at different dosages are in progress. The results suggest that chronic stimulation _in vivo_ at nerve terminals by such neurotropic drugs merits investigation as a means of producing improvement in dystrophic muscle.

This work is supported by the Muscular Dystrophy Group of Great Britain and by the Wellcome Trust.

References

1. Thesleff, S.(1980) Neuroscience 5, 1413.
2. Barnard, E. A. and Barnard, P. J. (1979) Ann. N.Y. Acad. Sci 317, 374.

# Comparison of the Actions of Dendrotoxin, A Facilitatory Neurotoxin, and 3,4-Diaminopyridine on Neuromuscular Transmission

## A. L. Harvey

Department of Physiology and Pharmacology, University of Strathclyde, Glasgow G1 1XW, UK

Dendrotoxin (DTx), a small polypeptide isolated from the venom of the Eastern green mamba, augments neuromuscular transmission by increasing acetylcholine release (Harvey & Karlsson, 1980). Some effects of DTx and 3,4-diaminopyridine (3,4-AP) have now been compared on isolated nerve-muscle preparations.

When added to chick biventer cervicis preparations, both DTx and 3,4-AP increased responses to indirect stimulation without affecting responses to acetylcholine, carbachol or KCl. 3,4-AP, but not DTx, produced 10-50% increase in the height of directly elicited twitches. In indirectly stimulated preparations, the maximum effects of DTx were seen after 1-2 hours. 3,4-AP was much more rapid in onset, its effects reaching a maximum within 30 min. DTx was approximately 500 times more potent than 3,4-AP: $2 \times 10^{-7}$ M DTx produced about 200% twitch augmentation whereas $10^{-4}$ M 3,4-AP was required to produce the same effect. However, the maximum twitch augmentation produced by 3,4-AP (about 300%) was greater. Moreover, 3,4-AP could still cause augmentation in preparations maximally stimulated by DTx.

Electrophysiological studies were performed using conventional intracellular recording methods on magnesium-paralysed amphibian sciatic nerve-sartorius muscle preparations. Both DTx and 3,4-AP increased the average quantal content. Again, DTx was more potent though slower acting: $10^{-8}$ M DTx caused a 20 fold increase in quantal content after 2 hours.

To demonstrate whether a common site of action for DTx and aminopyridines is involved, competition experiments were performed on the chick biventer cervicis preparation with the presynaptic blocking toxin, β-bungarotoxin. The blocking action of β-bungarotoxin was not affected by the presence of 3,4-AP but was significantly reduced by pretreatment with DTx.

In conclusion, both DTx and 3,4-AP facilitate neuromuscular transmission by increasing the evoked release of acetylcholine. However, it is unlikely that they act at the same site. Since DTx is extremely potent and long acting, it is worth further study in attempts to elucidate the physiological processes involved in neurotransmitter release.

A.L. Harvey & E. Karlsson (1980). Dendrotoxin from the venom of the green mamba, Dendroaspis angusticeps. A neurotoxin that enhances acetylcholine release at neuromuscular junctions. Naunyn-Schmiedeberg's Arch. Pharmac. 312, 1-6.

# Effects of Aminopyridines on Parasympathetic Neuro-effector Transmission in the Heart

W. Weide, R. Lindmar and K. Löffelholz

Department of Pharmacology, University, Obere Zahlbacher Strasse 67, D-6500 Mainz, Federal Republic of Germany

The release of acetylcholine (ACh) was determined in isolated, perfused chicken hearts. In the absence of aminopyridines (APs), stimulation of both vagus nerves (20 Hz, 1.8 mM $[Ca^{++}]_o$) increased the output of ACh into the perfusate from 24 to 280 pmol/g min, when an anticholinesterase agent was not present. 4-Aminopyridine (4-AP) or 3,4-diaminopyridine (3,4-DAP) enhanced the evoked release of ACh. When, under control conditions, the ACh release was maximal (high frequency of stimulation and/or high $[Ca^{++}]_o$), the APs were ineffective or much less effective (less than 2-fold increase) than at a low rate of release (up to 10-fold increase). The potency of 3,4-DAP was about 10-fold higher than that of 4-AP. As was expected from the AP-evoked facilitation of ACh release, the two compounds markedly increased the negative and chronotropic effects of vagal stimulation predominantly at low frequencies (0.3-3 Hz) in isolated atria of various species. The compounds did not alter force and rate of contraction at concentrations that maximally facilitated transmitter release. Only at concentrations above $10^{-3}$ M, 3,4-DAP enhanced force of contraction (cat and guinea pig atria), an effect that was unaltered by $3 \times 10^{-7}$ M propranolol. - Both, inhibition of ACh release observed in the presence of tetracaine ($10^{-7}$ - $10^{-4}$ M) and of pentobarbital ($10^{-5}$ - $10^{-3}$ M) was antagonized by 4-AP. Plotting the concentration of the inhibitors versus percent inhibition of release, however, revealed a parallel shift by 4-AP of the concentration-response curve only in the case of pentobarbital which is assumed to inhibit ACh release by a reduction of $Ca^{++}$ uptake. - It is concluded that 4-AP and 3,4-DAP in the μmolar range increased the parasympathetic neuro-effector transmission in the heart exclusively by a pre-synaptic action. Only part of the facilitation phenomenon seemed to be due to an increase in the maximum amount of ACh available for release, because the effect of APs was weak, or virtually absent, at maximum rates of release and was markedly enhanced by reducing transmitter release. Finally the results obtained on the heart support the general view that APs increase the transmitter release by facilitating neuronal $Ca^{++}$ uptake.

# Effects of 4-Aminopyridine on Endocrine Cells

O. Sand, K. Hove, S. Ozawa, K. Gautvik and E. Haug

Department of Physiology, Veterinary College of Norway, Oslo,
Department of Animal Nutrition, Agricultural University of Norway,
Ås and Institute of Physiology, University of Oslo, Norway

Exocytosis of secretory granules from most endocrine cells is triggered by Ca influx. The partially Ca dependent action potentials in several types of endocrine cells may play a key role in the stimulus-secretion coupling, in a similar way as for release of neurotransmitter. We have studied the electrophysiology and effects of 4-aminopyridine (4-AP) on three different groups of endocrine cells, secreting prolactin (PRL), calcitonin (CT) and parathyroid hormone (PTH).

PRL producing cells: The experiments were performed on the $GH_3$ strain of rat pituitary tumour cells. The electrophysiology of the cells has been described in detail by Ozawa & Miyazaki (Jap.J.Physiol.29: 411.1979). We have previously shown (Sand et al. Acta Physiol.Scand. 108:247.1980) that 4-AP inhibits the late K current in the cells, causing prolongation of the repolarizing phase and increased firing rate of the partially Ca dependent action potentials. These effects increase the Ca influx through voltage sensitive Ca channels. 4-AP caused a dose-dependent increase of prolactin release from $GH_3$ cells, with maximal stimulation (2 fold) at $10^{-4}$M. This increase of PRL release was similar to that obtained with thyroliberin (TRH). 4-AP had no effect on PRL synthesis, which was doubled in $10^{-6}$M TRH solution.

CT producing cells: Intracellular recordings were obtained from CT secreting cells from a rat medullary thyroid carcinoma. The cells displayed action potentials depending on both Ca and Na. The effects of 4-AP on CT release was measured during local in vivo infusions in 3 goats, causing a thyroid plasma concentration of $10^{-4}$M 4-AP. This increased the CT secretion rate by a factor of 2.5. Infusions of Ca in the same animals increased the secretion rate by a factor of 4.5.

PT cells: The electrophysiology of goat PT cells was studied in primary tissue culture, and our data show the existence of voltage sensitive Ca channels and a marked delayed rectification. Action potentials were not recorded, but current injection caused graded, regenerative responses. We suggest that exocytosis of stored PTH depends on Ca influx as in other secretory cells. A suppressive effect of plasma Ca on the membrane permeability to Ca could then explain the inverse relationship between the plasma Ca level and the PTH release. Local in vivo infusions in 2 goats, causing a parathyroid plasma concentration of $1.5 \times 10^{-4}$M 4-AP, increased the PTH secretion rate by 60-70%. Adrenergic β-blockade could not abolish this effect.

# An Electroencephalographic Study of 4-Aminopyridine in Conscious Volunteers

R. L. Sia, S. Boonstra, P. Westra, H. T. M. Haenen
and H. Wesseling

Institutes of Anaesthesiology and Clinical Pharmacology and
Department of Clinical Neurophysiology, State University of
Groningen, Oostersingel 59, 9713 EZ Groningen, The Netherlands


The renewed interest in the pharmacological properties and clinical usage of 4-AP prompted us to examine the effects of this drug upon central nervous system in conscious volunteers in the presence or absence of a sedative.
The EEG effects of 4-AP given intravenously in therapeutic doses was studied in four volunteers.
4-AP (0.2 mg kg$^{-1}$) caused an increase of the occipital α peak frequency of 0.4 to 1.0 Hz. In the dose range of 0.2-0.3 mg kg$^{-1}$ there was neither evidence for epileptic activity in the EEG nor were any clinical side effects observed. Pretreatment of the volunteers with 4-AP was also found to antagonize diazepam induced sleep. In the clinical situation 4-AP also reduced significantly the action of diazepam. The summarized results are listed below.

| No. | Dose of 4-AP (mg/kg) | Mode of administration of 4-AP (i.v.) | Control level of occipital α peak freq. (Hz) | Increase of occipital α peak freq. (Hz) after 4-AP | Level of consciousness during Diazepam after 4-AP | Level of consciousness after Diazepam only |
|---|---|---|---|---|---|---|
| 1 | 0.2 | quick bolus (< 10") | 10.7 | 0.5 | awake | asleep |
| 2 | 0.2 | " | 10.2 | 0.8 | awake | asleep |
| 3 | 0.2 | " | 10.0 | 0.4 | awake | asleep |
| 4 | 0.2 | " | 11.0 | 1.0 | awake | asleep |
| 1 | 0.3 | slow bolus (2') | 10.7 | 0.5 | - | |
| 2 | 0.3 | " | 11.5 | 0 | - | |
| 3 | 0.2 | " | 9.8 | 1.2 | - | |
| 4 | 0.2 | " | 11.3 | 1.0 | - | |

- no Diazepam

# DISCUSSION OF THE EIGHTH SESSION.

Dr. Bowman: Dr. Fastier, you refer to the blocking action of ruthenium red on the action of S-methylthiouronium. Can you tell us something about the mechanism of action of ruthenium red?

Dr. Fastier: I have found that the stimulant action of S-methylthiouronium on isolated rabbit intestinal strips can be blocked by salts of manganese and lanthanum which are supposed to have little ability to penetrate the membrane. I used ruthenium red as an other agent of this type. The antagonistic action of this agent seemed at the time to indicate that S-methylthiouronium was acting on the surface of the membrane. However, it now seems likely that they affect the response to S-methylthiouronium indirectly by interfering with $Ca^{2+}$ entry into the cell, thereby negating the action of S-methylthiouronium on $K^+$ flux.

Dr. Bergmann: Dr. Glover, in your experiments on the chick biventer cervicis muscle you showed that 2-amino-4-methylpyridine enhances the effect of ACh but reduces the effect of carbachol. How do you explain this difference?

Dr. Glover: The response to carbachol was smaller in this particular instance but this probably was due to random variation and it was not seen constantly.

Dr. Edman: I noticed that your aminopyridine compound enhanced contraction in chicken muscle in response to indirect stimulation at the same time as there was a marked depression of the response to direct stimulation. This seems at first sight to be difficult to fit together provided you have used supramaximal stimulation for tetanization in both cases.

Dr. Glover: There are two possible explanations. One is that the effect of the drug in decreasing contractility is more than compensated for by its effect in enhancing transmission. The other is that the stronger electrical stimulus used (longer pulse duration) to stimulate the muscle directly may drive more of the 2-amino-4-methylpyridine into the fibre. Perhaps Dr. Harvey would also like to comment on this.

Dr. Harvey: In response to the question of Dr. Edman on why 2-amino-4-methylpyridine can increase twitches to indirect stimulation and decrease responses to direct stimulation I should like to suggest that probably the effect on indirect stimulation would be greater but is reduced by a form of physiological antagonism. A similar effect could probably be mimicked by a mixture of e.g. 4-aminopyridine and dantrolene.

Dr. Durant: Have you investigated the effects of 2-amino-4-methylpyridine on Na release induced by agents such as the amphetamines?

Dr. Glover: No, but that would certainly be worth investigating.

Dr. Löffelholz: Our studies on the release of ACh in the perfused heart indicate that the potencies of various aminopyridines to increase spontaneous and evoked ACh release are different. For example, 3,4-diaminopyridine, in contrast to 4-aminopyridine, did not affect spontaneous ACh release but exhibited a strong facilitation of the evoked release of ACh.

Dr. Galvan: Dr. Sand your observation that 4-aminopyridine releases peptide type hormones leads to the possibility that the peptides themselves modulate cell excitability. What does prolactine or parathyroid hormone do to cell excitability?

Dr. Sand: We have not tested the two peptides you mentioned. However, a concentration of 4-aminopyridine of less than 10 μM enhances hormone secretion in our system. It is therefore reasonable to assume that the 4-aminopyridine concentrations used in many of the experiments reported in this Symposium may increase the release of different hormones and parahormones. Many of the peptides which thus may be released as a side effect of 4-aminopyridine are likely to influence cell excitability and transmitter release.

Dr. Bergmann: I want to ask Dr. Barnard if there are any observations of changes in the thymus of these dystrophic animals?

Dr. Barnard: No, this has not been reported in the chicken with inherited muscular dystrophy.

Dr. Marshall: As you know aminopyridines are not very effective in increasing contractility in certain chicken muscles in relation to their effects on neuromuscular transmission. In order to analyse if the effects you measure are due to direct or indirect effects have you considered making use of a combination of aminopyridines and TEA which have been shown to have a synergistic effect in chicken muscle?

Dr. Barnard: We are aware of this, and we do not know whether there could be any major contribution from direct effects on contractility to the beneficial effects of aminopyridines in the dystrophic chicken. We have not considered administering TEA because pharmacologically active concentrations of this compound are very high, as you are aware, and we doubted whether we could maintain such levels *in vivo*.

Dr. Lundh: Did you make any recordings of EMG in your chickens?

Dr. Barnard: We do not measure this parameter during the course of our treatments. We wish to avoid highly invasive procedures and to keep the treated group intact during the entire course of the treatment. We use the parameters I have illustrated, which are readily quantitated, but we also measure at the level of the muscle itself. These are 1) the amounts of the various molecular forms of cholinesterases, which are greatly perturbed in the dystrophic chicken muscle and can be changed towards the normal content by an effective drug treatment (Lyles and co-workers, J. Neurochem., 1979 and Barnard and co-workers, N.Y. Acad. Sci., 1979). 2) the changes in muscle structure expressed as a set of quantitative indices in the histological changes which develop in the affected muscles of untreated dystrophic chickens. Both of these analysis of the muscle can be obtained from small biopsy samples taken during the treatment and at the end of treatment. These analysis require a much longer period to complete after the period of treatment and they will be reported in due course.

Dr. Thesleff: Could you say something about the pharmacokinetics of aminopyridine in the chicken?

Dr. Barnard: There is no reported data on this. We intend to measure the lifetime of the drug to obtain the most effective regime for treating the dystrophic chickens.

Dr. Marshall: I should like to ask Dr. Harvey, do you get a blocking effect of high concentrations of DTx on indirectly stimulated preparations? Are there effects on spontaneous transmitter release and/or on action potentials? What is the $Ca^{2+}$ dependence of the increase in quantal content?

Dr. Harvey: There is some evidence that high concentrations of DTx do not cause as marked facilitatory responses but the mechanism is unclear. Miniature endplate potential frequency decreases and there is the appearance of giant spontaneous potentials. Effects on action potentials have not been measured although there was no sign of DTx changing the nerve terminal spike measured with an extracellular electrode. The calcium dependence has not been studied directly but DTx can increase twitch responses to indirect stimulation in the presence of 1/10 normal $Ca^{2+}$ (0.25 mM).

Dr. Thesleff: Is the onset of action of DTx frequency dependent as is that of β-bungarotoxin? Does DTx have phospholipase $A_2$ activity?

Dr. Harvey: The action of DTx does not seem to share the same frequency dependence as β-bungarotoxin. DTx still increases quantal content in preparations that were stimulated only intermittently. In the chick biventer cervicis nerve-muscle prepa-

## Discussion

ration stimulation at 1 Hz instead of 0.1 Hz suppresses the effect of DTx. The facilitatory effect is immediately restored by decreasing the rate of stimulation. There is no phospholipase $A_2$ activity of DTx. DTx is homologous with protease inhibitors, as is the β-chain of β-bungarotoxin. However, DTx is not acting in the venom as a "chaperone" for a phospholipase molecule as the crude venom has no phospholipase activity.

Dr. Barnard: Can the action of DTx be reversed by washing?

Dr. Harvey: The action of DTx is only very slowly reversed by washing.

Dr. Yanagisawa: Dr. Weide, have you checked the effect of $Ca^{2+}$-antagonists like verapamil on the release of ACh?

Dr. Weide: The antagonism between verapamil and 4-aminopyridine with respect to transmitter release in the heart is difficult or even impossible to study because the ACh and the NA release evoked by cardiac nerve stimulation is very resistant to blockade by verapamil.

Dr. Schiavone: In the sympathetic terminals of the spleen we have observed that 4-aminopyridine did reverse the blockade associated with a very low dose of tetracaine, but had no effect on blockade caused by higher doses of tetracaine. We presume this reflects the ability of tetracaine to specifically block $Ca^{2+}$-channels at very low concentrations. You have observed that 4-aminopyridine does not antagonize the blockade of parasympathetic nerves by low concentrations of tetracaine. Does this suggest that low tetracaine concentrations have differential effects at sympathetic and parasympathetic terminals?

Dr. Weide: We have studied the concentration-dependent inhibition of conduction in the vagal B- and C-fibres of our preparation and found no significant differences in the potencies of tetracaine to inhibit ACh release and conduction. Thus, in our experiments the inhibition of ACh release was due to the local anaesthetic action of tetracaine and not to a specific block of $Ca^{2+}$-channels as has been shown for sympathetic nerve terminals with low concentrations of tetracaine.

Dr. Fastier: This is a question directed to Dr. Westra. We have recently shown that 4-aminopyridine and 2-amino-4-methylaminopyridine have very little ability to displace opiates from their receptors in the rat brain. I therefore doubt whether 4-aminopyridine is a competitive antagonist to morphine. A possible basis for the antagonism is the ability of 4-aminopyridine to raise intracellular $Ca^{2+}$ levels, because $Ca^{2+}$ can antagonize some actions of opiates.

Dr. Westra: Some experimental reports, e.g. in the guinea-pig ileum will support your opinion and in preliminary experiments we found that the action of 4-aminopyridine, as an unspecific antagonist to opiates, is highly $Ca^{2+}$ dependent.

Dr. Durant: 4-aminopyridine alone has been shown to increase spontaneous respiratory frequency in anesthetized animals. Do you consider the antagonism of the morphine-induced respiratory depression by 4-aminopyridine to be specific or rather to be nonspecific?

Dr. Westra: 4-aminopyridine antagonizes the pharmacological effects of morphine and is therefore rather nonspecific, especially when one looks at the structure of respectively 4-aminopyridine and that of morphine.

Dr. Lundh: Did diazepam antagonize all side-effects of 4-aminopyridine, even the peripheral ones, like paraestesia and the deep aching pain in the arm of injection?

Dr. Westra: Yes, at least partially. For this reason, in my opinion, diazepam is still the drug of choice for patients complaining about the central and peripheral side-effects of 4-aminopyridine.

# Conclusions

# Conclusions

W. C. Bowman

Department of Physiology and Pharmacology, University of
Strathclyde, Glasgow G1 1XW, UK


Members of the audience as well as the lecturers have explored in considerable depth the wide-ranging effects of aminopyridines, and similarly-acting compounds on biological systems. Whether the wide variety of effects can be ascribed essentially to a single basic mechanism, that is to blockade of voltage-dependent $K^+$ channels, to some extent remains a matter of controversy, but at any rate, it seems clear that aminopyridines are at least relatively clean and specific in their actions at membrane level, when compared with other kinds of drugs.

As Professor Lechat in his historical review, and several other speakers have pointed out, the whole now rapidly expanding subject was really started by the groundwork, first of Dohrn in 1925, then of Fastier and his colleagues in New Zealand in the forties and fifties, spurred on by the experiments of Lemeignan and Lechat in Paris in the sixties, and given added impetus by Paskov and Stoyanov and their colleagues in Bulgaria, who pioneered the use of 4-aminopyridine hydrochloride (or Pymadin as it is called) as an anticurare agent in anaesthetic practice in the sixties and early seventies. Then I think perhaps further catalysed in no small measure by the characteristically indefatigable international sorties of Francis Foldes, who awoke the interest of many of us in the subject. The result is the present snowballing growth of research, with the consequence that it is now difficult to find a current journal that does not contain one or more papers on 4-aminopyridine. And so, it gave pleasure to everyone present to have Professor Fastier at the symposium, all the way from New Zealand, and still making important contributions to the field. It was also gratifying that Professor Paskov from Bulgaria, another still active pioneer in the field, had been able to join in the meeting.

The fact that it had been found important to hold and to attend this symposium seems to be indicative of two things. One is that biological scientists need specific membrane ion channel blockers in order to study ion conductance and transmission mechanisms, and the other is that clinicians must need drugs with the ability to facilitate transmission, in the way that aminopyridines do.

Ulbricht, Dubois, Pichon, Llinas, Galvan, and Pelhate and their coworkers described experiments that elegantly show that aminopyridines, and some related compounds, block voltage-dependent, fast potassium channels in an all-or-nothing manner in a range of excitable membranes, including nodes of Ranvier in frog myelinated axons. Although the compound generally appears to block the channels in the closed form, Ulbricht's experiments indicate that transient opening of the

$K^+$ gates may be important to allow access to the receptor sites, at least in frog nodal membranes, in order that reblocking should occur. Potassium conductance is composed of several components (see also Thompson, 1977), the main ones being a fast and a slow phase. As Dubois showed, 4-aminopyridine blocks only the fast phase.

Many mammalian A fibre nodes of Ranvier possess only very few, if any, $K^+$ channels, and so the action potentials of such fibres are not prolonged by aminopyridines, as described at the symposium by Mallart and Brigant for mouse motor nerves and by Galvan, Grafe and Bruggencate for guinea-pig vagal A fibres. As pointed out by Meves, potassium channels become exposed in mammalian myelinated fibres when the myelin is damaged or removed. Sherratt and his coworkers in London demonstrated this after removing the myelin with diphtheria toxin. Under these circumstances, aminopyridines then prolonged the action potentials and thereby facilitated conduction. These observations led Sherratt and his coworkers to propose that aminopyridines might therefore be of value for improving nerve conduction in the demyelinating diseases (Sherratt, Bostock and Sears, 1980; Bostock, Sears and Sherratt, 1981).

Although aminopyridines may not be absolutely specific in their action on voltage-dependent $K^+$ channels(see, for example, the papers by Lamel and Mandreck, Martinez de Muñoz and Vital-Brazil), they are, nevertheless, a highly useful neuro-biological tool for blocking fast potassium conductances. They have no action on transmitter-operated $K^+$ channels. However, as Jenkinson described, some of these transmitter-operated $K^+$ channels, in particular some that are triggered by a rise in cytosol calcium ion concentration, are blocked by the toxin apamin from bee venom. It would be interesting to know perhaps if the aminopyridine-resistant, calcium-activated, potassium channels of the uterine smooth muscle membrane, described at the symposium by Savineau, are blocked by apamin.

Fig. 1, from an experiment by Dr. Anne Bowman, simply repeats some of Jenkinson's observations, but on a different tissue - the rabbit isolated ileum from which pendular movements were recorded. The lower records show that apamin ($5 \times 10^{-9}$ molar) has no effect on β-adrenoceptor mediated inhibition produced by isoprenaline but it blocks the α-adrenoceptor mediated component of the inhibition produced by adrenaline, and the similar kind of response (although not of course mediated by α-receptors) produced by ATP. In the rabbit ileum, the inhibitory response produced by noradrenaline is, perhaps surprisingly, often due more to β-receptor stimulation than to α-receptor stimulation (Bowman and Hall, 1970), and in accordance with this the response to noradrenaline was relatively little affected by apamin. With adrenaline it is the other way round, the α-receptors being the more affected.

The upper records of Fig. 1 show the responses of an adjacent segment of ileum to stimulation of the periarterial sympathetic nerves (5, 10 and 20 Hz). Again the α-receptor mediated component is reduced or blocked by apamin (especially at 10 Hz). 4-Aminopyridine is not especially active on this preparation but it can be seen that in the continued presence of apamin, it has the opposite effect to apamin. That is, it tends to overcome the apamin block, presumably by increasing the release of noradrenaline from the nerves. (4-Aminopyridine has no effect on the responses of the tissue to added catecholamines.) And so apamin, together with aminopyridines and tetraethylammonium, provides us with another important tool to study the behaviour of different kinds of $K^+$ Channels.

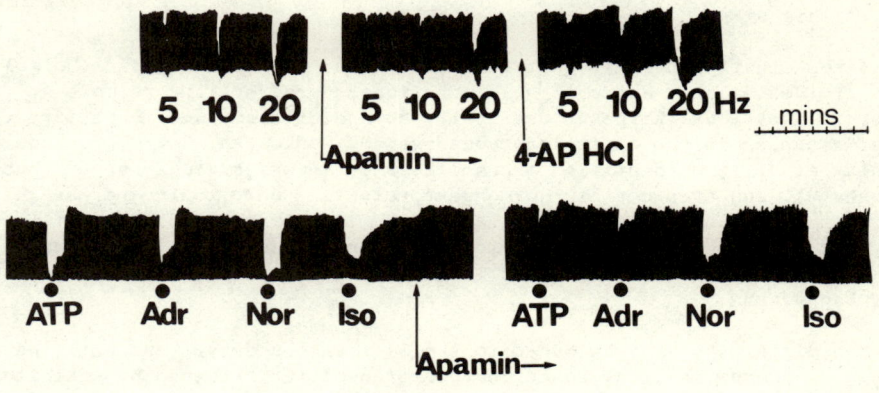

Fig. 1. Isolated segments of rabbit ileum suspended in Krebs solution. Pendular movements were recorded isometrically. The upper records show the responses to stimulation of the periarterial sympathetic nerves at 5, 10 and 20 Hz for 10 sec. Apamin ($5 \times 10^{-9}$M), added at the arrow and present for the remainder of the experiment, reduced the responses to nerve stimulation (i.e. blocked the α-receptor mediated component). 4-Aminopyridine hydrochloride (4-AP HCl, $1.5 \times 10^{-5}$M) added in the continued presence of apamin largely restored the responses to nerve stimulation. The lower records (from an adjacent segment of the same ileum) show, on the left, comparable inhibitory responses to ATP ($10^{-7}$M), adrenaline (Adr, $6 \times 10^{-8}$M), noradrenaline (Nor, $8 \times 10^{-8}$M) and isoprenaline (Iso, $7 \times 10^{-8}$M). On the right, additions of the same concentrations were repeated in the continued presence of apamin ($5 \times 10^{-9}$M). Responses to ATP and adrenaline were largely blocked, the response to noradrenaline was slightly reduced, and that to isoprenaline was unaffected. (From an unpublished experiment by Dr. Anne Bowman)

Prolongation of the action potentials of non-myelinated nerve terminals by 4-aminopyridine, as demonstrated by Mallart and Brigant at the mouse neuromuscular junction, and by Molgó, must allow the entry into the nerve endings of more calcium ions to activate the release mechanism. Whether, in addition, there is a direct facilitatory action on calcium ion transport, as first suggested by Lundh and Thesleff, remains controversial. The experiments of Llinas on the squid giant synapse indicate that the only direct effect in this tissue is blockade of $K^+$ conductance, effects on $Ca^{2+}$ flux being secondary to this action. However, indirect evidence from other tissues by other workers suggests the possibility of an additional direct action on nerve terminal calcium channels or on other components of the calcium-dependent process (see, for example, the paper by Maeno) Be that as it may, the influx of calcium ions, by whatever mechanism, is sufficient to explain the great enhancement of evoked transmitter release produced by 4-aminopyridine. Again the compound provides a useful tool, this time for studying transmitter release mechanisms, as discussed by Thesleff and Molgó. Here the work of Dunant and Israel on *Torpedo* electric organs might be mentioned, because in this tissue the evidence is persuasive, to say the least, that it is *non*-vesicular acetylcholine that is released. Additionally, the experiments of Dreyer and Schmitt are of especial interest because the use of 4-aminopyridine enabled a clear distinction to be made between the action of botulinum toxin and the *peripheral* action of tetanus toxin, which were previously thought to act in the same way at this site.

Aminopyridines clearly increase acetylcholine release at both somatic (Molgó) and autonomic (Foldes et al., Weide et al.) junctions, noradrenaline release at noradrenergic junctions (Kirpekar and Prat), both excitatory and inhibitory transmitters at synapses in the central nervous system (Jankowska, Saade, Corradetti et al., Gogolak et al.), unidentified transmitters at invertebrate synapses (Hue et al., Shimahara), and even certain hormones (prolactin, calcitonin and parathyroid hormone) from endocrine cells (Sand et al.). In this last connection, it is of interest that in unpublished experiments, B.L. Furman has shown that 4-aminopyridine also increases the release of immunoreactive insulin from isolated islets of Langerhans.

Another transmitter that may be added to the list is the as yet unidentified nonadrenergic, noncholinergic, nonpurinergic transmitter released by inhibitory nerve stimulation to the smooth muscle of the bovine retractor penis. In the experiment illustrated in Fig. 2, a constant number of 10 stimuli was applied at different frequencies. 4-Aminopyridine greatly augmented the inhibitory responses especially (as is usual) at low frequencies of stimulation. Compare, for example, the response to stimulation at 0.1 Hz before and after 4-aminopyridine in Fig. 2.

It thus seems that aminopyridines nonspecifically enhance almost any evoked process that is ultimately dependent on an action potential whose declining phase is due to fast channel potassium ion conductance. Such processes may include the contractile mechanisms in some skeletal muscles (as Edman and others have described), in cardiac muscle, at least of some species (as Yanagisawa and others have described), and in some smooth muscles. In general, effects on muscle membranes require higher doses than effects on transmission. Furthermore, in the case of skeletal muscle there may not only be a species difference with regard to sensitivity to 4-aminopyridine, but even a muscle difference within the same species (see for example, Bowman et al., 1979; Agoston et al., 1981). As far as cardiac muscle is concerned, Rodger and Shahid stressed the importance of controlling the pH in studies on isolated preparations. 4-Aminopyridine base is an extremely alkaline substance, and a rise in pH, by itself, has a powerful inotropic action.

An important question is whether there is any difference in the sensitivity or responsiveness of the various synaptic and junctional transmission processes to 4-aminopyridine, and this question cannot yet be fully answered, because different experimental conditions (such as stimulation frequency, ionic milieu, presence or absence of other drugs and so on) used for studying different systems, can give an erroneous impression of different sensitivities. However, despite the probable nonspecificity of action of 4-aminopyridine, Glover's experiments with 4-methyl-2-aminopyridine indicate that it may be possible to synthesise compounds with greater selectivity for particular types of synapse or junction. Such selectivity, if it can be achieved, need not of course depend on differences in the properties of fast potassium channels at different sites, but may merely reflect different pharmacokinetic properties of the compounds that allow them to reach some sites more easily than others.

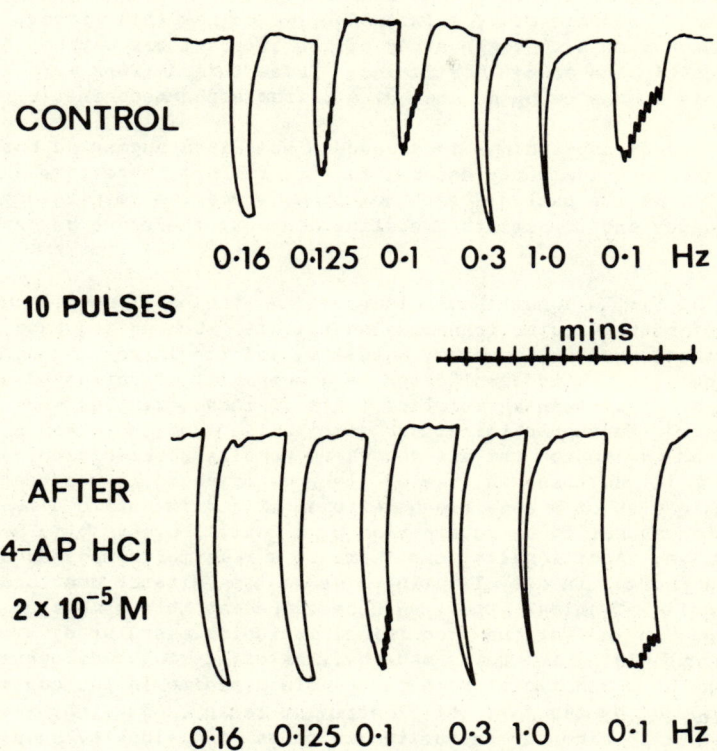

Fig.2. Isolated strip of bovine retractor penis muscle set up as described by Gillespie and Martin, 1980, and stimulated to relax through its nonadrenergic, noncholinergic, nonpurinergic nerves. Ten stimuli were applied at different frequencies (0.16, 0.125, 0.1, 0.3, 1.0 Hz) as indicated. The upper records show inhibitory responses before the addition of 4-aminopyridine, and the lower records show augmented responses (especially at the lower frequencies) in the presence of 4-aminopyridine ($2 \times 10^{-5}$M). From a previously unpublished experiment by Dr. Anne Bowman)

One of the problems with a drug that facilitates transmission in the way that 4-aminopyridine does is that mobilisation of transmitter from the reserve store to the readily-releasable position may not be able to keep up with the demands of the enhanced release process. The consequence of this at the neuromuscular junction is that there is pronounced tetanic rundown of endplate potentials after the first augmented one. This has been clearly demonstrated in the past with 4-amino-pyridine by Thesleff, Lundh and Molgó and their coworkers, and with 4-hydroxy-pyridine at the present symposium by Montoya et al. The mechanical counterpart of this effect is that when 4-aminopyridine is used as an anticurare agent, tetanic fade is not improved. In fact, as Gibb et al. illustrated at this symposium, tetanic fade may be enhanced by aminopyridines. They are of the opinion that tubocurarine and related drugs exaccerbate the situation by interfering with transmitter mobilisation. In any event, for the most effective use of aminopyridines as anticurare agents, they should be given in combination with a substance that enhances mobilisation or that in some other way improves the maintenance of tetanic tension. The Bulgarian anaesthetists often mix 4-aminopyridine with the anticholinesterase drug, galantamine, which has this effect, and Miller et al. (1979) have made a thorough study of the interactions between 4-aminopyridine and neostigmine or pyridostigmine. These interactions were also discussed at this symposium by Agoston et al. from a pharmacokinetic point of view.

The inability of 4-aminopyridines to produce a sustained augmented contraction or train of endplate potentials may account for its failure to restore breathing adequately in Dr. Ball's patients with botulism, since the respiratory drive is of a high frequency and transmitter mobilisation must therefore be especially important.

There seems to be little doubt that aminopyridines can be clinically useful in certain types of neuromuscular transmission failure, such as the Eaton-Lambert syndrome, myasthenia gravis, possibly botulism, and the infrequent occasions in which neuromuscular block is complicated by a component of action of excess magnesium ions or by certain antibiotics. All of these examples were discussed at this symposium. Further clinical use might arise from the clear antagonistic action, described by Agoston and his coworkers, against benzodiazepines and ketamine, especially ketamine in view of its growing abuse as a street drug. And one might speculate about a possible beneficial effect in senile dementia, since the condition is thought to be accompanied by a central presynaptic defect in a cholinergic system. Additionally, can there be a role for compounds of this type in Huntington's chorea, in demyelinating diseases (as already mentioned) and, in view of the results of animal experiments described at this symposium by Paskov and the Barnards, in the various myopathies, including muscular dystrophy? It is also worth re-emphasising the point made by Thesleff during a discussion period, that there might be a beneficial role for 4-aminopyridine in the control of convulsions produced by the toxin of *Clostridium tetani*. It might seem paradoxical that a drug with a convulsant action in normal individuals, should be proposed for trial as an anticonvulsant in tetanus. However, the convulsions of tetanus are a consequence of reduced release of inhibitory transmitter in the spinal cord, and 4-aminopyridine acts to increase the release of transmitters, including central inhibitory transmitters. Furthermore, it acts more powerfully at synapses at which transmission is already depressed. Consequently, it is logical to test whether it increases the release of inhibitory transmitter in tetanus, and thereby suppressing the convulsions. In view of the results of Dreyer and Schmidt, 4-aminopyridine would not, however, be expected to antagonise the secondary neuromuscular depressant effect of tetanus toxin.

The main problems with the clinical use of 4-aminopyridine arise from the unwanted side-effects that stem mainly from concurrently enhanced autonomic and central transmission, leading, amongst other effects, to hypertension and convulsions with doses only slightly greater than those commonly used. Cardiovascular and other side-effects in cats and dogs have recently been described (Bowman et al., 1981). A great deal of important information on central actions of aminopyridines was reported at the symposium by Galvan, Saade, Westra, Tung, Gogolak and others. One of the central actions is antagonism of narcotic analgesics by 4-aminopyridine and this must also be regarded as a disadvantage if it occurs at the end of an operation.

As Marshall pointed out, until further improvements are made, it seems logical that 3,4-diaminopyridine should be the aminopyridine of choice for use in peripheral conditions, since on the whole it is the most potent in its peripheral actions, yet is relatively less active on the central nervous system.  4-Aminopyridine probably remains the drug of choice for central actions.  However, as reported by Marshall, Fastier et al., Glover, Ohta et al., and Sobek at this symposium, structure:action data are now beginning to accumulate, and so it is to be hoped that medicinal chemists may soon devise compounds that are more selctive in their actions.  Possibly a family of compounds can be designed each with a relatively selective action on a particular tissue.  At any rate, the field remains an exciting one, and there is a great deal of further work to be done. One cannot ask more of a symposium than that it should fan the enthusiasm of its participants for further work; it is safe to say that this one succeeded in this aim.

While officially closing the meeting, Professor Bowman thanked Professor Lechat and his colleagues, Madeleine Lemeignan and Jorge Molgó, on behalf of himself, Professor Thesleff and all the participants, for their extraordinary skill and effort in organising a symposium that from every aspect - scientific, environmental and gastronomic - had been an outstanding success.  He also thanked the speakers, the discussants and the audience for their enthusiastic participation.

## REFERENCES

Agoston, S., Bowman, W.C., Houwertjes, M.C., Rodger, I.W. and Savage, A.O. (1981) *Clin. Exp. Pharmacol. Physiol.* in the press

Bostock, H., Sears, T.A. and Sherratt, R.M. (1981) *J. Physiol. (Lond.)*, 313, 305-315.

Bowman, W.C. and Hall, M.T. (1970) *Br. J. Pharmacol.*, 38, 399-415.

Bowman, W.C., Marshall, R.J., Rodger, I.W. and Savage, A.O. (1981) *Br. J. Anaesth.*, 53, 555-565.

Bowman, W.C., Rodger, I.W. and Savage, A.O. (1979) *Br. J. Pharmacol.*, 66, 466-467P.

Gillespie, J.S. and Martin, W. (1980) *J. Physiol. (Lond.)*, 309, 55-64.

Miller, R.D., Booij, L.H.D.J., Agoston, S. and Crul, J.F. (1979) *Anesthesiology*, 50, 416-420.

Sherratt, R.M., Bostock, H. and Sears, T.A. (1980) *Nature (Lond.)*, 283, 570-572.

Thompson, S.H. (1977) *J. Physiol. (Lond.)*, 265, 465-488.

# Index

A23187
  acetylcholine release 173
Acetylcholine
  chemiluminescent measurement of release 173
  evoked contraction 229
  heart release and aminopyridines 325
  parasympthetic transmission 127
  release and 4-AP 163, 213
  release and calcium antagonists 331
  release and tetracaine 331
2-Amino-4-methylaminopyridine
  opiate displacement 331
2-Amino-4-methylpyridine
  acetylcholine enhancement 329
  dopaminergic stereotype 212
Aminopyridine analogues 145
3-Aminopyridine
  pyramidal cell evoked activity 220
  squid synaptic transmission 81
4-Aminopyridine (4AP) 331
  acetylcholine release 173, 213, 331
  activities 43, 53
  in anaesthesia 303
  anaesthetic effects on myo-neurones 215
  analogues 226, 232, 321
  anti-curare action 232
  <u>Aplysia</u> pre-synaptic modulations 230
  blood brain passage and toxicity 222
  botulism therapy 297, 313
  brain effects 217
  brain protein synthesis 224
  carbachol desensitization 240
  cardiac muscle effects 261
  cardiotonic effects 278
  catecholamine release 183
  convulsive effects and morphine dependence 211
  cuneate and gracile neurone effects 239
  dose 117, 327
  EEG study 327
  endocrine cells 326
  facilitation of parasympathetic transmission 127
  ionic channel blocking 53
  ionic channels in cockroach 238
  isometric force - ($Ca^{++}$) relation in muscle 275
  kanamycin antagonism 234
  morphine analgesic reversal 233
  morphine antagonism 231, 331
  muscle contractility 249
  myopathic models 228
  neuromuscular transmission 95
  neurones of mammals 237
  noradrenaline output 183
  outward membrane currents smooth muscle 276
  pacemaker membrane currents 277
  parasympathetic transmission 127
  peptide hormones 127, 329
  pharmacokinetics 303, 330
  potassium currents 29, 43, 53
  presynaptic currents in motor endings 223
  pyramidal cell evoked activity 220

side effects 287, 297, 331
spinal cord transmission 117
squid axon, automatic activity 221
squid synaptic transmission 81
succinyldicholine neuromuscular block 241
therapeutic applications 287
toxin effects 214
Amino-2 pyridine
   pharmacological effects 3
4-Aminoquinoline
   cardiac effects 218
Amphetamines 329
Anaesthesia
   4AP applications 303
Anaesthetics
   myoneural activity and 4AP 215
Analogues
   4AP 226
Antibiotics 95
   aminoglycoside 232
   myoneural activity and 4AP 215
4AP see 4-Aminopyridine
Apamin
   bee venom 199
   potassium permeability 199
Aplysia californica
   presynaptic modulation and 4AP 230
Automatic activity
   squid axon and 4AP 221
Automatic facilitation 145
Axons, squid giant
   4AP effects 221
Axons, unmyelinated
   aminopyridine effects 53

Bicuculline 211
Blood-brain barrier
   aminopyridines and 222
Botulinum toxin 95
   action and 4AP 214
   type A in monkeys 313
Botulism
   4AP use 297
   3, 4-diaminopyridine use 313
Brain
   protein synthesis and 4AP 224

Caffeine
   anti-curare 232
Calcitonin cells
   4AP effects 326
Calcium
   antagonists 331
   -dependent potassium permeabilities 199
   potassium stimulated uptake 227
Carbachol
   diaphragm desensitization and 4AP 240
Cardiac effects
   4-aminopyridine 218
   4-aminoquinoline 218
Cardiac muscle
   4AP effects 261
Cardiotonic effect
   aminopyridines and pH 278
Catecholamine release
   4AP effects 183
Cerebellum
   4AP effects 217
Cerebral cortex
   acetylcholine release in rat and 4AP 213
Chemical modulators
   kinetics and characteristics 242
Chemiluminescence
   acetylcholine release 173
Cockroach
   abdominal ganglion synaptic transmission 218
Convulsant activity 145
   morphine dependence and 211
   in therapy 297
Curare
   4AP antagonism 232

Dendrotoxin 330, 331
   blocking effects 330
   3, 4-diaminopyridine comparison 324
   eastern green mamba 324
3, 4-Diaminopyridine
   blood-brain passage and toxicity 222
   in botulism 313
   dendrotoxin comparison 324
   potassium channel block 29
   pyramidal cell evoked activity 220
   tetanic fade and neuromuscular blockers 216
   therapeutic use 287
Diazepam 327
   4AP antagonism 331

Eaton-Lambert syndrome
   aminopyridine use 287
Electric Organ 163
Electroencephalopathy
   4AP in conscious volunteers 327
Electroplaque 163
Endocrine cells
   4AP effects 326

End plate potentials
  currents 95
  giant miniature 87
Enkephalins 127
Epinephrine 127

First isolation 3

Gramicidin 173

Heart see also cardiac
  parasympathetic neuroeffector
    transmission and amino-
      pyridines 325
Hexamethonium 127
Hippocampus
  4AP effects 217
  pyramidal cell layer, evoked
    activity and aminopyridines 2
    220
Histamine 127
History 3
Homatropine methylbromide 127
4-Hydroxypyridine
  neuromuscular transmitter
    release 225

Imidazole
  excitation of evoked trasmitter
    release 227
Inotropic action 145
Intramembrane particles 173
  P and E face 173
Ionic channels see also potassium
  aminopyridines 53
  cockroach and 4AP 238
Ionic currents
  aminopyridines 53

Kanamycin
  4AP antagonism 234
  depressant effects 234

Lanthanum 183
Lipid solubility
  aminopyridines activity 145

Membranes
  currents 53
  excitable and potassium
    currents 11
  nodal, aminopyridine effects 29
  postsynaptic, depolarisations 219
Mercaptopropionic acid 211
4-Methyl-2-aminopyridine
  4AP differences 322
S-Methylthiouronium
  potassium channel block 321

Models myopathic and 4AP 228
Morphine
  antagonists 231, 331
Morphine analgesia
  4AP reversal 233
Morphine dependence
  effects of 4-aminopyridine 211
Motor endings
  presynaptic currents and
    aminopyridines 223
Muscle see also cardiac muscle
  contractility and 4AP 249
  delayed potassium outward
    current 11
  isometric force $-$ ($Ca^{++}$) relation
    and 4AP 275
  skinned 275
Muscle, smooth
  outward membrane currents and
    4AP 276
Muscular distrophy 330
  avian and aminopyridines 323
Myasthenia gravis 323
  aminopyridine treatment 287
Myenteric plexus 127
Myopathic states
  4AP effects on models 228

Naloxone 127
  morphine antagonism in rabbits
    231
Neomycin 242
Nerve
  delayed potassium outward
    current 11
  terminals, motor 95
  terminals, properties 87
Neuromuscular transmission
  aminopyridines 95
  block and 4AP 241
  blocking agents 216
  disease, aminopyridine use
    287
  facilitation 145
Neurones
  cuneate and gracile with 4AP 239
  peripheral and central, 4AP
    effects 237
Nicotine 127, 183
Node of Ranvier 29, 43
Noise
  analysis 53
  ionic channel in unmyelated
    axons 53
Normorphine 127

Pace maker
  4AP and membrane currents 277

Parasympathetic transmission
  4-aminopyridine 127
Parathyroid cells
  4AP effects 326
Pentylenetetrazol 211
pH
  and cardiotonic effects 278
Physostigmine
  morphine antagonism 231
Picoline 3
Potassium channels
  4-aminopyridine block 29, 53
  3, 4-diaminopyridine block 29
  selective blocking 29
  S-methylthiouronium block 321
Potassium conductance 43, 95
  inhibition 145
Potassium currents
  aminopyridine effects 29
  excitable membranes 11
  frog myelinated nerve 29, 43
  time course 11
Potassium permeability
  apamin and aminopyridines 199
  calcium-activated 199
Prolactin cells
  4AP effects 326
Protein synthesis
  brain and 4AP 224
Purkinje fibres
  4AP and pace maker membrane
    currents 277
Pyridine
  frog muscle effects 229
Pyrocatechin 232

Ruthenium red
  blocking action 329

Sino-atrial node
  neurotransmitter release and
    4AP 261
Spike frequency adaptation 43
  motor and sensory fibres 43
Spinal cord
  aminopyridine and transmission
    117
Spinal reflexes 117
Spleen
  noradrenaline output and
    4AP 183
Stereotype
  dopaminergic and 2-amino-4-
    methylpyridine 212

Streptomycin 242
Structure-activity
  relationships 145
Strychnine 211
Succinyldicholine
  4AP and neuromuscular block 241
Superior cervical ganglion
  237
Synapses
  excitatory and inhibitory and
    4AP 117
Synaptic transmission
  facilitation by 4AP in cockroach
    219
  nerve-electroplaque 163
  principles 87
Synaptosomes
  calcium uptake 227
  chemiluminescence 173

Tetanic fade
  3, 4-diaminopyridine effects 216
Tetanus toxin
  action and 4AP 214
Tetraethylammonium (TEA) 11,
  330
  anti-curare 232
  motor ending presynaptic currents
    223
Therapeutic applications 287-303
<u>Torpedo marmorata</u>
  nerve-electroplaque function
    163
Toxicity
  aminopyridine and blood brain
    barrier 227
Transmission
  parasympathetic 127
  spinal cord, 4-aminopyridine
    117
Transmitter release 87
  active zones 87
  evoked 95
  facilitation 87
  4-hydroxypyridine 225
  imidazole excitation 227
  spontaneous 95
  types 87
2, 4, 6-Triaminopyrimidine
  cardiotonic effects 278
Tubocurarine 216

Verapamil 331
Voltage clamp experiments 29, 53